# Neonatal Neural Rescue:
# A Clinical Guide

# Neonatal Neural Rescue: A Clinical Guide

Edited by

## A. David Edwards FMedSci

Professor of Paediatrics and Neonatal Medicine and Director,
Centre for the Developing Brain, King's College, London;

Associate Director,
NIHR Medicines for Children Research Network, London, UK

## Denis V. Azzopardi FMedSci

Professor of Neonatal Medicine,
Imperial College, London, and King's College, London;

Consultant Neonatologist Queen Charlotte's and Chelsea Hospital,
London, and St Thomas' Hospital, London, UK

## Alistair J. Gunn FRSNZ

Professor of Physiology and Paediatrics,
Faculty of Medical and Health Sciences, Auckland University;

Consultant Paediatrician,
Starship Children's Hospital, Auckland, New Zealand

Foreword by

## Joseph J. Volpe MD

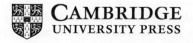

CAMBRIDGE
UNIVERSITY PRESS

CAMBRIDGE UNIVERSITY PRESS
Cambridge, New York, Melbourne, Madrid, Cape Town,
Singapore, São Paulo, Delhi, Mexico City

Cambridge University Press
The Edinburgh Building, Cambridge CB2 8RU, UK

Published in the United States of America by Cambridge University Press, New York

www.cambridge.org
Information on this title: www.cambridge.org/9781107681606

First published 2013

Printed and bound in the United Kingdom by the MPG Books Group

*A catalogue record for this publication is available from the British Library*

*Library of Congress Cataloguing in Publication data*
Neonatal neural rescue : a clinical guide / edited by David Edwards, Denis V. Azzopardi, Alistair J. Gunn.
    p. ; cm.
Includes bibliographical references and index.
ISBN 978-1-107-68160-6 (hardback)
I. Edwards, David, 1952–   II. Azzopardi, Denis V.   III. Gunn, Alistair J.
[DNLM:  1. Brain Injuries – therapy.   2. Asphyxia Neonatorum – therapy.   3. Hypothermia, Induced.
4. Infant, Newborn. WS 340]
617.4′81044–dc23

                                                                      2012031827

ISBN 978-1-107-68160-6 Hardback

# Contents

*List of contributors*   *page* vii
*Foreword, by Joseph J. Volpe*   ix

## Section 1: Scientific background

1. **Neurological outcome after perinatal asphyxia at term**   1
David Odd and Andrew Whitelaw

2. **Molecular mechanisms of neonatal brain injury and neural rescue**   16
Pierre Gressens and Henrik Hagberg

3. **The discovery of hypothermic neural rescue therapy for perinatal hypoxic–ischaemic encephalopathy**   33
A. David Edwards

4. **Clinical trials of hypothermic neural rescue**   40
A. David Edwards and Denis V. Azzopardi

5. **Economic evaluation of hypothermic neural rescue**   53
Dean A. Regier and Stavros Petrou

## Section 2: Clinical neural rescue

6. **Challenges for parents and clinicians discussing neuroprotective treatments**   65
Peter Allmark, Claire Snowdon, Diana Elbourne and Su Mason

7. **The pharmacology of hypothermia**   73
Alistair J. Gunn and Paul P. Drury

8. **Selection of infants for hypothermic neural rescue**   85
Ericalyn Kasdorf and Jeffrey M. Perlman

9. **Hypothermia during patient transport**   95
Susan E. Jacobs

10. **Whole body cooling for therapeutic hypothermia**   107
Abbot R. Laptook

11. **Selective head cooling**   119
Paul P. Drury, Laura Bennet and Alistair J. Gunn

12. **Hypothermic neural rescue for neonatal encephalopathy in mid- and low-resource settings**   128
Nicola J. Robertson and Sudhin Thayyil

13. **Cerebral function monitoring and EEG**   142
Lena Hellström-Westas

14. **Magnetic resonance imaging in hypoxic–ischaemic encephalopathy and the effects of hypothermia**   153
Mary A. Rutherford and Serena Counsell

15. **Novel uses of hypothermia**   166
Seetha Shankaran and Rosemary Higgins

16. **Neurological follow-up of infants treated with hypothermia**   172
Charlene M. T. Robertson and Joe M. Watt

17. **Registry surveillance after neuroprotective treatment**   182
Robert H. Pfister, Jeffrey D. Horbar and Denis V. Azzopardi

## Section 3: The future

18. **Novel neuroprotective therapies**   195
Sandra E. Juul, Donna M. Ferriero
and Mervyn Maze

19. **Combining hypothermia with other therapies
for neonatal neuroprotection**   208
Faye S. Silverstein and John D. Barks

20. **Biomarkers for studies of neuroprotection
in infants with hypoxic–ischaemic
encephalopathy**   219
Denis V. Azzopardi and A. David Edwards

*Index*   229

The colour plates can be found between pages 134 and 135.

# Contributors

**Peter Allmark BSc MA PhD**
Center for Health and Social Care Research, Sheffield Hallam University, Sheffield, UK

**Denis V. Azzopardi MD FRCPCH FMedSci**
Centre for the Developing Brain, King's College, London, UK and Institute of Clinical Sciences, Imperial College, London, UK

**John D. Barks MD**
Division of Neonatal-Perinatal Medicine, University of Michigan, C. S. Mott Children's Hospital, Ann Arbor, Michigan, USA

**Laura Bennet PhD**
Faculty of Medical and Health Sciences, University of Auckland, Auckland, New Zealand

**Serena Counsell PhD**
Centre for the Developing Brain, King's College, London, UK

**Paul P. Drury BSc(Hons)**
Faculty of Medical and Health Sciences, University of Auckland, Auckland, New Zealand

**A. David Edwards MA MBBS DSc MRCR FRCP FRCPCH FMedSci**
Centre for the Developing Brain, King's College, London, UK

**Diana Elbourne BSc MSc PhD**
Medical Statistics Unit, London School of Hygiene and Tropical Medicine, London, UK

**Donna M. Ferriero MD MS**
Department of Pediatrics, University of California, San Francisco, San Francisco, California, USA

**Pierre Gressens MD PhD**
U 676, Inserm & Paris Diderot University, Paris, France and Centre for the Developing Brain, King's College, London, UK

**Alistair J. Gunn FRACP PhD FRSNZ**
Faculty of Medical and Health Sciences, Auckland University, New Zealand

**Henrik Hagberg MD PhD**
Perinatal Center, Sahlgrenska Academy, Gothenburg, Sweden and Centre for the Developing Brain, King's College, London, UK

**Lena Hellström-Westas MD PhD**
Department of Women's and Children's Health, Uppsala University, Uppsala, Sweden

**Rosemary Higgins MD**
NICHD Neonatal Research Network, Eunice Kennedy Shriver National Institute for Child Health and Human Development, Bethesda, MD, USA

**Jeffrey D. Horbar MD**
Vermont Oxford Network, Burlington, VT, USA

**Susan E. Jacobs MBBS MD FRACP**
Neonatal Services, Royal Women's Hospital, Melbourne, Australia

**Sandra E. Juul MD PhD**
Division of Neonatology, University of Washington, Seattle, WA, USA

**Ericalyn Kasdorf MD**
Division of Newborn Medicine, Weill Cornell Medical College, and New York Presbyterian Hospital, New York, NY, USA

**Abbot R. Laptook MD**
Department of Pediatrics, Warren Alpert Medical School, Brown University, Providence, RI, USA

**Su Mason BNurs PhD**
Clinical Trials Unit, University of Leeds Institute of Molecular Medicine, Leeds, UK

**Mervyn Maze MD**
Department of Anesthesia and Perioperative Care,
University of California, San Francisco, CA, USA

**David Odd MD FRCPCH**
Department of Neonatology, Southmead Hospital,
Bristol, UK

**Jeffrey M. Perlman MBChB**
Division of Newborn Medicine, Weill Cornell Medical
College and New York Presbyterian Hospital,
New York, NY, USA

**Stavros Petrou PhD**
National Perinatal Epidemiology Unit, University of
Oxford, Oxford and Division of Health Sciences,
Warwick Medical School, Coventry, UK

**Robert H. Pfister MD**
Vermont Children's Hospital at the University of
Vermont, Burlington, VT, USA

**Dean A. Regier PhD**
Canadian Centre for Applied Research in Cancer
Control, British Columbia Cancer Registry,
Vancouver, British Columbia, Canada

**Charlene M. T. Robertson MD**
Pediatric Rehabilitation Outcomes Unit, Glenrose
Rehabilitation Hospital, Edmonton, Alberta, Canada

**Nicola J. Robertson MBChB FRCPCH PhD**
Department of Neonatology, Institute for Women's
Health, University College London, London, UK

**Mary A. Rutherford FRCR FRCPCH**
Centre for the Developing Brain, King's College,
London, UK

**Seetha Shankaran MD**
Department of Pediatrics, Wayne State University
School of Medicine, Detroit, MI, USA

**Faye S. Silverstein MD**
Departments of Pediatrics and Neurology, University
of Michigan, Ann Arbor, MI, USA

**Claire Snowdon BA MA PhD**
Centre for Family Research, University of Cambridge,
Cambridge, UK

**Sudhin Thayyil MD DCH FRCPCH PhD**
Department of Neonatology, Institute for
Women's Health, University College London,
London, UK

**Joseph J. Volpe MD**
Department of Neurology, Boston Children's
Hospital, Harvard Medical School, Boston,
MA, USA

**Joe M. Watt MBBS FRCPC**
Pediatric Neuromotor Programs, Syncrude
Center for Motion and Balance, Glenrose
Rehabilitation Hospital, Edmonton, Alberta,
Canada

**Andrew Whitelaw MD FRCPCH**
School of Clinical Science, University of Bristol,
Bristol, UK

# Foreword

Joseph J. Volpe, MD

The overall intent of this book is to elucidate the scientific underpinnings of neonatal neural rescue, especially hypothermia, to synthesize the critical evidence supporting its clinical value and to describe the means of implementation of hypothermia, including important practical considerations. The intent, thus, is ambitious and challenging. The clinical focus is the preservation of neurological structure and function in the infant exposed to perinatal asphyxia. The work was led admirably by three pioneering figures in the field of neural rescue: Professors David Edwards, Denis Azzopardi and Alistair Gunn.

An appropriate query might be raised at the outset – why address an entire book, with more than 20 chapters, to the problem of brain injury secondary to perinatal asphyxia? Some prominent clinicians and the "guidelines" of several scientific societies have stated that perinatal asphyxia with its associated hypoxic–ischaemic brain injury is an uncommon condition. This declaration is decidedly incorrect. The advent of MRI in the study of the newborn with neurological signs referable to the central nervous system has led to the discovery, clearly documented in multiple publications, that the topographic signature of hypoxic–ischaemic brain injury is common in the context of clinical signs consistent with perinatal asphyxia. In developed countries, infants brain-injured by perinatal asphyxia yearly account for cumulative totals measured in the many thousands. Even more dramatically, in underdeveloped countries, the yearly numbers are of the order of a million or more. Thus, the focus of this book, the prevention of hypoxic–ischaemic brain injury related to perinatal asphyxia, is extraordinarily important and timely.

The remarkable advances in recent years in neonatal neural rescue, especially with hypothermia, are synthesized in this outstanding book. The first section provides the scientific background of hypoxic–ischaemic brain injury and the likely mechanisms mediating the beneficial effects of hypothermia. The second section is focused principally on hypothermia and its implementation in the neonatal intensive care unit. Such important clinical issues as obtaining parental consent for neuroprotective therapies, criteria for selection of infants, specific modes of hypothermia, management of related neurological phenomena, e.g., seizures, and neurological/cognitive follow-up are addressed. The concluding section looks to the future and explores such critical topics as other potential novel neuroprotective interventions, especially those that interact favourably with hypothermia, and the search for biomarkers and facilitators of early phase studies.

Each chapter is written by one or more experts in the field and is well-organized, lucid and highly informed. The reference lists are broad and deep and, alone, are a great resource. Overall, the book is a tour de force and will be of enormous value to neonatologists, neurologists, paediatricians, neonatal nurses and indeed, anyone involved in the care of the asphyxiated infant.

Hypothermia for treatment of neonatal hypoxic–ischaemic brain injury represents the first consistently useful neuroprotective intervention in management of the asphyxiated infant. Upon the foundation of hypothermia, additive and synergistic therapies hopefully will be added. This book sets the stage for this next level of intervention in a field that until now has been desperately lacking. Professors Edwards, Azzopardi and Gunn have set a high bar for future scholarship in neonatal neural rescue and deserve great credit for their accomplishments with this volume.

Section 1 **Scientific background**

Chapter **1**

# Neurological outcome after perinatal asphyxia at term

David Odd and Andrew Whitelaw

## Introduction

It was nearly 150 years ago that an association between perinatal events and brain injury was first reported, claiming that "the act of birth does occasionally imprint upon the nervous and muscular systems of the infantile organism very serious and peculiar evils" [1]. While a great deal is now known about this association and the pathophysiology behind it, the quantification of these "evils" is still uncertain. While the World Health Organisation estimates that 25% of neonatal and 8% of all deaths under 5 years in low-income countries are due to birth asphyxia [2], there remains no agreed definition; therefore, the reported prevalence varies. Consequently, the number of infants exposed is unknown, although approximately 7% of term infants require resuscitation after birth [3]. It is well recognized that only a small proportion of these infants will go on to develop neurological signs in the neonatal period and an estimated 2 per 1000 births in the developed world [4] will develop neonatal encephalopathy.

While encephalopathy is, therefore, relatively uncommon, the outcome can be devastating to the infant and family and it remains a major cause of death and long-term disability with a substantial burden on the community as a whole. It is estimated that each infant with complex neurological sequelae will cost the state over 1 million US dollars (800,000 Euros) in health care, social support and lost productivity throughout their lifetime [5]. In addition, unmeasured impacts on behaviour, school failure and psychiatric disease are likely all to have additive effects. As well as the direct costs, other population impacts are also likely. Increasingly literature suggests a causal link between IQ and lifespan [6] and the true cost to society of perinatal asphyxia is likely to be extensive.

## Perinatal asphyxia and hypoxic–ischaemic encephalopathy

Central to any discussion on perinatal asphyxia is the distinction between perinatal asphyxia, which refers to poor condition at birth, and hypoxic–ischaemic encephalopathy, which refers to acute brain dysfunction following critical lack of oxygen. The first does not automatically lead to the second and while the International Classification of Disease (10th revision) includes a diagnosis of "birth asphyxia", there is little agreement on how the diagnosis should be made [7]. Indeed, perhaps due to the difficulty in determining the timing of an asphyxial event, the phrase "perinatal asphyxia" is often used as a more general term [8].

## Measures of perinatal asphyxia

The concept of perinatal asphyxia is a critical lack of oxygen delivery during labour and/or delivery which is sufficiently severe to produce objectively measurable functional de-compensation. It is important to recognize that some degree of hypoxia–ischaemia occurs during normal labour. Every time the uterus contracts, the arteries bringing oxygen to the placental bed and so to the fetus, are constricted. The fetus can tolerate these short periods of hypoxia as they tend to be brief (e.g., less than a minute) and are followed by a longer period of uterine relaxation during which oxygen delivery is resumed. Furthermore, the fetus can tolerate brief periods of hypoxia by switching energy production to anaerobic glycolysis. This production of lactic acid and subsequent acidaemia while indicating hypoxia do not immediately indicate there is energy failure at a cellular level. Indeed, the level of physiological compromise believed to represent a pathological state remains unclear and there is no agreed "gold standard" measure for the diagnosis of perinatal asphyxia.

*Neonatal Neural Rescue*, ed. A. David Edwards, Denis V. Azzopardi and Alistair J. Gunn. Published by Cambridge University Press. © Cambridge University Press 2013.

**Table 1.1.** Individual components of the Apgar score

| Component | Score | | |
|---|---|---|---|
| | **0** | **1** | **2** |
| Heart rate (pulse)* | No pulse felt | Less than 100 | Greater than 100 |
| Respiratory effort | Apnoea | Irregular, shallow ventilation | Breathing/crying |
| Reflex irritability (grimace)* | No response to stimulation | Grimace/feeble cry when stimulated | Sneeze/cough/pulls away when stimulated |
| Muscle tone (activity)* | Flaccid | Good tone | Spontaneous movement |
| Colour (appearance)* | Blue/white | Partially pink | Entirely pink |

*The Apgar mnemonic introduced as a teaching tool in 1963 by Dr Joseph Butterfield.

Despite the lack of a valid and reliable test, a pragmatic definition of perinatal asphyxia is required in the assessment of causes and outcomes and in the trial of novel therapies. To diagnose perinatal asphyxia, several indicators are used. Impaired physiology is often documented by the Apgar score and abnormal biochemistry by acid–base measures in neonatal blood while others have used the presence of antenatal risk factors, meconium stained liquor, or the need for resuscitation. These measures are sometimes used individually, but more commonly are combined into a more complex diagnostic criterion. The recent trials of therapeutic hypothermia [9–11] all used a range of criteria to define infants with encephalopathy following perinatal asphyxia.

### Acidosis

Acidaemia is one of the most commonly used diagnostic measures of perinatal asphyxia: measured in blood from the scalp capillary beds, the umbilical vessels of the infant immediately after birth, or blood taken within a few minutes of birth. While acidaemia can result from $CO_2$ retention it is perhaps lactic acidosis, as indicated by base deficit, that represents more unambiguous evidence of hypoxia. Opinion concerning the level at which acidosis is considered pathological varies, although severe acidosis is often defined as a pH of less than 7 or a base deficit $\geq 16$ mEq/L [12] in the umbilical cord blood. Around 2.5% of infants have a low pH (by these criteria) at delivery [12] and this finding underlines the point that brief periods of anaerobic metabolism can still support vital organs.

### The Apgar score and birth condition

Despite advocates for the use of pH as the "best" measure of perinatal hypoxia, the most commonly used measure of birth condition remains the Apgar score and consequently it is often used in studies of perinatal asphyxia (Table 1.1). Proposed in 1953 by Virginia Apgar, it was suggested that a combined score to assess the status of newborn infants in the first few minutes of life would provide "clear classification or "grading" of newborn infants which can be used as a basis for discussion and comparison of the results of obstetric practices, types of maternal pain relief and the effects of resuscitation" [13]. While other scores have been suggested since [14], none have been widely accepted.

While it provides an ordinal measure of the clinical status of the infant, little agreement exists as to what a "low" or "normal" score should be. Like measures of acidosis, many studies have proposed a "cut-off" value (and specified the time at which the infant should have achieved it) to identify infants likely to have been exposed to perinatal asphyxia. There is currently little evidence in the literature on which to base these judgements and little consensus on what a "low" or "normal" score should be, or what a particular score suggests for an individual infant. The American Academy of Pediatrics suggest that a score of 7 or above should be considered a normal value, with a score of 3 or below severely low [15]. Virginia Apgar suggested 8 or above as an appropriate "normal" score [16], while others have suggested a cut-off value of 6 [7]. The number of infants with low Apgar scores, therefore, differs

**Table 1.2.** The Sarnat grading of encephalopathy

| Measure | Sarnat grade | | |
|---|---|---|---|
| | 1 | 2 | 3 |
| Conscious level | Hyperalert | Lethargic | Stupor |
| Muscle tone | Normal | Hypotonic | Profound hypotonia |
| Posture | Mild distal flexion | Strong distal flexion | Decerebrate |
| Stretch reflexes | Normal | Overactive | Overactive |
| Moro reflex | Strong | Incomplete | Absent |
| Suck reflex | Normal | Weak | Absent |
| Tonic neck reflex | Slight | Strong | Absent |
| Pupils | Dilated | Constricted | Poorly reactive |
| Gut motility | Normal | Increased | Variable |
| Seizures | Uncommon | Focal or multifocal | Generalized |

between studies, although one large population study reported a prevalence of 0.70% [17] for a 5-minute score below 7. In view of the variability in consistently defining a low Apgar score, the need for resuscitation may be considered a "gestalt" indicator that, in the view of the clinician on the spot, the infant had not established regular breathing, circulation and activity.

Not surprisingly, these measures are closely correlated, with coefficients between pH and the Apgar score reported as 0.3–0.4 [18,19], while sensitivity (0.40 vs. 0.48) and specificity (0.88 vs. 0.96) were similar for both a low pH and Apgar score in predicting neonatal morbidity (defined as needing admission to a neonatal unit) [19]. Interestingly this has led to clinicians calling for both the Apgar score [20] and umbilical pH measurements [19] to be discontinued in favour of the other measure.

## Diagnosis of hypoxic–ischaemic encephalopathy

Irrespective of the definition used, only a proportion of infants exposed to perinatal asphyxia will develop signs of neurological impairment in the newborn period and be diagnosed as having hypoxic–ischaemic encephalopathy (HIE). It is this group of infants in which most of the evidence of long-term outcomes exists. These infants are commonly described using a three-point grading system of mild, moderate and severe encephalopathy. First proposed by Sarnat and Sarnat in 1976 [21] (Table 1.2), the grading system has since been modified and while different interpretations of it are used, it remains a common classification in the literature. A particular strength of Sarnat's system is that it combines clinical examination with electroencephalogram (EEG) and in recent years the value of continuous amplitude-integrated EEG (aEEG) has been well demonstrated to document the depth of brain dysfunction and its change over hours and days [22]. However, while this ordinal grading is extensively used, the clinical picture of hypoxic–ischaemic encephalopathy seen is often complex and the underlying pattern of cerebral damage likely to be just as complex. The pioneering work of Myers in the pregnant monkey has, for example, shown that acute total asphyxia produced by cord clamping tends to injure the basal ganglia, thalamus and brain stem while prolonged partial asphyxia produced by high-dose halothane to the mother over hours tended to produce watershed injury in the frontal and occipital cortex and sub-cortex [23].

## Long-term outcome after perinatal asphyxia

The neurological outcome of infants who are exposed to perinatal asphyxia has important impacts on the population as a whole, guides discussion with parents and influences the immediate neonatal management. It is also critical to the assessment of new therapies. While the literature for perinatal asphyxia is extensive (a PubMed MeSH search for "asphyxia neonatorum" returns over 6,000 results), the data on long-term, pragmatic outcomes are surprisingly scarce and heterogeneous in nature. Studies are often small and have limited power to identify modest, but important effects. Indeed, while there is overwhelming evidence for an association between perinatal asphyxia and death, cerebral palsy (CP) or impaired cognition, the quantification and prediction of these outcomes is complex and several questions remain difficult to answer.

Many studies concentrate on the outcome of infants with moderate or severe HIE, but even here the outcomes are often restricted to short-term follow-up. While appropriate for objective and persistent measures of outcome such as mortality or CP, long-term impairments in cognition or behaviour and in particular pragmatic measures of function are less well reported. Data from work involving preterm infants suggest that the burden of neuropathological disabilities may increase as the child gets older (and is expected to perform more complex cognitive processes) and that even certain diagnoses believed to be robustly identified during infancy, such as CP, may alter in prevalence over time [24]. A further caveat of these studies remains: these studies can only show association and not causation. While less of a concern for major (and otherwise rare) outcomes such as death or CP, subtle deficits in IQ are socially patterned, as is the risk of perinatal asphyxia [25]. The possibility of residual or uncontrolled confounding is likely and may result in distorting the apparent strength of any associations found. Bias may also be a concern and even in studies where follow-up is complete (minimizing selection bias), the initial cohort may not represent the population as a whole: an increasing concern in randomized control trials.

However, infants with evidence of a substantial perinatal asphyxia insult represent a group of infants in whom substantial risks for poor outcomes exist and consequently the outcome of infants with moderate or severe HIE is considered separately to the larger population of infants likely exposed to milder levels of perinatal asphyxia.

# Outcome of infants with moderate or severe HIE

## Mortality

Many infants who develop moderate or severe HIE are likely to die in the neonatal period and this is well reported in the recent randomized controlled trials (RCT) of therapeutic hypothermia [9–11]. These infants (enrolled between 1999 and 2006) represent a group of term infants who received intensive care support after a perinatal asphyxial insult sufficient to produce moderate or severe encephalopathy. While entry criteria differed between the studies, all recruited infants with some evidence of perinatal asphyxia who then developed clinical and, in two trials, electroencephalopathic evidence, of encephalopathy. Mortality was, not surprisingly, substantial, with between 27% [9] and 38% [11] of the infants in the control groups dying before 18 months of age. A composite estimate from the three studies suggested the pooled mortality would be 33%. It should be noted that a major cause of mortality is likely to be active withdrawal of care in infants believed to have poor neurological outcomes: dependent on the clinicians' perception of the probable outcome and potentially reinforcing certain prognostic factors. The long-term mortality is likely to be higher than these estimates and data from Finland suggest that a further 2% of infants with encephalopathy who survive the neonatal period may die before their 14th birthday [26].

## Cerebral palsy

Next to neonatal death, cerebral palsy is arguably the most recognized consequence of perinatal asphyxia and while specifically a defect of motor development, it remains a strong risk factor for the development of deficits in cognitive functioning later in life [27]. The most common pattern of CP in infants with HIE remains dyskinetic or spastic quadriplegia [4] (consistent with basal ganglia damage) and the recent RCTs have reported rates of CP in survivors (at 18 months) between 30% [11] and 41% [9]. A pooled estimate from all three control groups would suggest that 35% of survivors have identifiable CP at 2 years of age, although the proportion after moderate HIE is likely to be lower than after severe disease (e.g., 28% vs. 43% [10]).

## Cognitive Impairment

Cognitive impairment has also been well established as a consequence of perinatal asphyxia but the quantification of any impact remains elusive. Again, perhaps the most rigorously followed up group of infants in recent years is the infants enrolled in trials of neuroprotective hypothermia. At 18 months of age, the recent RCTs suggested rates of poor cognition (Bayley Mental Development Index < 70) were around 36% of survivors in the control groups.

However, longer term measures of IQ are likely to be more important and only a handful of studies have successfully measured cognition beyond 2 years of age. Many of these studies were able to report only on a small number of infants, while the inclusion criteria, length of follow-up and outcomes measured and reported differ between studies. While some have reported outcomes compared to a contemporaneous group of "control" infants, others have no such group, or compare to established "normal ranges" [27,28]. Overall, there is strong evidence that infants who survive encephalopathy have lower IQ scores than their peers. In one population-based study, infants with all grades of HIE had an IQ deficit of approximately 10 points compared with a control group of infants with no evidence of perinatal compromise [3]. Which infants are at risk of developing cognitive impairment is still debated and some have suggested that only those infants in whom the perinatal event was substantial enough to cause noticeable cerebral palsy [15] are at risk, although there is a growing body of evidence suggesting otherwise [29,30]. A consequence of this debate is that many recent studies report only the cognitive outcome of infants who otherwise appear to have escaped a substantial movement disorder, leaving it difficult to apply the data to an infant in the neonatal period before it is known if they are destined to develop CP or not.

In general, the IQ of infants with severe HIE is likely to be lower than their peers, although Marlow (who recruited infants with any encephalopathy in the first 7 days and not just HIE infants) estimated the mean score to be as high as 103 in survivors without CP [30]. In contrast, the IQ score of survivors with CP after severe HIE was estimated as only 48 by Robertson at 8 years of age [31]. Infants with moderate HIE (again, without obvious CP) have been reported to have mean IQ scores either similar to their peers (Marlow et al: 112 vs. 114, $P = 0.57$ [30]) or slightly lower (Robertson et al: 102 vs. 112, $P < 0.001$ [31], Viggedal el al: 106 vs. 116 [32]). Van Handel reported a low mean IQ of 87 (SD 22) in infants who survived moderate HIE without developing severe motor, sensory or developmental delay [33].

Papers that have combined the outcome of all infants with mild, moderate or severe HIE have also reported evidence for lower IQ measures, but again the difference between studies makes conclusions difficult (Table 1.3). Some studies have preferred to report the risk of developing a low IQ score rather than assuming that there is a shift in the population mean. The "cut-off" points used to define a low (and perhaps importantly low) score differ, but below 70 (2 standard deviations [SD] from the mean) is commonly reported. Robertson reported the risk of a low score (≤70) at the age of 5 years as increasing from 1.8% in infants with mild encephalopathy through to 83% in infants with severe disease [27], although peer comparison data were not presented.

While childhood IQ is strongly associated with longer term cognitive measures, it also tends to be more influenced by social and environmental factors than adult-age measures of cognition which should perhaps be considered the gold-standard. Not surprisingly, these are rarely measured, although Lindstrom et al have reported that the majority (71%) of infants with moderate neonatal encephalopathy who do not develop CP have some degree of cognitive impairment as teenagers [29].

## Differential cognitive impairment

IQ, while a reliable measure of cognition, fails to tell the whole story and if survivors of HIE do develop cognitive impairment, is it global or are specific domains, perhaps associated with high-risk areas of the brain known to be at risk of perinatal asphyxia, selectively damaged? Interpretation of the data is complicated as the localization of specific brain functions to specific anatomic areas is often difficult. Working memory in children has been shown to be more localized in the caudate nucleus and anterior insula than in the dorsolateral prefrontal cortex as in adults [34], while comprehension has not been consistently localized to one area [35,36] and any study looking at specific function would have to consider the possibilities that different profiles of ischaemic damage are likely to involve different areas of the newborn brain [23].

**Table 1.3.** IQ beyond 2 years of age

| Paper | Category of HIE | Age at outcome (years) | Measure | HIE infants | | Control infants | | Evidence for difference (reported $P$ values) |
|---|---|---|---|---|---|---|---|---|
| | | | | n | IQ | n | IQ | |
| Barnett [53] | Mild, moderate or severe without CP | 5–6 | WPPSI | 53 | 102 (16) | – | – | – |
| Marlow [30] | Moderate without motor disability | 7 | BAS-II | 32 | 112 (11) | 49 | 114 (14) | 0.57 |
| | Severe without motor disability | | | 18 | 103 (13) | 49 | | <0.01 |
| Odd [3] | Mild, moderate or severe (CP included) | 8 | WISC-III | 26 | 95 (20) | 5461 | 105 (16) | 0.007 |
| Robertson [31] | Mild | 8 | WISC-R | 56 | 106 (13) | 155 | 112 (13) | >0.05 |
| | Moderate (all) | | | 84 | 95 (23) | 155 | | <0.001 |
| | Moderate (non-impaired) | | | 66 | 102 (17) | 155 | | <0.001 |
| | Moderate (impaired) | | | 18 | 68 (27) | 155 | | <0.001 |
| | Severe | | | 5 | 48 (21) | 155 | | – |
| Van Handel [33] | Mild (without severe motor, sensory or developmental delay) | 9–10 | WISC-III | 33 | 98 (12) | 46 | 109 (12) | <0.001 |
| | Moderate (without severe motor, sensory or developmental delay) | | | 47 | 86 (22) | | | |
| George [28] | Mild | 12 | MISIC | 41 | 87 (14) | – | – | – |
| | Moderate or severe | | | 5 | 72 (11) | – | – | – |
| Viggedal [32] | Mild (without known neuro-developmental disability) | 25 | WAIS-R | 20 | 107 (IQR 96–116) | 18 | 116 (IQR 105–132) | >0.05 |
| | Moderate (without known neuro-developmental disability) | | | 11 | 106 (IQR 100–113) | 18 | | >0.05 |

WPPSI, Wechsler Preschool and Primary Scale of Intelligence; BAS, British Ability Scales; MISIC, Malin's Intelligence Scale for Indian Children; WISC, Wechsler Intelligence Scale for Children; WAIS, Wechsler Adult Intelligence Scale.

However, certain studies have reported differential effects of perinatal asphyxia on cognitive domains. There are data to suggest that watershed brain injury (likely caused by more chronic, partial hypoxic insults) may selectively affect verbal skills [37]. Steinman [37] reports the outcome of 81 term infants with HIE and suggested that evidence of damage in the watershed areas is associated with lower verbal IQ scores in infants at 4 years of age (independent of basal ganglia injury). Small studies have also suggested that the cognitive impairment from more acute asphyxial insults may result in part from selective memory deficits, with hippocampal injury a recognized consequence of HIE [38]. Consistent with this, Marlow et al [30] followed up 65 infants with encephalopathy to 7 years and reported increased risks of attention and memory problems [30] although the effect size seen was relatively modest for those with moderate HIE (approx. 0.5 SD) and more pronounced in those after severe HIE (around 1 SD). Lindstrom et al have also reported that infants suffering neonatal encephalopathy had a much higher risk of problems with short-term memory (64% vs. 13%, $P < 0.002$) at age 15–19 years. However, other studies have found little evidence of any differential effect, with data suggesting more global impairment of function [3,28,39].

## Visual and hearing impairment

As well as movement and cognitive function, critical neuronal pathways involved in vision and hearing are also affected by perinatal asphyxia. Survivors of moderate or severe HIE also have reportedly higher rates of sensori-neuronal hearing loss, with rates in recent trials suggesting prevalence at 18 months is around 6% [9–11]. These same studies suggest a prevalence of visual impairments of around 13% [9–11]. The long-term visual and hearing disability impact is not clear, although increased risks of more subtle dysfunction, such as myopia and strabismus, have been reported [40].

## Epilepsy and other neurological disorders

While neonatal seizures are common in infants with moderate or severe HIE (indeed for some diagnostic groups they are required), the development of epilepsy in childhood occurs less frequently. At 18 months, the prevalence of seizure disorders is likely to be around 15% [9–11], although longer term prevalence and severity of seizures are less clearly defined. At 3.5 years, 7% of moderate or severe HIE survivors had

developed poorly controlled epilepsy, having daily or weekly seizures [41]. However, a Norwegian study suggested that infants who had low (0–3 at 5 minutes) Apgar scores and then developed neurological signs in the neonatal period had only a 5% chance of a diagnosis of epilepsy by the time they were 8–13 years old [40].

In addition to the risks of epilepsy, other neurological disorders may also be more common in survivors of HIE. Work has suggested that the prevalence of autistic spectrum disorder is around 4% in survivors of moderate/severe encephalopathy compared with less than 1% in the control group [42]. Others have reported that non-disabled survivors of HIE scored higher in measures of hyperactivity than controls [27,33], although this has not been found in all studies [29]. Interestingly even if measures of attention or hyperactivity are worse, it remains unclear if the rates of attention deficit hyperactivity disorder (ADHD) itself are higher. Some studies have suggested an increased risk [40], while others (who reported worse scores in several measures of social function and attention) found little evidence for increased risk of defined neuro-psychiatric disorders (including ADHD) [33].

Other less well defined psychiatric disorders may also be more common in the survivors of HIE and more general behavioural problems have also been reported. Van Handel reported poorer functioning in measures of anxiety/depression as well as social problems in survivors of moderate encephalopathy [33], while George et al reported that there were behavioural problems in 15% of infants who had had mild HIE and 57% of those who survived moderate or severe HIE although no peer comparison group was assessed [28].

If these associations truly exist, it seems entirely reasonable that these other neuro-psychiatric problems are directly caused by an asphyxial insult to the developing cerebrum. However, they are also all more common in infants with learning difficulties and so these associations (while real) may simply be dependent on the cognitive problems already described above.

## Educational performance

Given the raft of potential neurological impairments that may develop in infants who survive encephalopathy, perhaps a better functional measure of neurophysiological outcomes is that of school performance. Likely to be dependent on cognitive, movement, and sensory functions and behaviour, it is not surprising that educational failure is common in survivors of

HIE. Robertson *et al* reported on the school performance of survivors of neonatal encephalopathy at age 8. They reported that all infants with severe HIE were receiving additional educational support (compared to 20% in their peer group) and all were functioning at least 1 grade below that which they were expected to [31]. The effect on survivors of moderate encephalopathy was less severe, but still 38% were receiving additional help and there was a substantial chance of performing worse than their peers: more noticeable in infants with motor disability. Marlow reported on several educational measures and suggests again that even non-disabled survivors of encephalopathy have worse performance at several school measures and that this increases as the degree of encephalopathy worsens [30].

In the Avon Longitudinal Study of Parents and Children (ALSPAC) cohort based in the United Kingdom, infants who had moderate or severe HIE were 6 times more likely than controls to need support at school [43].

## Composite and social outcomes

While mean differences in summary IQ values (for example) are important for objective assessment of outcome and new therapies, all too often after the birth and resuscitation of an infant who develops HIE, the question that parents ask is "Will my baby be normal"? As discussed above, it is likely that infants with moderate or severe HIE who survive will have some degree of cognitive impairment and increased risk of CP. Several other pathologies appear to be more common in these infants, many of which are poorly quantified as yet, while new burdens may develop as the infant develops into adulthood. However, these outcomes are likely to be inter-dependent; i.e., it is those infants with CP, low IQ and epilepsy that will need support at school and a proportion of infants is likely to have a "normal" life.

To this end, many studies report pragmatic outcomes such as "death or disability". Definitions vary, but in short-term follow-up (e.g., preschool) this definition often includes death, severe low IQ (<70 points), CP or severe visual or hearing impairment. Overall (and dependent on definitions), the risk of a poor outcome tends to be reported between 53% [9] and 66% [11]. These more recent values are higher than some others reported. Badawi *et al* suggested (using similar criteria) that 39% of infants had a poor

outcome in early childhood (compared with 2.7% of control subjects) [39].

Longer term outcomes than these are, again, less commonly reported. Marlow *et al* [30] reported outcome on 65 infants who had encephalopathy of any type in the first week and suggested that 6% of infants with moderate encephalopathy and 42% with severe encephalopathy had evidence of major disability at 7 years of age. A large population study in Finland followed over 12,000 infants born in 1966 [26] and using a composite measure of probable perinatal asphyxia and encephalopathy, it was estimated that 20% of 14-year-old survivors had an IQ of less than 71, CP or epilepsy.

Perhaps the most pragmatic measure of outcome is that of social functioning: a complex process and dependent on multiple competencies. While it seems likely that many infants with severe encephalopathy will (if they survive) have cognitive or movement deficits that will have a functional impact on social and educational performance, the outcome of infants with moderate encephalopathy is less clear. Despite increased risks of disability and uncertainty over long-term problems (and in particular disabling neuro-psychiatric disease) many of these infants are likely to have normal range IQ and school and social performance and this proportion is likely to improve with the advent of novel therapies.

However, quantification of these measures is difficult, although the few studies that have reported measures of social performance suggest (not surprisingly) that important levels of functional deficits exist. Lindstrom *et al* have reported that following neonatal encephalopathy 36% of infants had problems interacting with peers [29] compared with none of the controls ($P < 0.01$). Kjellmer *et al* [44] reported that infants with moderate encephalopathy were more likely to be living with parents (44% vs. 17%) and be unemployed (19% vs. 7%) than their peers in adult life, although the study was based on small numbers and the results correspondingly imprecise. In a study using the Swedish birth registry, survivors of HIE appeared to be less likely to have attended university (32% vs. 43%), to be earning money (71% vs. 89%) and to be employed (62% vs. 86%) and more likely to be living with their parents in early adulthood (23% vs. 11%) [48]. However, of note, a third of infants who survived encephalopathy did attend university, while over half were in employment.

# Outcome of mild or clinically silent neurological damage

## The continuum of reproductive casualty

While some imprecision remains about the likely outcome of moderate or severe encephalopathy, very few data exist on the outcome of infants with mild or clinically silent perinatal asphyxia. While any long-term effects of perinatal asphyxia are likely to be less pronounced (if they exist at all), these infants represent a much larger proportion of infants than those with moderate or severe encephalopathy (and hence they may have an important population impact). The pathophysiological threshold needed to produce persistent, functional, neurological deficits is unknown. Indeed, it may be that no threshold exists at all. In 1862, Little suggested that "the greater or smaller the impairment of intellect may safely be attributed to the greater or less mischief inflicted upon the cerebrum" [1]. The concept has been referred to in the literature repeatedly and in 1956 Pasamanick *et al.* more formally postulated that a "continuum of reproductive casualty" existed [45]; such that while profound perinatal events cause death or obvious neurological deficit, milder insults may cause subtle defects in functioning only detectable as the child grows older. However, a robust test of this hypothesis has proved difficult to carry out and surprisingly few data have been produced to either refute or support the theory, although it is widely reported that clinically important brain damage leading to learning disability can only occur if the asphyxial insult around birth is significant enough to produce moderate or severe encephalopathy in the neonatal period [8,15].

## Specific studies of mildly asphyxiated infants

While much of the published outcome data have reported on infants with moderate or severe HIE, some work exists on the outcome of infants believed to have developed only mild encephalopathy. In Robertson's papers, infants with mild HIE had outcomes similar to their peers [27,31]. Similar findings have been presented by others [32], although a brief report from India reported a mean IQ score of 87 at 12 years of age in infants who developed mild HIE [28], but did not recruit any comparison group. Van Handel recently reported reduced IQ scores compared with a peer group in children at 10 years who had developed mild HIE after birth (98 vs. 109) [33]. However, numbers of infants in these studies have

been small and any effect of mild (or clinically silent HIE) is likely to be only modest.

Few papers have attempted to assess the outcome of infants who after an episode of perinatal asphyxia do not go on to develop any obvious signs of neurological impairment. While some have found little evidence of an association [46], there is often limited power/precision to identify a small association, which due to the much larger number of infants exposed may still be of importance.

Two recent papers have reported data from large population based studies capable of excluding infants who develop neurological signs and have specifically reported the outcomes of infants in poor condition at birth who did not develop noticeable encephalopathy. In one, infants born in the 1970s with low Apgar scores (<7 at 5 minutes) but no history of neonatal pathology were investigated using an IQ test administered during military conscription (at age 18 years) [25]. There appeared to be an increase in the risk of a low score (less than 80) when compared to those in good condition at birth (odds ratio [OR], 1.35 (1.07 to 1.69)). In another paper based on the ALSPAC cohort study, infants found to have needed resuscitation at birth (but who did not develop encephalopathy symptoms) were found to have higher risk of a low IQ score (<80) than a group of non-resuscitated peers (OR, 1.65 (1.13 to 2.43)) [3].

As with infants with encephalopathy, less information is available on the long-term educational and social outcomes of infants likely exposed to mild degrees of perinatal asphyxia. Medniek *et al* [47] reported the outcome of 24 infants who had transient (< 8 days) neonatal symptoms. When compared to matched controls, they had similar IQ measures, but had lower scores in a measure of social maturity ($P < 0.05$). Van Handel reported worse scores in measures of behaviour at age 10 compared to peers in infants who survived mild HIE, although no obvious increase in psychiatric diagnoses (including ADHD) [33]. Finally, in a study using the Swedish birth registry, infants born in poor condition without neurological symptoms appeared to be less likely to have attended university (39% vs. 43%) or be earning an income (87% vs. 89%) than a control group in early adulthood [48].

# Other evidence of poor outcomes

As well as being analysed for the more commonly measured outcomes, some large linkage studies have been used to provide additional evidence for an impact of perinatal asphyxia on other long-term morbidities. These papers tend to investigate the association between a measure of perinatal asphyxia (often the Apgar score) and a variety of outcome measures. While the lack of neonatal clinical data does restrict the interpretation of any potential causal pathway, it does provide supportive evidence for other effects. Studies using techniques such as these have reported increased risks of psychiatric symptoms [49] and schizophrenia [50] for infants born with signs of perinatal asphyxia. While the size of these studies often makes the associations unlikely to be due to chance, the possibility of important residual confounding limits interpretation. Whether these infants have increased risks of mental health issues, what that increased risk is and if this is in addition to that expected from the cognitive impacts of HIE still needs to be clarified.

# Predictors of outcomes

If the data reviewed above allow broad conclusions to be drawn about the overall effects of perinatal asphyxia, the prediction of outcome for the individual infant is far more problematic. Over the years, several clinical predictors have been proposed and while many factors (including the Apgar score) are strongly associated with outcome, their predictive value is often too poor to be of clinical use. While the intensity and duration of the asphyxial insult is likely to be an important predictor of outcome, the extent of neuronal damage is also dependent on other (mostly unmeasured, or unmeasurable) factors as well: polymorphisms in certain candidate genes have been implicated, while concomitant clinical conditions such as infection, pyrexia and inflammation may also increase the risk of permanent neurological injury in the presence of similar asphyxial insults. Despite these and other limitations, prediction of outcome remains important in clinical practice to guide management, provide advice to parents and in targeting of novel therapies. In common with the studies reporting outcome discussed earlier in the chapter, many studies considered below are relatively small and so imprecision is a concern: confidence intervals around the point estimates are rarely presented for measures of sensitivity or specificity, while the development of the predictors is often performed using short-term outcomes and they are often not validated in an independent population.

There is also the possibility that measures derived early in the neonatal course (e.g., in the first 24 hours)

may become self-fulfilling while recent changes in the treatment of HIE may alter the predictive value by differentially affecting the marker over the outcome. This is a particular concern when looking at the clinical grade of HIE where the clinical grade of encephalopathy is unlikely to be affected by therapeutic hypothermia or other novel treatments despite potentially improving outcomes.

## Encephalopathy grade, clinical examination and biochemical measures

The development and severity of the encephalopathy is perhaps the most commonly used predictor of long-term outcome and consequently many of the outcome data listed above have been presented with this in mind. Infants with mild (or indeed no) measurable encephalopathy are likely to have similar rates of CP and death to the general population [46,51] although the potential impact on other measures is discussed above. Infants with moderate HIE have a substantial risk of death, CP and cognitive impairment. However, even infants within this clinical category have varied outcomes: the risk of a composite "poor" outcome at 18 months was reported as 66% in a recent RCT [9]. The overall outcome of infants with severe disease is often considered more certain, with earlier studies reporting death or impairment in all infants [31]. However, it appears that even in infants with severe disease outcome may be variable; one recent RCT reported a composite poor outcome of only 2% higher than the moderate group (68% [9]) and Badawi suggested only 62% of surviving infants with severe encephalopathy had a poor outcome at 2 years (compared with 25% with moderate disease (and 2.1% of controls)) [52]. In one paper assessing the variance in outcome in a cohort of infants with mild to severe HIE, grade of encephalopathy accounted for less than 20% of the variance seen in reading skills (in comparison with maternal social-demographic measures which accounted for over 30% [31]).

In addition to the encephalopathy severity, changes in neurological signs over time also have important prognostic significance. Sarnat and Sarnat in their original study found that encephalopathic infants who normalized by 5 days did not go on to develop cerebral palsy [21]. One study looked at neurological status at discharge and found good correlation (r = 0.65) with neuro-developmental outcome at 24 months (sensitivity 77% and specificity 83%) [53], while infants taking longer than 7 days to establish sucking feeds had a poor outcome at 2 years. In general, repeated examinations revealing the rate (or lack) of recovery of normal neurological signs appear more informative than single examinations. Barnett showed how motor examination before 2 years of age helped predict outcome at 5 years, although a normal score before 2 years still did not preclude infants developing cognitive abnormalities later [54].

In addition to these clinical measures, attempts have been made to validate more objective (often laboratory based) predictors of outcome and many other "bedside" tests have been proposed as prognostic indicators. Some data on biochemical measurements of perinatal asphyxia, such as lactate production, exist but predictive (rather than diagnostic) value appears limited [55]. Studies looking at levels of lactate dehydrogensase (LDH) (commonly measured as a diagnostic measure of perinatal asphyxia) suggest it may also provide some prognostic information [56] while biochemical indices in the CSF have also been advocated [57]. As yet none are commonly used in clinical practice.

### Cerebral blood flow velocity

The use of routine head ultrasound examination has become common in clinical practice and can provide important prognostic information. Using pulse Doppler, it is relatively easy to record cerebral blood flow velocity wave forms on the major intracranial arteries. A low resistance index (RI) (resistance index = peak systolic velocity minus end-diastolic velocity divided by peak systolic velocity) in the anterior cerebral artery has been advocated as a good prognostic measure in infants with moderate or severe HIE. Levene *et al* [58] found that a resistance index below 0.55 from 24 hours of age had a sensitivity of 100% and specificity of 81% for death or developmental delay, although this technique was found to be less predictive in hypothermic encephalopathic infants [59].

### Cerebral function monitors, EEG and neuro-imaging

Several other modalities have been proposed as indicators of outcome in infants with moderate or severe HIE. In particular, several aEEG devices designed to summarize single, or dual channel electroencephalography have become popular in clinical practice over the past decade and are commonly used as both diagnostic and prognostic tools, with the changes in aEEG over time being shown to be a very useful indicator of prognosis. The time to (or lack of) recovery of normal amplitude aEEG appears more informative than a single EEG

recording. The routine imaging of the cerebrum (and in particular early MR scanning) has also become more common and provides a wealth of prognostic information. Both EEG and neuro-imaging are discussed in detail later in this book.

## Conclusion

First, the application of the results discussed above to clinical practice is problematic. Two of the main limitations are imprecise results and relatively short-term outcome data. Infants rarely fit into categories perfectly and studies which exclude infants who develop other "confounding" pathology (in particular cerebral palsy) in later childhood make outcome prediction difficult when faced with an asphyxiated infant in the neonatal period (and no idea if the infant will, or will not develop cerebral palsy at that point).

Second, infants with mild (or clinically silent) encephalopathy may have long-term consequences of their perinatal compromise. There is now evidence that measures of IQ and more specific cognitive measures are worse than in their peers. However, the effects in the individual infants may well be small and there is little evidence of functional deficits or pragmatic worse outcomes for these infants. Infants with moderate encephalopathy have an extremely varied outcome. Some will die in the neonatal period, or progress to develop serious motor or cognitive impairment. For those without severe impairment, increasing evidence exists for substantially lower scores in neurophysiological testing and an increased need for educational and social support. The outcome of infants with severe encephalopathy appears even worse, although IQ in those who escape early death or profound intellectual impairment (while lower than their peers) is variable and some may have acceptable functional outcomes.

Third, the prediction of an individual infant's outcome with moderate or severe disease is difficult. A combination of repeated clinical examination, continuous aEEG, cerebral Doppler measures from 24 hours and MR imaging at 6 to 14 days is relatively good at identifying infants who will develop CP but, at present, maternal education levels may still remain the best predictor of school performance [31].

Fourth, an overarching limitation of the literature is the relevance of these results to modern perinatal practice. In many ways, the data discussed are already obsolete. We have concentrated on infants who did not

**Table 1.4.** IQ beyond 2 years of age (binary outcome)

| Paper | Category of HIE | Age at outcome (years) | Measure | Cut-off used | Proportion with low IQ | | Evidence for difference (reported P values) |
|---|---|---|---|---|---|---|---|
| | | | | | HIE infants | Controls | |
| Odd [3] | Mild, moderate or severe (CP included) | 8 | WISC-III | <80 | 6/26 (23%) | 354/5461 (6%) | 0.009 |
| Robertson [27] | Mild | 5.5 | Stanford-Binet-III | >1 SD below mean | 1.8% | – | – |
| | Moderate (non-disabled) | | Stanford-Binet-III | >1 SD below mean | 18.3% | – | – |
| | Moderate (disabled) | | Stanford-Binet-III | >1 SD below mean | 56.3% | – | – |
| | Severe | | Stanford-Binet-III | >1 SD below mean | 83.3% | – | – |
| George [28] | Mild | 12 | MISIC | <=70 | 4/41 (10%) | – | – |
| | Moderate or severe | | MISIC | <=70 | 2/5 (40%) | – | – |
| Barnett [54] | Mild to severe without CP | 5–6 | WPPSI | <=85 | 8/53 (10%) | | |

WPPSI, Wechsler Preschool and Primary Scale of Intelligence; MISIC, Malin's Intelligence Scale for Indian Children; WISC, Wechsler Intelligence Scale for Children.

receive therapeutic hypothermia to make the data as homogenous as possible and the impact of this and other new treatments on prognosis will be discussed later in this book. The data discussed here are based on infants born over many decades and the impact of changing obstetric and neonatal care (outside specific neuro-protective treatments) on long-term outcomes is mostly unknown. Even very recent changes, such as the use of room air rather than oxygen during resuscitation attempts may have important impacts, as may changes in clinicians' attitudes to withdrawal of care in these infants. Paradoxically, the best quality outcomes (in the oldest survivors) are perhaps the least applicable to our modern practice.

Fifth, while the published data are able to provide broad "brushstokes" around the outcome of these infants a substantial degree of uncertainty is likely to remain in all but the very well, or very unwell, infants and clinical follow-up of all infants at risk for many months or years remains essential (Table 1.4).

# References

1. Little W. On the influence of abnormal parturition, difficult labours, premature birth and asphyxia neonatorum, on the mental and physical condition of the child, especially in relation to deformities. *Trans London Obstet Soc* 1862;**3**:193–325.

2. Bryce J, Boschi-Pinto C, Shibuya K, et al. WHO estimates of the causes of death in children. *Lancet* 2005;**365**:1147–52.

3. Odd D, Odd DE, Lewis G, Whitelaw A, Gunnell D. Resuscitation at birth and cognition at 8 years of age: a cohort study. *Lancet* 2009;**9**:1615–22.

4. Thornberg E, Thornberg E, Thiringer K, Odeback A, Milsom I. Birth asphyxia: incidence, clinical course and outcome in a Swedish population. *Acta Paediatr* 1995;**84**:927–32.

5. Kruse M, Michelsen SI, Flachs EM, Bronnum-Hansen H, Madsen M, Uldall P. Lifetime costs of cerebral palsy. *Dev Med Child Neurol* 2009;**51**:622–8.

6. Deary IJ, Batty GD. Commentary: pre-morbid IQ and later health – the rapidly evolving field of cognitive epidemiology. *Int J Epidemiol* 2006;**35**:670–2.

7. Levene MI, Sands C, Grindulis H, Moore JR. Comparison of two methods of predicting outcome in perinatal asphyxia. *Lancet* 1986;**1**:67–9.

8. MacLennan A. A template for defining a causal relation between acute intrapartum events and cerebral palsy: international consensus statement. *BMJ* 1999;**319**:1054–9.

9. Azzopardi DV, Strohm B, Edwards AD, et al. Moderate hypothermia to treat perinatal asphyxial encephalopathy. *N Engl J Med* 2009;**361**:1349–58.

10. Gluckman PD, Wyatt JS, Azzopardi D, et al. Selective head cooling with mild systemic hypothermia after neonatal encephalopathy: multicentre randomised trial. *Lancet* 2005;**365**:663–70.

11. Shankaran S, Laptook AR, Ehrendranz RA, et al. Whole-body hypothermia for neonates with hypoxic-ischemic encephalopathy. *N Engl J Med* 2005;**353**:1574–84.

12. Goldaber KG, Gilstrap LC III, Leveno KJ, Dax JS, McIntire DD. Pathologic fetal acidemia. *Obstet Gynecol* 1991;**78**:1103–7.

13. Apgar V. A proposal for a new method of evaluation of the newborn infant. *Curr Res Anesth Analg* 1953;**32**:260–7.

14. Chamberlain G, Banks J. Assessment of the Apgar score. *Lancet* 1974;**2**:1225–8.

15. ACOG Committee Opinion. Number 333, May 2006 (replaces No. 174, July 1996): The Apgar score. *Obstet Gynecol* 2006;**107**:1209–12.

16. Apgar V. The newborn (Apgar) scoring system. Reflections and advice. *Pediatr Clin North Am* 1966;**13**: 645–50.

17. Moster D, Lie RT, Irgens LM, Bjerkedal T, Markestad T. The association of Apgar score with subsequent death and cerebral palsy: A population-based study in term infants. *J Pediatr* 2001;**138**:798–803.

18. Valentin L, Ekman G, Isberg PE, Polberger S, Marsal K. Clinical evaluation of the fetus and neonate. Relation between intra-partum cardiotocography, Apgar score, cord blood acid-base status and neonatal morbidity. *Arch Gynecol Obstet* 1993;**253**:103–15.

19. Josten BE, Johnson TR, Nelson JP. Umbilical cord blood pH and Apgar scores as an index of neonatal health. *Am J Obstet Gynecol* 1987;**157** (Pt 1):843–8.

20. Is the Apgar score outmoded? *Lancet* 1989;**1**:591–92.

21. Sarnat HB, Sarnat MS. Neonatal encephalopathy following fetal distress. A clinical and electroencephalographic study. *Arch Neurol* 1976;**33**:696–705.

22. Eken P, Toet MC, Groenendaal F, de Vries LS. Predictive value of early neuroimaging, pulsed Doppler and neurophysiology in full term infants with hypoxic-ischaemic encephalopathy. *Arch Dis Child Fetal Neonatal Ed* 1995;**73**:F75–80.

23. Myers RE, Two patterns of perinatal brain damage and their conditions of occurrence. *Am J Obstet Gynecol* 1972;**112**:246–76.

24. Marlow N, Wolke D, Bracewell MA, Samara M. Neurologic and developmental disability at six years of age after extremely preterm birth. *N Engl J Med* 2005;**352**:9–19.

25. Odd DE, Rasmussen F, Gunnell D, Lewis G, Whitlaw A. A cohort study of low Apgar scores and cognitive outcomes. *Arch Dis Child Fetal Neonatal Ed* 2008;**93**: F115–20.

26. Rantakallio P, von Wendt L, Koivu M. Prognosis of perinatal brain damage: a prospective study of a one year birth cohort of 12,000 children. *Early Hum Dev* 1987;**15**:75–84.

27. Robertson CM, Finer NN. Educational readiness of survivors of neonatal encephalopathy associated with birth asphyxia at term. *J Dev Behav Pediatr* 1988;**9**:298–306.

28. George B, Padmam MS, Nair MK, Indira MS, Syamalan K, Padmanohan J. Hypoxic ischemic encephalopathy developmental outcome at 12 years. *Indian Pediatr* 2009;**46**(Suppl):s67–70.

29. Lindstrom K, Lagerroos P, Gillberg C, Fernell E. Teenage outcome after being born at term with moderate neonatal encephalopathy. *Pediatr Neurol* 2006;**35**:268–74.

30. Marlow N, Rose AS, Rands CE, Draper ES. Neuropsychological and educational problems at school age associated with neonatal encephalopathy. *Arch Dis Child Fetal Neonatal Ed* 2005;**90**: F380–7.

31. Robertson CM, Finer NN, Grace MG. School performance of survivors of neonatal encephalopathy associated with birth asphyxia at term. *J Pediatr* 1989;**114**:753–60.

32. Viggedal G, Lundalv E, Carlsson G, Kjellmer I. Follow-up into young adulthood after cardiopulmonary resuscitation in term and near-term newborn infants. II. Neuropsychological consequences. [See comment]. *Acta Paediatr* 2002;**91**:1218–26.

33. van Handel M, Swaab H, de Vries LS, Jongmans MJ. Behavioral outcome in children with a history of neonatal encephalopathy following perinatal asphyxia. *J Pediatr Psychol* 2010;**35**:286–95.

34. Scherf KS, Sweeney JA, Luna B. Brain basis of developmental change in visuospatial working memory. *J Cogn Neurosci* 2006;**18**:1045–58.

35. Karunanayaka PR, Holland SK, Schmithorst VJ, et al. Age-related connectivity changes in fMRI data from children listening to stories. *Neuroimage* 2006;**34**: 349–60.

36. Vannest J, Karunanayaka PR, Schmithorst VJ, Szaflarski JP, Holland SK. Language networks in children: evidence from functional MRI studies. *AJNR Am J Roentgenol* 2009;**192**:1190–6.

37. Steinman KJ, Gomo-Tempini ML, Glidden DV, et al. Neonatal watershed brain injury on magnetic resonance imaging correlates with verbal IQ at 4 years. *Pediatrics* 2009;**123**:1025–30.

38. Gadian DG, Aicardi J, Watkins KE, Porter DA, Mishkin M, Vargha-Khadem F. Developmental amnesia associated with early hypoxic-ischaemic injury. *Brain* 2000;**123**(Pt 3):499–507.

39. Dixon G, Badawi N, Kurinczuk JJ, et al. Early developmental outcomes after newborn encephalopathy. *Pediatrics* 2002;**109**:26–33.

40. Moster D, Lie RT, Markestad T. Joint association of Apgar scores and early neonatal symptoms with minor disabilities at school age. *Arch Dis Child Fetal Neonatal Ed* 2002;**86**:F16–21.

41. Robertson C, Finer N. Term infants with hypoxic-ischemic encephalopathy: outcome at 3.5 years. *Dev Med Child Neurol* 1985;**27**:472–84.

42. Badawi N, Dixon G, Felix JF, et al. Autism following a history of newborn encephalopathy: more than a coincidence? *Dev Med Child Neurol* 2006;**48**:85–9.

43. Odd DE, Whitelaw A, Gunnell D, Lewis G. The association between birth condition and neuropsychological functioning and educational attainment at school age. A cohort study. *Arch Dis Child* 2011;**96**:30–7.

44. Kjellmer I, Beijer E, Carlsson G, Hrbek A, Viggedal G. Follow-up into young adulthood after cardiopulmonary resuscitation in term and near-term newborn infants. I. Educational achievements and social adjustment. *Acta Paediatr* 2002;**91**:1212–7.

45. Pasamanick B, Rogers ME, Lilienfeld AM. Pregnancy experience and the development of behavior disorders in children. *Am J Psychiatry* 1956;**112**:613–8.

46. Handley-Derry M, Low JA, Burke SO, Waurick M, Killen H, Derrick EJ. Intrapartum fetal asphyxia and the occurrence of minor deficits in 4- to 8-year-old children. *Dev Med Child Neurol* 1997;**39**:508–14.

47. Mednick BR, Michelsen NM. Neurological and motor functioning of 10–12-year-old children who showed mild transient neurological symptoms in the first five days of life. *Acta Neurol Scand* 1977;**56**: 70–8.

48. Odd DE, Gunnell D, Lewis G, Rasmussen F. Long-term impact of poor birth condition on social and economic outcomes in early childhood. *Pediatrics* 2011;**127**: e1498–504.

49. Zammit S, Odd D, Horwood J, et al. Investigating whether adverse prenatal and perinatal events are associated with non-clinical psychotic symptoms at age 12 years in the ALSPAC birth cohort. *Psychol Med* 2009;**39**:1457–67.

50. Dalman C, Thomas HV, David AS, Gentz J, Lewis G, Allebeck P. Signs of asphyxia at birth and risk of schizophrenia. Population-based case-control study. *Br J Psychiatry* 2001;**179**:403–8.

51. Gonzalez FF, Miller SP. Does perinatal asphyxia impair cognitive function without cerebral palsy? *Arch Dis Child Fetal Neonatal Ed* 2006;**91**:F454–9.

52. Badawi N, Felix JF, Kurinczuk JJ, et al. Cerebral palsy following term newborn encephalopathy: a population-based study. *Dev Med Child Neurol* 2005;**47**:293–8.

53. Murray DM, Bala P, O'Connor CM, Ryan CA, Connolly S, Boylan GB. The predictive value of early neurological examination in neonatal hypoxic-ischaemic encephalopathy and neurodevelopmental outcome at 24 months. *Dev Med Child Neurol* 2010;**52**: e55–9.

54. Barnett AL, Guzzetta A, Mercuri E, et al. Can the Griffiths scales predict neuromotor and perceptual-motor impairment in term infants with neonatal encephalopathy? *Arch Dis Child* 2004;**89**:637–43.

55. Oh W, Perritt R, Shankaran S, et al. Association between urinary lactate to creatinine ratio and neurodevelopmental outcome in term infants with hypoxic-ischemic encephalopathy. *J Pediatr* 2008;**153**:375–8.

56. Thoresen M, Liu X, Jary S, Brown E, Sabir H, Stone J, Cowan F, Karlsson M. Lactate dehydrogenase in hypothermia-treated newborn infants with hypoxic-ischaemic encephalopathy. *Acta Paediatr* 2012; **101**:1038–44.

57. Oygür N, Sonmez O, Saka O, Yegin O. Predictive value of plasma and cerebrospinal fluid tumour necrosis factor-alpha and interleukin-1 beta concentrations on outcome of full term infants with hypoxic-ischaemic encephalopathy. *Arch Dis Child Fetal Neonatal Ed* 1998;**79**:F190–3.

58. Archer LN, Levene MI, Evans DH. Cerebral artery Doppler ultrasonography for prediction of outcome after perinatal asphyxia. *Lancet* 1986;**2**:1116–8.

59. Elstad M, Whitelaw A, Thoresen M. Cerebral Resistance Index is less predictive in hypothermic encephalopathic newborns. *Acta Paediatr* 2011;**100**:1344–9.

**Chapter 2**

# Molecular mechanisms of neonatal brain injury and neural rescue

Pierre Gressens and Henrik Hagberg

## Introduction

Perinatal brain injury is a common cause of life-long neurological deficits and there is an urgent need to better understand its pathophysiology and to find strategies for prevention and treatment. The etiology is complex and multifactorial but hypoxia–ischaemia (HI), infection/inflammation and excitotoxicity (see below) are considered important causes or precipitating insults of preventable/treatable forms of perinatal brain injury. In this review, we will focus on mechanisms of brain injury in response to acute sterile insults in the developing brain that occur in term (e.g., neonatal encephalopathy) or preterm infants.

Genetic background, developmental age, sex and brain maturity affect vulnerability and the mechanisms of brain injury [1,2]. Furthermore, antecedents such as infection/inflammation, intrauterine growth restriction or pre-exposures to hypoxia can modulate brain vulnerability in response to acute insults [3–5]. Brain injury evolves over time and different mechanisms are critical during the primary, secondary and tertiary phases (Figure 2.1). Indeed, recent experimental data suggest that interventions can be effective if administered hours, days or even weeks after the primary insult [6,7].

The aim of the present review is to describe the critical mechanisms of brain injury during the secondary and tertiary phases after an acute insult and to present some therapeutic strategies that may have potential for clinical translation.

## Concept of secondary brain injury

In experimental studies, cerebral HI of sufficient severity to deplete tissue energy reserves (primary insult) is often

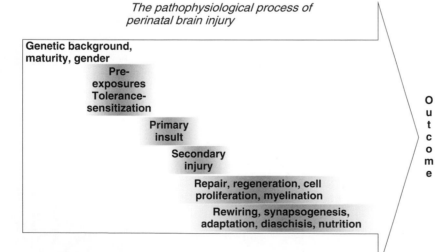

*The pathophysiological process of perinatal brain injury*

Genetic background, maturity, gender

Pre-exposures Tolerance-sensitization

Primary insult

Secondary injury

Repair, regeneration, cell proliferation, myelination

Rewiring, synapsogenesis, adaptation, diaschisis, nutrition

Outcome

**Figure 2.1.** Multiple factors occurring alone or in combination prior, during and after the acute perinatal insult determine outcome. Injurious and reparative processes are operative both during the secondary phase shortly after as well as during the tertiary phase day-weeks after exposure.

followed by transient but complete restoration of glucose usage, ATP and phosphocreatine upon reperfusion/reoxygenation [8–10]. Thereafter, a secondary decrease of high-energy phosphates occurs in parallel with a decrease in tissue glucose metabolism and development of cell injury [8–10]. Similarly, infants with neonatal encepalopathy show characteristic abnormalities in cerebral energy metabolism, which is frequently normal soon after birth, but shows a progressive decline in [PCr]/[Pi] some hours later [11]. Infants displaying this phenomenon develop severe neurodevelopmental impairment or die and there is a close relationship between the magnitude of the late decline in [PCr]/[Pi], reduced brain growth and the severity of neurodevelopmental impairment 4 years later [12].

These findings suggest that most of the injury after HI evolves over time *after* rather than during the insult. There are many examples of successful post-treatment after HI in animals, suggesting a therapeutic window following HI before the secondary phase of tissue deterioration. Hypothermia following HI reduces secondary energy failure and brain injury in experimental studies [13] and was later proven to be an effective neuroprotective treatment in newborns with neonatal encephalopathy [14]. However, the mechanisms involved in secondary brain injury are incompletely understood and such information is critical for development of the next generation of therapies for preterm infants or to be combined with hypothermia in severely

asphyxiated infants at term, hopefully, to further reduce serious disability in children and adults.

## Mechanisms of secondary brain injury

The deficit in high-energy phosphates induced by HI leads to a primary failure to maintain transmembrane ionic gradients, release of neuroactive compounds into the extracellular compartments, accumulation of intracellular $Ca^{2+}$ and the activation of a series of mechanisms that if sustained will lead to immediate cell death. If the individual is resuscitated, these acute alterations are completely or partly reversed but the complex process has been started in which multiple interrelated factors may produce secondary brain injury.

The precise mechanisms of damage are incompletely understood but some components of the process have been elucidated. Excitatory amino acids (EAAs), mitochondrial impairment, intracellular calcium regulation, generation of reactive oxygen species (ROS), including nitric oxide (NO), apoptotic/necrotic mechanisms, changes in the availability of trophic factors and the immuno-inflammatory system, are all implicated in the process (Figure 2.2).

### Excitotoxicity

Glutamate and aspartate are the main excitatory transmitters in the brain, but they are known to exert toxic effects (excitotoxicity) if applied in excess to the nervous

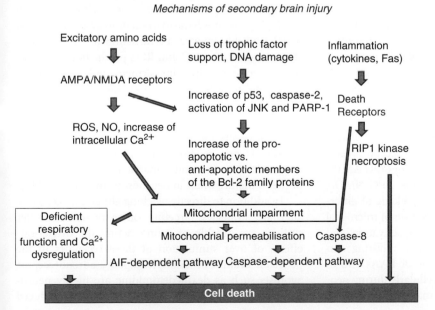

*Mechanisms of secondary brain injury*

**Figure 2.2.** Summary of injury mechanisms during the secondary phase.

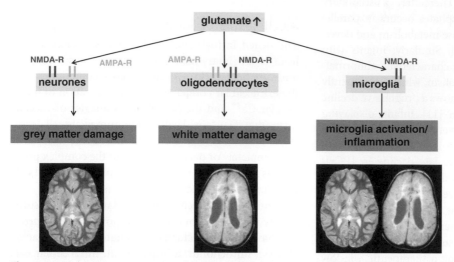

**Figure 2.3.** Schematic representation of the expression of glutamate receptors on neural cells in the perinatal brain.

system. Both N-methyl-D-aspartate (NMDA) and α-amino-3-hydroxy-5-methyl-4-isoxazole-propionic acid (AMPA)/kainate receptors are expressed on neurons and oligodendroglial precursors (preferentially on somata) in vulnerable areas of grey and white matter [15–17]. The expression of EAA receptors is upregulated in the immature human brain, which reflects the critical role of these receptors for brain development. Hence, the immature brain is also more vulnerable to excitotoxicity (especially NMDA) than the adult [18], affecting both white and grey matter [19].

There is considerable evidence for a role of EAAs in the process leading to HI brain injury. EAA receptors are expressed by all types of neural cells. In particular, neurons [16] and oligodendrocyte precursor cells (OPCs) [20] express NMDA and AMPA receptors, while microglia [21] have been recently shown to express NMDA receptors (Figure 2.3). NMDA receptors have also been described on endothelial cells [22]. Excess activation of neuronal NMDA or AMPA receptors leads to neuronal cell death. Excess activation of OPC AMPA receptors leads to OPC cell death while OPC NMDA receptor activation seems to lead to blockade of differentiation rather than cell death. Activation of microglial NMDA receptors leads to microglial activation and release of factors potentially toxic for neighbouring neural cells. Extracellular concentrations of EAAs and to some extent glycine increase extracellularly during neonatal HI in mixed grey and white matter of fetal sheep

[23] and is followed by a secondary increase during reperfusion [24,25]. EAAs also increase markedly in the cerebrospinal fluid (CSF) of newborns with neonatal encephalopathy and the levels are associated with the degree of encephalopathy and short-term outcome [26].

Blocking NMDA receptors before or after HI reduces subsequent neuronal damage [27] and during "*in vitro* ischaemia", NMDA receptor activation results in $Ca^{2+}$-dependent injury of oligodendroglial processes [17]. AMPA blockade reduces grey and white matter damage when given after HI or excitotoxic insult [15,27,28]. The mechanism of excitotoxicity in response to HI probably involves perturbation of $Ca^{2+}$ homeostasis, triggering of NO and ROS production with subsequent mitochondrial impairment and activation of lipases and proteases (Figure 2.2). Some NMDA receptor antagonists (e.g., dizocilpine, xenon) can, however, induce apoptosis in the immature brain [29,30] which may complicate the use of such drugs for cerebroprotection. There are, however, other NMDA receptor antagonists like memantine that do not induce apoptosis in the immature brain in neuroprotective dosages [31].

In addition to directly blocking glutamate receptors, alternate strategies targeting other neurotransmitter systems are capable of counteracting the deleterious effects of over stimulation of these receptors in the perinatal brain. For example, alpha-2-adrenoreceptor agonists such as dexmedetomidine are highly neuroprotective in a model of neonatal excitotoxicity induced by an NMDA agonist [32,33]. Accordingly, dexmedetomidine is also neuroprotective against a neonatal HI insult [34]. In addition endocannabinoids protect the newborn brain against an AMPA-kainate receptor-mediated neonatal excitotoxic injury [35].

## Calcium regulation

Calcium ($Ca^{2+}$) is an intracellular second messenger, acting as key regulator of numerous cellular functions [36]. To allow efficient $Ca^{2+}$ dependent signalling, the intracellular $Ca^{2+}$ concentration ($Ca^{2+}ic$) is strictly regulated at a low level of 100 nM, i.e., 10,000 times lower than the extracellular concentration [36]. The large electrochemical gradient is upheld through ATP-requiring processes at the level of the cell membrane (Na+/Ca2+ exchange and Na+/K+ ATPase, Ca2+ ATPase), mitochondria and endoplasmic reticulum [36]. In the adult brain, transmembrane ionic gradients cannot be maintained once ATP has been depleted and a rapid depolarization occurs after a few minutes of complete anoxia or ischaemia with a concomitant rise of $Ca^{2+}ic$. A marked rise of $Ca^{2+}ic$ may trigger several toxic processes like activation of calpains, ROS, apoptosis, phospholipases, endonucleases and NO production [37].

Intracellular calcium regulation is thus considered to play an important role in the cellular response to injury. However, its significance in immature brain injury is less clear. In studies *in vitro*, the rise of $Ca^{2+}ic$ tends to be slower and less pronounced in immature neurons [38]. However, $Ca^{2+}$ accumulates to some extent in the brain tissue during HI [39] and calcium-dependent enzymes such as calpains and phospholipase C are activated [40], which offers some indirect information in support of an increase of $Ca^{2+}ic$ in the immature brain during HI.

It is equally unclear exactly what happens to $Ca^{2+}ic$ after delayed injury. Five to 72 hours following a period of HI there is a delayed accumulation of calcium in regions with brain injury [39]. In stroke models in adult rodents, there are waves of NMDA receptor-dependent depolarizations (spreading depression) in border-zone areas accompanied by neuronal uptake of $Ca^{2+}$. In the immature brain, spreading depression occurs at a slower rate and the degree of $Ca^{2+}$ influx appears to be lower than in the adult counterpart [41]. There is also a pronounced accumulation of calcium in axons and neuronal mitochondria detected by pyroantimonate technique/electron microscopy [42]. The pathophysiological role of these $Ca^{2+}$ elevations is yet unknown but could theoretically contribute to NMDA receptor-dependent excitoxicity during the reperfusion phase.

## Mitochondrial impairment

There seems to be a shift towards a more juxta-nuclear mitochondrial localization [42,43] and a progressive accumulation of calcium in the mitochondrial matrix of neurons 0.5–3 hours after HI [42]. Some mitochondria developed a considerable degree of swelling, reaching a diameter of several micrometers at 3 hours of reperfusion, whereas the majority of mitochondria appeared only moderately affected. Chromatin condensation was observed in the nuclei of many cells with severely swollen mitochondria with calcium deposits.

During early recovery after HI, high-energy phosphates in the cerebral cortex are restored as previously mentioned [9,10,44]. During this phase, the 2-deoxyglucose (2-DG) usage is increased, which correlates with increased levels of tissue lactate and a depression of mitochondrial respiration [44]. Post-HI administration of an NMDA receptor antagonist normalized 2-DG usage and lactate levels, improved mitochondrial respiration and attenuated cortical brain injury [10,44]. These data suggest that NMDA-receptor activation in the early recovery phase suppresses mitochondrial respiration with a compensatory increase of anaerobic glucose cycling to lactate, which precedes development of cortical brain injury. Interestingly, a similar pattern of increased glucose use occurred in the central nervous system (CNS) of asphyxiated infants, particularly in brain regions that were subsequently injured [45]. Such an increase in glucose usage occurred in parallel with marked elevations of glutamate in the CSF [26], suggesting that HI brain injury in post-asphyxiated infants is also preceded by a phase of mitochondrial impairment related to activation of EAA receptors.

Mitochondrial impairment could, if persistent, have severe consequences on recovery of calcium regulation [36] and mitochondrial ATP production after HI. Furthermore, mitochondrial swelling and/or outer mitochondrial membrane permeabilization lead to release of killer proteins that may lead to apoptotic-like execution of cell death (below).

## Apoptotic mechanisms

### Apoptosis in the immature brain

Cell death is often classified as apoptotic or necrotic based on biochemical or morphological criteria [46].

Necrotic cell death is triggered by an acute insult resulting in severe primary energy failure, complete loss of membrane integrity and leaking of cytoplasmic contents into the extracellular matrix leading to an inflammatory response. Apoptotic cells do not lose membrane integrity and the organelles remain largely intact until the final stages when cell fragments bud off as apoptotic bodies, which are subsequently phagocytosed by microglia or healthy neighbouring cells. In morphological terms, mixed apoptotic–necrotic phenotypes predominate in HI and recent data suggest apoptotic, necroptotic and necrotic pathways are all important [46].

Apoptosis was initially recognized for its role in development. In some brain regions, half of the neurons die by apoptosis during normal brain development. Therefore, it is entirely appropriate that many apoptosis-related factors are upregulated in the immature brain, such as caspase-3, Apaf-1, Bcl-2 and Bax [47,48]. Multiple apoptotic pathways converge on caspase-3, so this protease is critical in the execution of neuronal apoptosis both during brain development and after acute injury [49]. Caspase-3 appears to be particularly important in the brain, because mice devoid of caspase-3 through genetic targeting displayed a hyperplastic, disorganized brain, whereas other organs appeared normal [49]. The constitutive levels of caspase-3 and the activation after injury are several-fold more pronounced in the immature brain [50,51]. In summary, due to ongoing apoptotic processes during brain development, the apoptotic biochemical machinery is highly upregulated in the immature brain, which may confer heightened vulnerability.

### Caspase-dependent cell death and apoptosis-inducing factor (AIF) in HI

Studies suggest that mitochondria regulate apoptotic cell death through their capacity to undergo mitochondrial membrane permeabilization (MP) and release of proapoptotic proteins [52]. Cytochrome C (Cyt C) and other apoptogenic proteins, such as AIF, endonuclease G, SMAC/Diablo and HtrA2/Omi, are released from the mitochondrial intermembrane space. Bax, Bad, Bid and other members of the Bcl-2 family are involved in the regulation of mitochondrial release of proapoptotic proteins. Cyt C interacts with APAF-1, ADP and pro-caspase-9 to form the heptameric apoptosome, leading to activation of caspase-9, which in turn cleaves and activates pro-caspase-3 [52].

AIF, on the other hand, promotes apoptosis in a caspase-independent manner [52]. In addition, the downstream activation of executioner caspases, such as caspase-3, can be triggered through Fas receptor-mediated activation of caspase-8 without involvement of mitochondria, the so-called extrinsic pathway.

Apoptosis is found in the brains of infants who die after intrauterine insults or perinatal HI [53] and ample evidence supports the concept that apoptotic mechanisms are critically involved [54].

Caspase-3 is markedly activated after HI in the immature brain [50,55] and cells with the cleaved active form of caspase-3 colocalize with markers of DNA fragmentation in injured brain regions [55]. Caspase-3 inhibitors [50] as well as transgenic overexpression of X-linked inhibitor of apoptosis (XIAP) [56] attenuate caspase-3 activation and provide a considerable degree of neuroprotection in the neonatal setting in some [50] but not in all studies [57].

There are data to suggest that the extrinsic pathway is activated in response to HI [58] and Fas receptor deficiency seems to confer some degree of protection in neonatal HI [59]. Most data, however, suggest that activation of the intrinsic pathway is the key event in the immature brain. Assembly of the apoptosome is easily induced in homogenates from the immature brain [60], Cyt C is released to the cytosol in response to HI [43], caspase-9 is activated [61] and inhibition of APAF-1 reduces HI brain injury [62]. In addition, other proapoptotic proteins, such as AIF [63], SMAC/Diablo [56] and HtrA2/Omi [56], translocate from the mitochondria to a nuclear localization, suggesting that proapoptotic proteins are indeed released during the early recovery phase after HI. Cells with immunohistochemical translocation of Cyt C and AIF often exhibit signs of DNA fragmentation and nuclear condensation and these cells are preferentially localized in regions with early loss of the neuronal marker MAP-2 [55].

Development of brain injury in immature mice after HI depends on AIF [63]. The distribution of AIF translocation matches the accumulation of poly (ADP-ribose) (PAR), suggesting that activation of poly(ADP-ribose) polymerase (PARP) might trigger AIF release from mitochondria [64]. AIF is released to the cytosol, binds to another protein, cyclophilin A (CyA) [65], and the AIF-CyA complex translocates to the nucleus and triggers DNA degradation. The release of pro-apoptotic proteins from mitochondria depends on induction of MP. In the mature brain, MP is mediated by cyclophilin D-dependent opening of the mitochondrial permeability transition pore. However, in the immature brain, MP depends on Bax/Bak that most likely forms a pore in the outer mitochondrial membrane [66,67]. Bax gene deficiency or Bax inhibitory peptide confers substantial neuroprotection after HI [67,68]. These data suggest that Bax-dependent MP and subsequent activation of caspase- and AIF-dependent processes is critical in HI injury in the immature brain. The mechanisms of triggering of MP are partly unknown but a shift in the pro- versus anti-apoptotic bcl-2 family balance is probably important.

### Bcl-2 family proteins in HI

Transgenic mice overexpressing human Bcl-xL postnatally were resistant to neonatal HI [69]. Using a site-specific antibody for phosphorylation of Bcl-2 at serine-24 (PS24-Bcl-2), the number of cells positive for PS24-Bcl-2 increased during 3–24 hours of reperfusion in all investigated brain areas after neonatal HI [61]. Phosphorylation of Bcl-2 coincided with Cyt C translocation and co-localized with, but preceded, caspase-3 activation. In summary, Bcl-2 is phosphorylated (and probably inactivated) and translocated to the nucleus, concomitant with increased mitochondrial Bax immunoreactivity, Cyt C release and activation of caspase-3. Furthermore, following HI, mice deficient in the BH3 only proteins Bad or Bim exhibited reduced activated caspase-3 and decreased parenchymal loss, suggesting that these BH3 only proteins are also involved [70].

The protein p53 is a tumour suppressor that triggers apoptosis by means of multiple pathways: it causes cell cycle arrest, inhibits or stimulates autophagy [71] through transactivating pro-apoptotic and repressing antiapoptotic genes. p53 also has cytoplasmic actions at the mitochondrial level through interaction with bcl-2 family proteins and can promote Bax-dependent MP [71]. Recently, it was shown that p53 translocates to mitochondria after HI and a peptide (pifithrin-α) that selectively blocks the p53 interaction with mitochondria, reduces Cyt C release, caspase-3 activation and attenuates HI injury, whereas inhibition of p53 transactivation was less protective [72].

### C-Jun N-terminal kinase 3 (JNK3) in neonatal HI

JNK3 is a member of the stress-activated group of mitogen-activated protein kinases (MAPK). The JNK isoform 3 (JNK3) is specifically expressed in the CNS and stress-induced JNK3 contributes to brain injury; hence, JNK3 deficiency renders adult mice resistant to excitotoxicity [73] and attenuates HI damage in newborn mice [74]. JNK3 deletion decreased caspase-3 cleavage and Bim/PUMA expression, coupled with an up-regulation of AKT/FOXO3a levels [74], suggesting that the primary mode of JNK3 action is to promote apoptosis and that JNK3 is acting upstream of mitochondria (Figure 2.2).

### Calpains

Calpains are cysteine proteases involved in signal transduction cascades, which differ from caspases as activity is calcium dependent and the proteolysis does not require an aspartic acid residue [75]. A high concentration of calcium can contribute to uncontrolled activation of calpains. They have been implicated in both apoptosis and necrosis, axonal degeneration and cytoskeletal disruption [76].

Calpain activity is high in the developing brain, especially in the white matter [75]. HI activates and relocates calpain to the membrane fraction [40] and inactivates the endogenous calpain inhibitor calpastatin in vulnerable brain regions [40,47]. Calpain cleavage products accumulate during delayed cerebral injury, especially in white matter [40]. Furthermore, synergistic activation of caspase-3 and m-calpains suggests a link between the two death signaling systems following HI [47]. The involvement of calpains is further supported by the neuroprotective efficacy of the calpain inhibitor MDL28170 [77].

### Necroptosis and autophagy

Necroptosis is a cellular mechanism of necrotic cell death that can be induced in the absence of intracellular apoptotic signalling. It is triggered by death receptor engagement by TNF-α (or other ligands), leading to the activation of death domain receptor-associated adaptor kinase RIP1 [78]. Allosteric inhibition of RIP1 with necrostatin-1 attenuates delayed mouse ischaemic brain injury in the adult [78]. Recently, it was shown that necrostatin-1 inhibits brain injury also in the immature brain subjected to HI, specifically in male mice [79].

Autophagy is a process involving degradation of cytoplasmic macromolecules and organelles in mammalian cells by means of the lysosomal system and can be induced during starvation and normal growth control to maintain cellular homeostasis and survival [80,81]. It has also been suggested that autophagy can trigger a type of cell death distinct from apoptosis.

Autophagy, as judged by the autophagosome-related marker LC-3 II, was induced after HI in both immature and adult brain [51] and was not different in male and female animals [82]. To investigate the importance of autophagy in neonatal HI, Atg7 gene-deficient mice (*Atg7flox/flox*; nestin-*Cre*) were used. Atg7 is critical in autophagy as, together with Atg3, it conjugates phosphatidyl ethanolamine to the C-terminal glycine residue of LC3-I, forming the membrane-bound form, LC3-II. Indeed, both caspase-dependent and caspase-nondependent cell death in hippocampus were substantially reduced in Atg7-deleted mice [83], suggesting that autophagy is a detrimental response. However, Atg7 may also take part in apoptosis, which complicates the interpretation [84]. In another study, beclin 1, a Bcl-2-interacting protein required for autophagy, was shown to increase in neurons after neonatal HI. Further enhancement of beclin 1 by pharmacological means reduced injury, implying that autophagy is protective [85]. Such a beneficial role of autophagy is further supported by its potential role in hypoxic or ischaemic preconditioning [85,86].

Additional studies are needed to further understand the importance of necroptosis and autophagy in perinatal brain injury and how these processes interact with apoptotic mechanisms.

## Reactive oxygen species (ROS)

ROS are molecules that contain one or more unpaired electrons [87], which makes free radicals highly reactive and able to disrupt the molecular structure of lipids and proteins with devastating consequences for cellular function [87]. Depending on the cellular energy balance, ROS can induce both necrosis and apoptosis by mechanisms that involve mitochondrial alterations following perinatal brain damage.

There are several pathways whereby ROS are produced in the brain [87]. The superoxide radical ($O2.-$) is produced by: (1) electron leakage from the electron transport chain in mitochondria, (2) oxidation of hypoxanthine to xanthine and urate by xanthine oxidase (mainly in endothelial cells), (3) degradation of free fatty acids by phospholipase A2 into arachidonic acid and subsequent oxidation of arachidonic acid by cyclooxygenase and lipooxygenase and (4) NADPH oxidase activity in macrophages, neutrophils and microglia.

The $O2.-$ radical has a relatively low reactivity and does not easily cross cell membranes. However, $O2.-$ can react with $Fe^{2+}$ ions and form hydroxyl radicals (.OH) which react with almost every molecule in the presence of transition metals such as $Fe^{2+}$ ions and exert toxic effects on DNA, activating poly(ADP-ribose)polymerase and depleting cellular NAD+ and ATP. The .OH radical initiates lipid peroxidation in a self perpetuating reaction which disrupts membrane function. Thiol-groups on enzymes and structural proteins are oxidized with loss of enzyme function and cytoskeletal disruption [87].

There are several defence systems in the brain to reduce the formation of OFRs and several pathways for their inactivation. The $O2.-$ adduct is dismutated by superoxide dismutase (SOD) into hydrogen peroxide ($H_2O_2$), which is converted to water and oxygen by either catalase or glutathione peroxidase. Compounds like vitamin E (α-tocopherol) act as lipid soluble scavengers, which inhibit lipid peroxidation. Chelation of transition metals such as iron is another endogenous protective mechanism against excessive formation of ROS. Intracellular concentrations of glutathione may be particularly important and immature oligodendrocytes are especially prone to ROS-induced death because of limited glutathione stores [88].

There is evidence for increased hypoxanthine levels, free radical formation and lipid peroxidation during reperfusion after HI in neonatal mice, newborn piglets, immature rats and fetal sheep [54].

The neuroprotective strategy of use of free radical inhibitors and scavengers has been evaluated experimentally. Treatment with the 21-aminosteroid tirilazad mesylate, a lipid peroxidation inhibitor, after hypoxia–ischaemia in 7-day-old rats reduces brain damage [89]. Allopurinol and its metabolite oxypurinol, being inhibitors of xanthine oxidase and ROS scavengers in high concentrations, reduce brain damage when administered before or after HI [90]. Furthermore, the iron chelator deferoxamine attenuates hypoxic–ischaemic brain damage [91]. Recently several antioxidants, such as ascorbic acid, pyrrolydine dithiocarbamate, tanshionine and melatonin have been shown to be neuroprotective [92–96]. Other experimental data support the concept that ROS production has an important impact on the HI responses mediated by hypoxia-inducible factor-1 (HIF-1) and cyclooxygenase-2 (COX-2) [97,98].

In adult ischaemia, neutrophils are a major source of free radical production following ischaemia and the major site of action for some neuroprotective free radical scavengers appears to be at the blood–brain barrier [99]. The role of neutrophils and NADPH expressed mainly in neutrophils appears to be less prominent in the immature brain [100,101].

## Nitric oxide (NO)

As a second messenger NO is involved in distinct biological processes such as maintainance of blood pressure, defense against microorganisms and cancer, and neurotransmission. On the other hand NO is involved in brain injury as inhibition of NO synthesis attenuates NMDA neurotoxicity [102]. Production of NO, first identified as the endothelium-derived relaxing factor, occurs through conversion of arginine to citrulline by three different nitric oxide synthases (NOS): neuronal NOS (nNOS), endothelial NOS (eNOS) and macrophage or inducible NOS (iNOS) [103]. Both eNOS and nNOS are expressed constitutively, but all types of NOS can be induced in response to a variety of stimuli. Both eNOS and nNOS are dependent upon $Ca^{2+}$ binding for activation and nNOS is activated by NMDA receptor stimulation. The activity of iNOS is mainly expressed in inflammatory cells: it produces large amounts of NO and its activity is $Ca^{2+}$ independent [104]. NO and O2.- react very quickly to form peroxynitrite ($ONOO^-$), which is freely diffusible and oxidizes thiol groups, induces protein nitrosylation and causes mitochondrial impairment, thus contributing to brain damage (Figure 2.2) [105].

Investigations on the role of NO in ischaemic brain injury have yielded conflicting results and the effects of different subtypes of NOS have to be considered separately [104,106]. In many studies, eNOS confers protection through a beneficial vasodilator effect improving perfusion, while nNOS and iNOS enhance injury in response to focal ischaemia [106]. Recent data also suggest that immature brain behaves differently from adult tissue. As in the adult, NO is produced in increasing amounts during reperfusion [24,25] and some data support a role for NO and NOS in injury to the developing brain: selective lesion of cells with NOS activity before an HI insult decreased brain injury [107]; neonatal mice lacking the gene for nNOS develop smaller brain injury than wild-type mice following hypoxia–ischaemia [108]; and non-specific NOS inhibitors provide neuroprotection [109]; recently a neuronal NOS inhibitor prevented development of cerebral palsy-like motor deficits in a preterm model of injury in newborn rabbits [110]. However, tissue concentrations of iNOS are very low

in the immature rat brain and do not appear to be induced within 36 hours of HI, and NOS inhibition was unable to prevent secondary energy failure after HI in immature mice [111]. Equally, intracerebral injection of the NO donor nitroprusside at doses which inflict damage in the adult brain is not toxic to the neonatal brain [112], suggesting that the immature brain may be more resistant to NO toxicity. In addition, NO released from nipradilol, an NO donor, exerts a neuroprotective effect on neonatal neurons [113]. It was also recently shown that inhaled NO plays a key role in the myelination of the developing brain and is neuroprotective in a model of neonatal excitotoxic brain damage [114].

## Inflammation in neonatal brain injury

Non-infectious exposure to excitotoxicity [115], HI [116] or stroke [117] induces inflammation in the immature brain. Immuno-inflammatory cells, predominantly microglia/macrophages [21,118], but also polymorphonuclear cells [100], lymphocytes, NK-cells and mast [119] and astroglia [100] are activated by HI. The cellular changes are accompanied by altered expression of toll-like receptors (TLRs), cytokines, chemokines and reactive oxygen species [120–124]. The initiation of the microglial response is well studied in the infectious setting where microbial products bind to receptors (including TLRs) on the cell surface and activate the transcription factor NF-κB. The initial signals after sterile tissue damage are less well characterized, but once elicited the microglial response can be aggravated by pro-inflammatory cytokines including IL-1 [125]. Microglia/macrophages may contribute to secondary brain injury through the production of pro-inflammatory cytokines, proteases, complement factors and excitotoxic amino acids [126]. In addition, microglial cells can induce oxidative injury through the production of reactive oxygen species (ROS) and nitric oxide. There are data suggesting that the early pro-inflammatory phase aggravates injury after HI as inhibition of platelet activating factor (PAF) [127], the pro-inflammatory cytokines IL-1 [121] and IL-18 [123], caspase-1 (activating IL-1 and IL-18) [128] and the complement C1q [129] all worsen HI injury. Furthermore, IL-1beta, IL-6, IL-9, or TNF-alpha all enhance ibotenate excitotoxicity [4], whereas the anti-inflammatory cytokine IL-10 is protective [130]. Part of the mechanisms underlying the sensitizing effect of pro-inflammatory cytokines could be linked to an imbalance between pro- and anti-inflammatory responses in the brain [131]. Inflammatory cells and mediators are highly context and time dependent, e.g., both beneficial and detrimental effects have been reported for microglia/macrophages [132] and components of the complement system [133,134]. We yet lack information as to the mechanisms of resolution of the pro-inflammatory phase and how repair and regain of CNS functions are achieved. Contradictory results have been obtained with regard to ischaemia–reperfusion as both inhibition of microglial activation as well as addition of exogenous-activated microglia have been shown to reduce injury [135]. Similarly, minocycline, which is known to reduce microglial activation, has yielded conflicting results in models of HI or excitotoxic perinatal brain damage [115,136,137].

Another important issue is to what extent peripheral myeloid cells invade the brain parenchyma and contribute to the population of activated microglia/macrophages after ischaemia. A recent study suggests a small transfer of CD45high/Cd11b+ leukocytes (< 10%) at 24 hours after neonatal stroke and a slightly higher contribution (30%) at 48 hours, indicating that fewer macrophages are coming from the blood in the immature compared to the adult brain after stroke [134,138]. Similar results were obtained in a model of neonatal excitotoxicity [115]. The possibility remains that the phenotypic expression of cells coming from the periphery changes rapidly when these cells settle in the brain parenchyma and/or that a subpopulation of microglia residing in the brain before the insult are expressing the CD45high/Cd11b+ phenotypic markers giving the false impression of cell invasion.

## Delayed interventions

One key issue for protecting the perinatal brain is the available window for intervention. From a clinical point of view, the longer this window, the better the chance to be able to implement the treatment. For example, hypothermia has to be initiated within the first 6 hours of life to be protective in term infants with neonatal encephalopathy [139]. Such a short window does not allow us to apply this treatment to all neonates who might benefit from it.

In a schematic way, one could distinguish between strategies aiming at extending the window of opportunity from the acute phase to the sub-acute phase and strategies targeting more long-term events such as

chronic inflammation or post-lesional plasticity. Although this is still a field in its youth, strategies for implementing delayed interventions (beyond the acute phase) are being tested in experimental models and can have different rationale and/or targets (Figure 2.1).

## Delaying the acute phase

As mentioned above, experimental and human data strongly support the fact that hypothermia is neuroprotective in term infants if introduced within the first 6 hours after birth. Although different groups are currently testing, in animal models and/or in clinical trials, the combination of early hypothermia and drugs such as xenon or melatonin [140,141] in an add-on strategy to enhance the efficacy of hypothermia, some groups have been trying to extend the window of intervention of hypothermia by first giving an anti-epileptic drug before delayed hypothermia. Using the classical Rice-Vannucci P7 rat model, Liu et al. [142] have shown that a combination of low-dose topiramate administered 15 minutes after the hypoxic–ischaemic insult and 3-hour hypothermia initiated 3 hours after the insult was neuroprotective while topiramate alone or hypothermia alone had no significant effect. More recently, the same group showed that early phenobarbital also enhanced the efficacy of delayed hypothermia [143].

An alternative strategy would be to use early but short-term hypothermia to enhance the window of opportunity for a protective drug. This strategy could allow reduction of the duration of hypothermia. Accordingly, it was shown that fructose-1,6-biphosphate (FBP) was neuroprotective against neonatal excitotoxic cortical damage [144]. However, the drug had to be given in the first 8 hours to be neuroprotective. Interestingly, a moderate but transient (4 hours) cooling immediately after the insult extended the therapeutic window for FBP, as FBP administered 24 hours after the excitotoxic insult was still significantly neuroprotective in mouse pups.

## Stimulating/favouring M2 microglia

Activated microglia have been shown to be detrimental for the production of hippocampal neurons but microglia and macrophages can also be beneficial and support neurogenesis, progenitor proliferation, survival, migration and differentiation in other brain regions. Recent studies suggest that the phenotypic expression of macrophages can vary depending on the situation and pro-inflammatory macrophages (M1) can undergo transition into an anti-inflammatory-reparative (M2) phenotype. More recently, three activation states of microglia in CNS have been proposed: classical activation (tissue defense, pro-inflammatory), alternative activation (repair, anti-inflammatory, fibrosis, extracellular matrix reconstruction) and acquired deactivation (immunosuppression, phagocytosis of apoptotic cells) [135,145].

Strategies aiming at activating microglia when they have reached the M2 phase could be beneficial for facilitating repair and plasticity. Since early phases of microglial activation are mostly deleterious (M1 type of activation) for the brain, such interventions should be delayed. Alternatively, or in parallel, strategies aiming at accelerating the M1-M2 switch could also be of major interest. At this point it is not known if modulation of the activation state of microglia/macrophages can be used for development of novel therapeutic strategies in the developing brain but a recent report suggests that M2 (alternative activation/acquired deactivation) macrophage cell therapy can indeed provide protective effects in an animal model of multiple sclerosis [135].

## Targeting long lasting inflammation

A recent and intriguing study performed in preterm infants with cerebral palsy [146] suggests that, at least in some patients with perinatal brain damage, there could be a long-lasting inflammation as measured by increased TNF-alpha levels in the plasma and the supernatants of peripheral blood mononuclear cells after lipopolysaccharide stimulation. This long-lasting altered inflammatory response could have deleterious effects on the progression of disease and/or on the clinical symptoms. If such a pathophysiological event was confirmed, recognizing and blocking such persistent inflammation could be of therapeutic value.

Additional studies are necessary to confirm these new hypotheses and to determine whether or not there is a long-lasting CNS inflammatory process. Techniques such as PET with markers of microglia or MRI using ferromagnetic particles taken up by activated microglia could be instrumental in this perspective if concerns about safety and ethics can be solved.

## Promoting positive post-lesional brain plasticity with pharmacological agents

Fostering positive post-lesional plasticity appears to be a very promising strategy for delayed interventions aiming at improving long-term neurological and cognitive function. However, there is still limited knowledge about the cellular and molecular mechanisms underlying post-lesional brain plasticity.

Different growth factors, such as brain-derived neurotrophic factor (BDNF), nerve growth factor (NGF), insulin-like growth factor-1 (IGF-1), erythropoietin (EPO) and vasoactive intestinal peptide (VIP) have been shown to reduce delayed neuronal death in various animal models of perinatal brain damage [147–151]. As for hypothermia, the window for intervention, when tested, was rather restricted to the first hours after the insult. Beyond their potential capability to prevent neuronal cell death, growth factors appear to be good candidates to target mechanisms involved in plasticity such as proliferation of neuronal precursors, axonal growth and sprouting, or synaptogenesis and synaptic stabilization.

Accordingly, BDNF and VIP have been shown to promote axonal sprouting following excitotoxic injury of the periventricular white matter in newborn mice [150,151]. Although growth factors like BDNF are big molecules unlikely to easily cross the intact blood–brain barrier, ampakines, which are allosteric positive modulators of glutamatergic AMPA receptors, are small and diffusible molecules able to induce BDNF production in the brain when administered systemically. Interestingly, ampakines have been shown to mimic BDNF effects on axonal sprouting in the mouse model of excitotoxic white matter injury [152].

Similarly, melatonin was shown to promote plasticity using the same model of neonatal excitotoxic white matter damage [92]. Although melatonin did not prevent the initial appearance of white matter damage, it promoted repair of secondary lesion with axonal regrowth and/or sprouting. Recent data have shown that the window for intervention is at least 24 hours after the insult (Gressens P., personal communication). Behavioural studies support the hypothesis that melatonin-induced white matter histological repair is accompanied by improved learning capabilities. Neuroprotective properties of melatonin have been confirmed in several animal models of perinatal brain damage, including in fetal sheep [153]. Melatonin is a safe compound in newborns and adults [154] and it crosses the blood–brain barrier as well as the placenta. Based on these data, a clinical trial testing the neuroprotective effects of melatonin has been initiated in preterm infants at high risk of developing brain damage and neurological handicap.

Although this study needs to be replicated, an intriguing clinical study has recently shown that EPO, when given an average of 24 hours after birth, had very significant neuroprotective effects in human term infants with neonatal encephalopathy [155]. The precise mechanism for this neuroprotection is unknown, but the timing of intervention argues in favour of an effect of EPO on post-lesional plasticity although a direct effect on delayed neuronal cell death cannot be excluded.

## Promoting positive post-lesional brain plasticity with exogenous stem cells

The development of adequate protocols for stem cell culture and application has raised the possibility of the use of these cells for the repair of perinatal cerebral lesions. Some studies have shown a positive effect of neural or mesenchymal stem cell therapy on the lesion extent and/or cognitive or motor outcome following perinatal brain lesions [7,156]. Of interest, in some of these studies, positive effects were observed when stem cells were injected several days (up to 10 days) after the insult.

For example, the therapeutic potential of neural stem cells in acute neonatal brain injuries has been evaluated in a rodent excitotoxic model [156]. Early (4-hour) and late (72-hour) neural stem cell implantation significantly reduced brain lesion size. The implanted cells, modified *in vitro* before transplantation to the oligodendrocytic lineage, were capable of migrating toward the lesion site even when implanted contralaterally to the lesion. At the lesion site, the neural stem cells underwent transient differentiation into neurons and oligodendrocytes but not astrocytes, suggesting that fate specification was achieved by the culture conditions. In parallel with the reduction in lesion size, the injured mice displayed a persistent and marked improvement in temporal and spatial memory at 3 and 6 weeks of age compared to littermates given intracerebroventricular injections of saline or fibroblasts.

Similarly, it was recently shown that two administrations of bone marrow-derived mesenchymal stem cells to neonatal mice 3 and 10 days after unilateral right carotid artery occlusion on P9 produced a 46% improvement in sensorimotor function as observed in the cylinder rearing test and a 60% decrease in neuronal loss, compared to vehicle-treated animals [7]. Moreover, cellular proliferation and differentiation of the proliferated cells into cells expressing neuronal, oligodendroglial and astrocyte markers was observed. Interestingly, remodelling of the corticospinal tract correlated with sensorimotor improvement.

However, it is not clear yet whether the stem cells themselves or factors secreted by stem cells mediate the positive effect. If stem cell integration is important for their effect, these cells need to proliferate, find the site of lesion and differentiate into an adequate cell type (e.g., neuron, oligodendrocyte) and integrate into the tissue to be functional. The ethical problems associated with the use of human stem cells are less evident in mesenchymal stem cells or stem cells derived from cord blood. Such cells permit an autologous transplant and do not entail the problem of immune tolerance of the transplanted cells. A clinical study is currently being performed using stem cells in children with neonatal encephalopathy at the Duke University.

A further intriguing alternative to treatment with stem cells is to stimulate the production of endogenous neuronal stem cells. It has already been shown that stem cells accumulate in the subventricular zone following an acute brain lesion. These results open a new perspective: the stimulation of this stem cell population to support the physiological repair processes of a lesion. A variant of this strategy would be to redirect new cell production from astroglia to oligodendrocytes and neurons [157]. In any case, these newly produced cells will need to integrate and function correctly in the damaged tissue. Moreover, stimulation of stem cell proliferation bears the theoretical risk of cancer induction.

## Targeting epigenetic marks

Prenatal factors like inflammation or maternal stress have been shown to make the developing brain more sensitive (sensitization process) to a second insult taking place around birth. This generally leads to destructive brain lesions that can be indentified by brain imaging. There is emerging evidence suggesting that the same prenatal factors, in the absence of a secondary insult, can lead to long-term disturbances of brain development. Although this latter phenomenon does not lead to clastic brain damage, it can be accompanied by long-lasting cognitive, motor and/or behavioural impairments [158].

The underlying mechanisms could involve myelin deficit linked to blockade of oligodendrocyte maturation, impaired neuronal migration, increased neuronal cell death, impaired axonal growth or altered synaptogenesis [158,159]. At the molecular level, little is known but recent data suggest that modified epigenetic marks could be one of the underlying mechanisms. There is a rapidly growing knowledge about the epigenetic mechanisms and drugs specifically targeting epigenetic mechanisms are being developed and tested, raising hope for the future design of innovative treatments that could be implemented way beyond the perinatal insult.

## Acknowledgements

This work was supported by Medical Research Council strategic award (MRC; United Kingdom, P19381 to HH), Medical Research Council (VR, Sweden, 2006–3396 to HH), ALF-LUA (Sweden, ALFGBG2863 to HH), Wellcome Trust (Programme Grant WT094823MA to HH, PG), Inserm, Université Paris 7, APHP (Contrat d'Interface to Dr Pierre Gressens), Fondation Lecducq, Fondation Grace de Monaco and Fondation Roger de Spoelberch.

## References

1. Vannucci SJ, Hagberg H. Hypoxia-ischemia in the immature brain. *J Exp Biol* 2004;**207**:3149–54.

2. Johnston MV, Hagberg H. Sex and the pathogenesis of cerebral palsy. *Dev Med Child Neurol* 2007;**49**:74–8.

3. Gidday JM, Fitzgibbons JC, Shah AR, et al. Neuroprotection from ischemic brain injury by hypoxic preconditioning in the neonatal rat. *Neurosci Lett* 1994;**168**:221–4.

4. Dommergues MA, Patkai J, Renauld JC, et al. Proinflammatory cytokines and interleukin-9 exacerbate excitotoxic lesions of the newborn murine neopallium. *Ann Neurol* 2000;**47**:54–63.

5. Eklind S, Mallard C, Leverin AL, et al. Bacterial endotoxin sensitizes the immature brain to hypoxic-ischaemic injury. *Eur J Neurosci* 2001;**13**:1101–6.

6. Gonzalez FF, Ferriero DM. Neuroprotection in the newborn infant. *Clin Perinatol* 2009;**36**:859–80.

7. van Velthoven CT, Kavelaars A, van Bel F, et al. Repeated mesenchymal stem cell treatment after neonatal hypoxia-ischemia has distinct effects on formation and maturation of new neurons and oligodendrocytes leading to restoration of damage, corticospinal motor tract activity and sensorimotor function. *J Neurosci* 2010;**30**:9603–11.

8. Lorek A, Takei Y, Cady EB, et al. Delayed ('secondary') cerebral energy failure following acute hypoxia-ischaemia in the newborn piglet: continuous 48-hour studies by 31P magnetic resonance spectroscopy. *Pediatr Res* 1994;**36**:699–706.

9. Blumberg RM, Cady EB, Wigglesworth JS, et al. Relation between delayed impairment of cerebral energy metabolism and infarction following transient focal hypoxia-ischaemia in the developing brain. *Exp Brain Res* 1997;**113**:130–7.

10. Gilland E, Bona E, Hagberg H. Temporal changes of regional glucose use, blood flow and microtubule-associated protein 2 immunostaining after hypoxia-ischemia in the immature rat brain. *J Cereb Blood Flow Metab* 1998;**18**:222–8.

11. Azzopardi D, Wyatt JS, Cady EB, et al. Prognosis of newborn infants with hypoxic-ischemic brain injury assessed by phosphorus magnetic resonance spectroscopy. *Pediatr Res* 1989;**25**:445–51.

12. Roth SC, Baudin J, Cady E, et al. Relation of deranged neonatal cerebral oxidative metabolism with neurodevelopmental outcome and head circumference at 4 years. *Dev Med Child Neurol* 1997;**39**:718–25.

13. Thoresen M, Penrice J, Lorek A, et al. Mild hypothermia after severe transient hypoxia-ischemia ameliorates delayed cerebral energy failure in the newborn piglet. *Pediatr Res* 1995;**37**:667–70.

14. Edwards AD, Brocklehurst P, Gunn AJ, et al. Neurological outcomes at 18 months of age after moderate hypothermia for perinatal hypoxic ischaemic encephalopathy: synthesis and meta-analysis of trial data. *BMJ* 2010;**340**:c363.

15. Follett PL, Deng W, Dai W, et al. Glutamate receptor-mediated oligodendrocyte toxicity in periventricular leukomalacia: a protective role for topiramate. *J Neurosci* 2004;**24**:4412–20.

16. Johnston MV. Excitotoxicity in perinatal brain injury. *Brain Pathol* 2005;**15**:234–40.

17. Salter MG, Fern R. NMDA receptors are expressed in developing oligodendrocyte processes and mediate injury. *Nature* 2005;**438**:1167–71.

18. McDonald JW, Silverstein FS, Johnston MV. Neurotoxicity of N-methyl-D-aspartate is markedly enhanced in developing rat central nervous system. *Brain Res* 1988;**459**:200–3.

19. Marret S, Mukendi R, Gadisseux JF, et al. Effect of ibotenate on brain development: an excitotoxic mouse model of microgyria and posthypoxic like lesions. *J Neuropathol Exp Neurol* 1995;**54**:358–70.

20. Volpe JJ, Kinney HC, Jensen FE, et al. The developing oligodendrocyte: key cellular target in brain injury in the premature infant. *Int J Dev Neurosci* 2011;**29**:423–40.

21. Tahraoui SL, Marret S, Bodenant C, et al. Central role of microglia in neonatal excitotoxic lesions of the

murine periventricular white matter. *Brain Pathol* 2001;**11**:56–71.

22. Legros H, Launay S, Roussel BD, et al. Newborn- and adult-derived brain microvascular endothelial cells show age-related differences in phenotype and glutamate-evoked protease release. *J Cereb Blood Flow Metab* 2009;**29**:1146–58.

23. Hagberg H, Andersson P, Kjellmer I, et al. Extracellular overflow of glutamate, aspartate, GABA and taurine in the cortex and basal ganglia of fetal lambs during hypoxia-ischemia. *Neurosci Lett* 1987;**78**:311–7.

24. Tan WK, Williams CE, During MJ, et al. Accumulation of cytotoxins during the development of seizures and edema after hypoxic-ischemic injury in late gestation fetal sheep. *Pediatr Res* 1996;**39**:791–7.

25. Thoresen M, Satas S, Puka-Sundvall M, et al. Post-hypoxic hypothermia reduces cerebrocortical release of NO and excitotoxins. *Neuroreport* 1997;**8**:3359–62.

26. Hagberg H, Thornberg E, Blennow M, et al. Excitatory amino acids in the cerebrospinal fluid of asphyxiated infants: relationship to hypoxic-ischemic encephalopathy. *Acta Paediatr* 1993;**82**:925–9.

27. Hagberg H, Gilland E, Diemer NH, et al. Hypoxia-ischemia in the neonatal rat brain: histopathology after post-treatment with NMDA and non-NMDA receptor antagonists. *Biol Neonate* 1994;**66**:206–13.

28. Sfaello I, Baud O, Arzimanoglou A, et al. Topiramate prevents excitotoxic damage in the newborn rodent brain. *Neurobiol Dis* 2005;**20**:837–48.

29. Ikonomidou C, Bosch F, Miksa M, et al. Blockade of NMDA receptors and apoptotic neurodegeneration in the developing brain. *Science* 1999;**283**:70–4.

30. Cattano D, Williamson P, Fukui K, et al. Potential of xenon to induce or to protect against neuroapoptosis in the developing mouse brain. *Can J Anaesth* 2008;**55**:429–36.

31. Manning SM, Boll G, Fitzgerald E, et al. The clinically available NMDA receptor antagonist, memantine, exhibits relative safety in the developing rat brain. *Int J Dev Neurosci* 2011;**29**:767–73.

32. Laudenbach V, Mantz J, Lagercrantz H, et al. Effects of alpha-2 adrenoceptor agonists on perinatal excitotoxic brain injury: comparison of clonidine and dexmedetomidine. *Anesthesiology* 2002;**96**:134–41.

33. Paris A, Mantz J, Toner PH, et al. Effects of dexmedetomidine on perinatal excitotoxic brain injury are mediated by the alpha2A-adrenoceptor subtype. *Anesth Analg* 2006;**102**:456–61.

34. Ma D, Hossain M, Rajakumaraswamy N, et al. Dexmedetomidine produces its neuroprotective effect via the alpha 2A-adrenoceptor subtype. *Eur J Pharmacol* 2004;**502**:87–97.

35. Shouman B, Fontaine RH, Baud O, et al. Endocannabinoids potently protect the newborn brain against AMPA-kainate receptor-mediated excitotoxic damage. *Br J Pharmacol* 2006;**148**:442–51.

36. Miller RJ. The control of neuronal Ca2+ homeostasis. *Prog Neurobiol* 1991;**37**:255–85.

37. Siesjo BK. Calcium and ischemic brain damage. *Eur Neurol* 1986;**25**:45–56.

38. Bickler P, Gallego S. Hansen B. Developmental changes in intracellular calcium regulation in rat cerebral cortex during hypoxia. *J Cereb Blood Flow Metab* 1993;**13**:811–9.

39. Stein DT, Vannucci RC. Calcium accumulation during the evolution of hypoxic-ischemic brain damage in the immature rat. *J Cereb Blood Flow Metab* 1988;**8**:834–42.

40. Blomgren K, Kawashima S, Saido TC, et al. Fodrin degradation and subcellular distribution of calpains after neonatal rat cerebral hypoxic-ischemia. *Brain Res* 1995;**684**:143–9.

41. Takita M, Puka-Sundvall M, Miyakawa A, et al. In vivo calcium imaging of cerebral cortex in hypoxia-ischemia followed by developmental stage-specific injury in rats. *Neurosci Res* 2004;**48**:169–73.

42. Puka-Sundvall M, Gajkowska B, Cholewinski M, et al. Subcellular distribution of calcium and ultrastructural changes after cerebral hypoxia-ischemia in immature rats. *Brain Res Dev Brain Res* 2000;**125**:31–41.

43. Northington FJ, Ferriero DM, Flock DL, et al. Delayed neurodegeneration in neonatal rat thalamus after hypoxia-ischemia is apoptosis. *J Neurosci* 2001;**21**:1931–8.

44. Gilland E, Puka-Sundvall M, Hillered L, et al. Mitochondrial function and energy metabolism after hypoxia-ischemia in the immature rat brain: involvement of NMDA-receptors. *J Cereb Blood Flow Metab* 1998;**18**:297–304.

45. Blennow M, Ingvar M, Lagercrantz H, et al. Early [18F] FDG positron emission tomography in infants with hypoxic-ischaemic encephalopathy shows hypermetabolism during the postasphyctic period. *Acta Paediatr* 1995;**84**:1289–95.

46. Northington FJ, Chavez-Valdez R, Martin LJ. Neuronal cell death in neonatal hypoxia-ischemia. *Ann Neurol* 2011;**69**:743–58.

47. Blomgren K, Zhu C, Wang X, et al. Synergistic activation of caspase-3 by m-calpain after neonatal hypoxia-ischemia: a mechanism of "pathological apoptosis"? *J Biol Chem* 2001;**276**:10191–8.

48. Ota K, Yakovlev AG, Itaya A, et al. Alteration of apoptotic protease-activating factor-1 (APAF-1)-dependent apoptotic pathway during development of rat brain and liver. *J Biochem* 2002;**131**:131–5.

49. Kuida K, Zheng TS, Na S, et al. Decreased apoptosis in the brain and premature lethality in CPP32-deficient mice. *Nature* 1996;**384**:368–72.

50. Cheng Y, Deshmukh M, D'Costa A, et al. Caspase inhibitor affords neuroprotection with delayed administration in a rat model of neonatal hypoxic-ischemic brain injury. *J Clin Invest* 1998;**101**:1992–9.

51. Zhu C, Wang X, Xu F, et al. The influence of age on apoptotic and other mechanisms of cell death after cerebral hypoxia-ischemia. *Cell Death Differ* 2005;**12**:162–76.

52. Galluzzi L, Blomgren K, Kroemer G. Mitochondrial membrane permeabilization in neuronal injury. *Nat Rev Neurosci* 2009;**10**:481–94.

53. Edwards AD, Yue X, Cox P, et al. Apoptosis in the brains of infants suffering intrauterine cerebral injury. *Pediatr Res* 1997;**42**:684–9.

54. Blomgren K, Hagberg H. Free radicals, mitochondria and hypoxia-ischemia in the developing brain. *Free Radic Biol Med* 2006;**40**:388–97.

55. Zhu C, Wang, X, Hagberg H, et al. Correlation between caspase-3 activation and three different markers of DNA damage in neonatal cerebral hypoxia-ischemia. *J Neurochem* 2000;**75**:819–29.

56. Wang X, Zhu C, Hagberg H, et al. X-linked inhibitor of apoptosis (XIAP) protein protects against caspase activation and tissue loss after neonatal hypoxia-ischemia. *Neurobiol Dis* 2004;**16**:179–89.

57. Joly LM, Mucignat V, Mariani J, et al. Caspase inhibition after neonatal ischemia in the rat brain. *J Cereb Blood Flow Metab* 2004;**24**:124–31.

58. Felderhoff-Mueser U, Taylor DL, Greenwood K, et al. Fas/CD95/APO-1 can function as a death receptor for neuronal cells in vitro and in vivo and is upregulated following cerebral hypoxic-ischemic injury to the developing rat brain. *Brain Pathol* 2000;**10**:17–29.

59. Graham EM, Sheldon RA, Flock DL, et al. Neonatal mice lacking functional Fas death receptor are resistant to hypoxic stress. *Neurobiol Dis* 2004;**88**:1122–4.

60. Gill R, Soriano M, Blomgren K, et al. Role of caspase-3 activation in cerebral ischemia-induced neurodegeneration in adult and neonatal brain. *J Cereb Blood Flow Metab* 2002;**22**:420–30.

61. Hallin U, Kondo E, Ozaki Y, et al. Bcl-2 phosphorylation in the BH4 domain precedes caspase-3 activation and cell death after neonatal cerebral hypoxic-ischemic injury. *Neurobiol Dis* 2006;**21**:478–86.

62. Gao Y, Liang W, Hu X, et al. Neuroprotection against hypoxic-ischemic brain injury by inhibiting the apoptotic protease activating factor-1 pathway. *Stroke* 2010;**41**:166–72.

63. Zhu C, Wang X, Huang Z, et al. Apoptosis-inducing factor is a major contributor to neuronal loss induced by neonatal cerebral hypoxia-ischemia. *Cell Death Differ* 2007;**14**:775–84.

64. Hagberg H, Wilson MA, Matsushita H, et al. PARP-1 gene disruption in mice preferentially protects males from perinatal brain injury. *J Neurochem* 2004;**90**:1068–75.

65. Zhu C, Wang X, Deinum J, et al. Cyclophilin A participates in the nuclear translocation of apoptosis-inducing factor in neurons after cerebral hypoxia-ischemia. *J Exp Med* 2007;**204**:1741–8.

66. Wang X, Carlsson Y, Basso E, et al. Developmental shift of cyclophilin D contribution to hypoxic-ischemic brain injury. *J Neurosci* 2009;**29**:2588–96.

67. Wang X, Han W, Du X, et al. Neuroprotective effect of Bax-inhibiting peptide on neonatal brain injury. *Stroke* 2010;**41**:2050–5.

68. Gibson ME, Han BH, Choi J, et al. BAX contributes to apoptotic-like death following neonatal hypoxia-ischemia: evidence for distinct apoptosis pathways. *Mol Med* 2001;**7**:644–55.

69. Parsadanian AS, Cheng Y, Keller-Peck CR, et al. Bcl-xL is an antiapoptotic regulator for postnatal CNS neurons. *J Neurosci* 1998;**18**:1009–19.

70. Ness JM, Harvey CA, Strasser A, et al. Selective involvement of BH3-only Bcl-2 family members Bim and Bad in neonatal hypoxia-ischemia. *Brain Res* 2006;**1099**:150–9.

71. Moll UM, Wolff S, Speidel D, et al. Transcription-independent pro-apoptotic functions of p53. *Curr Opin Cell Biol* 2005;**17**:631–6.

72. Nijboer CH, Heijnen CJ, van der Kooij MA, et al. Targeting the p53 pathway to protect the neonatal ischemic brain. *Ann Neurol* 2011;**70**:255–64.

73. Yang DD, Kuan CY, Whitmarsh AJ, et al. Absence of excitotoxicity-induced apoptosis in the hippocampus of mice lacking the Jnk3 gene. *Nature* 1997;**389**:865–70.

74. Pirianov G, Brywe KG, Mallard C, et al. Deletion of the c-Jun N-terminal kinase 3 gene protects neonatal mice against cerebral hypoxic-ischaemic injury. *J Cereb Blood Flow Metab* 2007;**27**:1022–32.

75. Croall DE, DeMartino GN. Calcium-activated neutral protease (calpain) system: structure, function and regulation. *Physiol Rev* 1991;**71**:813–47.

76. Leist M, Nicotera P. Apoptosis, excitotoxicity and neuropathology. *Exp Cell Res* 1998;**239**:83–201.

77. Kawamura M, Nakajima W, Ishida A, et al. Calpain inhibitor MDL 28170 protects hypoxic-ischemic brain injury in neonatal rats by inhibition of both apoptosis and necrosis. *Brain Res* 2005;**1037**:59–69.

78. Degterev A, Huang Z, Boyce M, et al. Chemical inhibitor of nonapoptotic cell death with therapeutic potential for ischemic brain injury. *Nat Chem Biol* 2005;**1**:112–9.

79. Northington FJ, Chavez-Valdez R, Graham EM, et al. Necrostatin decreases oxidative damage, inflammation and injury after neonatal HI. *J Cereb Blood Flow Metab* 2011;**31**:178–89.

80. Shintani T, Klionsky DJ. Autophagy in health and disease: a double edged sword. *Science* 2004;**306**:990–5.

81. Marino G, Madeo F, Kroemer G. Autophagy for tissue homeostasis and neuroprotection. *Curr Opin Cell Biol* 2011;**23**:198–206.

82. Zhu C, Xu F, Wang X, et al. Different apoptotic mechanisms are activated in male and female brains after neonatal hypoxia-ischaemia. *J Neurochem* 2006;**96**:1016–27.

83. Koike M, Shibata M, Tadakoshi M, et al. Inhibition of autophagy prevents hippocampal pyramidal neuron death after hypoxic-ischemic injury. *Am J Pathol* 2008;**172**:454–69.

84. Kroemer G, Levine B. Autophagic cell death: the story of a misnomer. *Nat Rev Mol Cell Biol* 2008;**9**:1004–10.

85. Carloni S, Buonocore G, Balduini W. Protective role of autophagy in neonatal hypoxia-ischemia induced brain injury. *Neurobiol Dis* 2008;**32**:329–39.

86. Park HK, Chu K, Jung KH, et al. Autophagy is involved in the ischemic preconditioning. *Neurosci Lett* 2009;**451**:16–9.

87. Halliwell B. Reactive oxygen species and central nervous system. *J Neurochem* 1992;**59**:1609–23.

88. Wang H, Li J, Follett PL, et al. 12-Lipoxygenase plays a key role in cell death caused by glutathione depletion and arachidonic acid in rat oligodendrocytes. *Eur J Neurosci* 2004;**20**:2049–58.

89. Bågenholm R, Andine P, Hagberg H. Effects of the 21-amino steroid tirilazad mesylate (U-74006F) on brain damage and edema after perinatal hypoxia-ischemia in the rat. *Pediatr Res* 1996;**40**:399–403.

90. Palmer C, Towfighi J, Roberts R, et al. Allopurinol administered after inducing hypoxic-ischemia reduces brain injury in 7-day-old rats. *Pediatr Res* 1993;**33**:405–11.

91. Palmer C, Roberts RL, Bero C. Deferoxamine posttreatment reduces ischemic brain injury in neonatal rats. *Stroke* 1994;**25**:1039–45.

92. Husson I, Mesples B, Bac P, et al. Melatoninergic neuroprotection of the murine periventricular white matter against neonatal excitotoxic challenge. *Ann Neurol* 2002;**51**:82–92.

93. Plaisant F, Clippe A, Vander Stricht D, et al. The antioxidant peroxiredoxin-5 protects against excitotoxic brain lesions in newborn mice. *Free Radic Biol Med* 2003;**7**:862–72.

94. Xia WJ, Yang M, Fok TF, et al. Partial neuroprotective effect of pretreatment with tanshinone IIA on neonatal hypoxia-ischemia brain damage. *Pediatr Res* 2005;**58**:784–90.

95. Miura S, Ishida A, Nakajima W, et al. Intraventricular ascorbic acid administration decreases hypoxic-ischemic brain injury in newborn rats. *Brain Res* 2006;**1095**:159–66.

96. Nurmi A, Goldsteins G, Narvainen J, et al. Antioxidant pyrrolidine dithiocarbamate activates Akt-GSK signaling and is neuroprotective in neonatal hypoxia-ischemia. *Free Radic Biol Med* 2006;**40**:1776–84.

97. Domoki F, Perciaccante JV, Puskar M, et al. Cyclooxygenase-2 inhibitor NS398 preserves neuronal function after hypoxia/ischemia in piglets. *Neuroreport* 2001;**12**:4065–8.

98. Sheldon RA, Osredkar D, Lee CL, et al. HIF-1 alpha-deficient mice have increased brain injury after neonatal hypoxia-ischemia. *Dev Neurosci* 2009;**31**:452–8.

99. Hall ED. Inhibition of lipid peroxidation in central nervous system trauma and ischemia. *J Neurol Sci* 1995;**13**:79–83.

100. Bona E, Andersson AL, Blomgren K, et al. Chemokine and inflammatory cell response to hypoxia-ischemia in immature rats. *Pediatr Res* 1999;**45**:500–9.

101. Doverhag C, Keller M, Karlsson A, et al. Pharmacological and genetic inhibition of NADPH oxidase does not reduce brain damage in different models of perinatal brain injury in newborn mice. *Neurobiol Dis* 2008;**31**:133–44.

102. Dawson VL, Dawson TM, Bartley DA, et al. Mechanisms of nitric oxide-mediated neurotoxocity in primary brain cultures. *J Neurosci* 1993;**13**:2651–61.

103. Jaffrey SR, Snyder SH. Nitric oxide: A neural messenger. *Annu Rev Cell Dev Biol* 1995;**11**:417–40.

104. Iadecola C, Ross ME. Molecular pathology of cerebral ischemia: delayed gene expression and strategies for neuroprotection. *Ann N Y Acad Sci* 1997;**835**:203–17.

105. Crow JP, Beckman JS. The role of peroxynitrite in nitric oxide-mediated toxicity. *Curr Top Microbiol Immunol* 1995;**196**:57–73.

106. Huang Z, Huang PL, Panahian N, et al. Effects of cerebral ischemia in mice deficient in neuronal nitric oxide synthase. *Science* 1994;**265**:1883–5.

107. Ferriero DM, Sheldon RA, Black SM, et al. Selective destruction of nitric oxide synthase neurons with quisqualate reduces damage after hypoxia-

ischemia in the neonatal rat. *Pediatr Res* 1995;**38**:912–8.

108. Ferriero DM, Holtzman DM, Black SM, et al. Neonatal mice lacking neuronal nitric oxide synthase are less vulnerable to hypoxic-ischemic injury. *Neurobiol Dis* 1996;**3**:64–71.

109. Trifiletti RR. Neuroprotective effects of NG-nitro-L-arginine in focal stroke in the 7-day old rat. *Eur J Pharmacol* 1992;**218**:197–8.

110. Yu L, Derrick M, Ji H, et al. Involvement of neuronal nitric oxide synthase in ongoing fetal brain injury following near-term rabbit hypoxia-ischemia. *Dev Neurosci* 2011;**33**:288–98.

111. Blumberg RM, Taylor DL, Yue X, et al. Increased nitric oxide synthesis is not involved in delayed cerebral energy failure following focal hypoxic-ischaemic injury in the developing brain. *Pediatr Res* 1999;**46**:224–31.

112. Maragos WF, Silverstein FS. Resistance to nitroprusside neurotoxicity in perinatal rat brain. *Neurosci Lett* 1994;**172**:80–4.

113. Kakizawa H, Matsui F, Tokita Y, et al. Neuroprotective effect of nipradilol, an NO donor, on hypoxic-ischemic brain injury of neonatal rats. *Early Hum Dev* 2007;**83**:535–40.

114. Olivier P, Loron G, Fontaine RH, et al. Nitric oxide is a key factor for myelination of the developing brain. *J Neuropathol Exp Neurol* 2010;**69**:828–37.

115. Dommergues MA, Plaisant F, Verney C, et al. Early microglial activation following neonatal excitotoxic brain damage in mice: a potential target for neuroprotection. *Neuroscience* 2003;**121**:619–28.

116. Hagberg H, Rousset CI, Wang X, et al. Mechanisms of perinatal brain damage and protective possibilities. *Drug Discovery Today: Disease Mechanisms* 2006;**3**:397–407.

117. Derugin N, Wendland M, Muramatsu K, et al. Evolution of brain injury after transient middle cerebral artery occlusion in neonatal rats. *Stroke* 2000; **31**:1752–61.

118. McRae A, Gilland E, Bona E, et al. Microglia activation after neonatal hypoxic-ischemia. *Brain Res Dev Brain Res* 1995;**84**:245–52.

119. Jin Y, Silverman AJ, Vannucci SJ. Mast cells are early responders after hypoxia-ischemia in immature rat brain. *Stroke* 2009;**40**:3107–12.

120. Szaflarski J, Burtrum D, Silverstein FS. Cerebral hypoxia-ischemia stimulates cytokine gene expression in perinatal rats. *Stroke* 1995;**26**:1093–1100.

121. Hagberg H, Gilland E, Bona E, et al. Enhanced expression of interleukin (IL)-1 and IL-6 messenger RNA and bioactive protein after hypoxia-ischemia in neonatal rats. *Pediatr Res* 1996;**40**:603–9.

122. Silverstein FS, Barks JD, Hagan P, et al. Cytokines and perinatal brain injury. *Neurochem Int* 1997;**30**:375–83.

123. Hedtjarn M, Leverin AL, Eriksson K, et al. Interleukin-18 involvement in hypoxic-ischemic brain injury. *J Neurosci* 2002;**22**:5910–19.

124. Hedtjarn M, Mallard C, Hagberg H. Inflammatory gene profiling in the developing mouse brain after hypoxia-ischemia. *J Cereb Blood Flow Metab* 2004;**24**:1333–51.

125. Kim SU, de Vellis J. Microglia in health and disease. *J Neurosci Res* 2005;**81**:302–13.

126. Giulian D, Vaca K. Inflammatory glia mediate delayed neuronal damage after ischemia in the central nervous system. *Stroke* 1993;**24**:184–90.

127. Liu XH, Eun BL, Silverstein FS, et al. The platelet-activating factor antagonist BN 52021 attenuates hypoxic-ischemic brain injury in the immature rat. *Pediatr Res* 1996;**40**:797–803.

128. Liu XH, Kwon D, Schielke GP, et al. Mice deficient in interleukin-1 converting enzyme are resistant to neonatal hypoxic-ischemic brain damage. *J Cereb Blood Flow Metab* 1999;**19**:1099–1108.

129. Ten VS, Sosunov SA, Mazer SP, et al. C1q-deficiency is neuroprotective against hypoxic-ischemic brain injury in neonatal mice. *Stroke* 2005;**36**:2244–50.

130. Mesples B, Plaisant F, Gressens P. Effects of interleukin-10 on neonatal excitotoxic brain lesions in mice. *Brain Res Dev Brain Res* 2003;**141**:25–32.

131. Aden U, Favrais G, Plaisant F, et al. Systemic inflammation sensitizes the neonatal brain to excitoxicity through a pro-/anti-inflammatory imbalance: key role of TNF-alpha pathway and protection by etanercept. *Brain Behav Immun* 2010;**24**:747–58.

132. Imai F, Suzuki H, Oda J, et al. Neuroprotective effect of exogenous microglia in global brain ischemia. *J Cereb Blood Flow Metab* 2007;**27**:488–500.

133. Cowell RM, Plane JM, Silverstein FS. Complement activation contributes to hypoxic-ischemic brain injury in neonatal rats. *J Neurosci* 2003;**23**:9459–68.

134. Denker SP, Ji S, Dingman A, et al. Macrophages are comprised of resident brain microglia not infiltrating peripheral monocytes acutely after neonatal stroke. *J Neurochem* 2007;**100**:893–904.

135. Mikita J, Dubourdieu-Cassagno N, Deloire MS, et al. Altered M1/M2 activation patterns of monocytes in severe relapsing experimental rat model of multiple sclerosis. Amelioration of clinical status by M2

activated monocyte administration. *Mult Scler* 2011;**17**:2–15.

136. Arvin KL, Han BH, Du Y, et al. Minocycline markedly protects the neonatal brain against hypoxic-ischemic injury. *Ann Neurol* 2002;**52**:54–61.

137. Tsuji M, Wilson MA, Lange MS, et al. Minocycline worsens hypoxic-ischemic brain injury in a neonatal mouse model. *Exp Neurol* 2004;**189**:58–65.

138. Vexler ZS, Yenari MA. Does inflammation after stroke affect the developing brain differently than adult brain? *Dev Neurosci* 2009;**31**:378–93.

139. Thoresen M. Cooling the newborn after asphyxia - physiological and experimental background and its clinical use. *Semin Neonatol* 2000;**5**:61–73.

140. Ma D, Hossain M, Chow A, et al. Xenon and hypothermia combine to provide neuroprotection from neonatal asphyxia. *Ann Neurol* 2005;**58**:182–93.

141. Faulkner S, Bainbridge A, Kato T, et al. Xenon augmented hypothermia reduces early lactate/ N-acetylaspartate and cell death in perinatal asphyxia. *Ann Neurol* 2011;**70**:133–50.

142. Liu Y, Barks JD, Xu G, et al. Topiramate extends the therapeutic window for hypothermia-mediated neuroprotection after stroke in neonatal rats. *Stroke* 2004;**35**:1460–5.

143. Barks JD, Liu YQ, Shangguan Y, et al. Phenobarbital augments hypothermic neuroprotection. *Pediatr Res* 2010;**67**:532–7.

144. Rogido M, Husson I, Bonnier C, et al. Fructose-1, 6-biphosphate prevents excitotoxic cell death in the neonatal mouse brain. *Brain Res Dev Brain Res* 2003;**140**:287–97.

145. Colton CA. Heterogeneity of microglial activation in the innate immune response in the brain. *J Neuroimmune Pharmacol* 2009;**4**:399–418.

146. Lin CY, Chang YC, Wang ST, et al. Altered inflammatory responses in preterm children with cerebral palsy. *Ann Neurol* 2010;**68**:204–12.

147. Holtzman DM, Sheldon RA, Jaffe W, et al. Nerve growth factor protects the neonatal brain against hypoxic-ischemic injury. *Ann Neurol* 1996;**39**:114–22.

148. Johnston BM, Mallard EC, Williams CE, et al. Insulin-like growth factor-1 is a potent neuronal rescue agent after hypoxic-ischemic injury in fetal lambs. *J Clin Invest* 1996;**97**:300–8.

149. Gressens P, Marret S, Hill JM, et al. Vasoactive intestinal peptide prevents excitotoxic hypoxic-like cell death in the murine developing brain. *J Clin Invest* 1997;**100**:390–7.

150. Husson I, Rangon CM, Lelièvre V, et al. BDNF-induced white matter neuroprotection and stage-dependant neuronal survival following a neonatal excitotoxic challenge. *Cereb Cortex* 2005;**15**:250–61.

151. Osredkar D, Sall JW, Bickler PE, et al. Erythropoietin promotes hippocampal neurogenesis in in vitro models of neonatal stroke. *Neurobiol Dis* 2010;**38**:259–65.

152. Destot-Wong KD, Liang K, Gupta SK, et al. The AMPA receptor positive allosteric modulator, S18986, is neuroprotective against neonatal excitotoxic and inflammatory brain damage through BDNF synthesis. *Neuropharmacology* 2009;**57**:277–86.

153. Welin AK, Svedin P, Lapatto R, et al. Melatonin reduces inflammation and cell death in white matter in the 0.65 gestation fetal sheep following ombilical cord occlusion. *Pediatr Res* 2007; **61**:153–8.

154. Gitto E, Reiter RJ, Amodio A, et al. Early indicators of chronic lung disease in preterm infants with respiratory distress syndrome and their inhibition by melatonin. *J Pineal Res* 2004;**36**:250–5.

155. Zhu C, Kang W, Xu F, et al. Erythropoietin improved neurologic outcomes in newborns with hypoxic-ischemic encephalopathy. *Pediatrics* 2009;**124**: e218–26.

156. Titomanlio L, Bouslama M, Le Verche V, et al. Implanted neurosphere-derived precursors promote recovery after neonatal excitotoxic brain injury. *Stem Cells Dev* 2011;**20**:865–79.

157. Covey MV, Jiang Y, Alli VV, et al. Defining the critical period for neocortical neurogenesis after pediatric brain injury. *Dev Neurosci* 2010;**32**:488–98.

158. Favrais G, van de Looij Y, Fleiss B, et al. Systemic inflammation disrupts the developmental program of the white matter. *Ann Neurol* 2011;**70**:550–65.

159. Leviton A, Gressens P. Neuronal damage accompanies perinatal white matter damage. *Trends Neurosci* 2007;**30**:473–8.

## Chapter 3

# The discovery of hypothermic neural rescue therapy for perinatal hypoxic–ischaemic encephalopathy

A. David Edwards

## The pragmatic tradition

Cooling treatments are part of a noble pragmatic tradition which will try almost anything that might have medical value. There are records going back hundreds of years of physicians submerging newborn babies in cold water to animate them after delivery. Early hypothermic therapy for infants focused on resuscitation and re-animation, rather than neuroprotection. Indeed, no link was made between abnormal birth and later neurological problems until William Little's classic paper in 1861 [1] and even then it was controversial; Sigmund Freud, for example, famously disagreed.

The 20th century pioneers of infant hypothermia like Björn Westin and James Miller also reported their work more in terms of re-animation than neuroprotection [2], using the concepts and methods of physiology, the dominant contemporary medical science of the time [3–6] and although some children were conscientiously followed up, long-term neural function was not the central issue. The concepts and techniques needed for precise thinking about neuroprotection had yet to be developed.

## Lost interest

After this flowering of physiological research interest in therapeutic cooling waned. The problem of resuscitation was solved by mechanical ventilation and Silverman's influential controlled trial showing that preterm infants survived better if kept warm [7], together with observational [8] and experimental [9] data exposed the potential risks of cooling infants.

Studies of hypothermia in Europe and the United States were sporadic and often not encouraging [10–15]. However, in the Soviet Union, cooling was regarded as a successful therapy for birth asphyxia [16]. Unfortunately, a combination of the language barrier, cold war politics and the Russians' failure to carry out randomized trials contributed to an almost total ignorance of this work in the West and when Russian neonatologists visited the United Kingdom, prominent neonatologists who met them had little interest in their ideas on cooling (Peter Dunn, personal communication).

## A new generation of research

The rebirth of hypothermia studies was contingent less on a sudden re-evaluation of the healing power of cooling than on the arrival of a new conceptual framework which gave it relevance. A new generation of researchers addressed subtly different questions. They discussed neural cell death and long-term neurodevelopmental impairments using the language not of physiology but of the molecular and cellular sciences. They were aware of the powerful neuroprotective effect of *intra*-ischaemic hypothermia during cardiac surgery but came to the idea of *post*-insult hypothermic neural rescue from very different starting points.

Marianne Thoresen, who was working on cerebral perfusion, recalls being impressed that during the bitter Oslo winter children not infrequently fell through the ice and suffered prolonged drowning in iced water but emerged with preserved cerebral function. In Toronto clinicians had tried reducing cerebral metabolic rate with cooling and phenobarbitone to protect drowned brains after resuscitation [17]. These concepts were not successful, but the attempted neural rescue sparked an interest. Peter Gluckman and Tania Gunn in Auckland, New Zealand were interested in cooling for its effect on thyroid function. They began cooling fetal sheep for endocrine studies

*Neonatal Neural Rescue*, ed. A. David Edwards, Denis V. Azzopardi and Alistair J. Gunn. Published by Cambridge University Press. © Cambridge University Press 2013.

in 1983. Denis Azzopardi, John Wyatt and David Edwards, young researchers working for Osmund Reynolds at University College London, were struck by his group's astonishing Magnetic Resonance Spectroscopy (MRS) data showing that the infant brain is normal in the hours after asphyxia and dies only after a distinct delay [18,19]. This was one of a series of discoveries that opened new doors.

## Big new ideas

Delayed brain injury (called "*secondary energy failure*" by Reynolds) was a critical new idea. If brain cells are normal until secondary energy failure starts and the mechanism of delayed cell death could be unravelled, it opened the possibility of therapeutic intervention in what had previously seemed an impossible situation. Delayed injury was also reported at around this time by neuropathologists [20–22].

Edwards and Wyatt set about using Reynolds's sophisticated MRS approach to replicate secondary energy failure in piglets [23] and rat pups [24] so that they could test treatments to prevent it. In Gluckman's laboratory on the other side of the world Alistair Gunn and Chris Williams developed a simple and elegant biophysical method to do essentially the same thing in fetal sheep [25].

Delayed cell death was one component of the powerful new conceptual framework. A new and transforming concept developed from the seminal work of John Olney [26,27] and Brian Meldrum [28]. They discovered *excitotoxicity*, showing that at least some of the neural cell death caused by hypoxia–ischaemia was delayed and mediated by excess production of the excitatory neurotransmitter glutamate and that it could be blocked pharmacologically to provide good protection against hypoxic damage. The next critical idea was the discovery of apoptosis, first noted in the 1970s [29], but put on a firm molecular basis by Robert Horvitz [30], Martin Raff [31] and Gerard Evan [32] who showed that it could be triggered by cellular insults. The radical idea that hypoxia–ischaemia triggered a delayed biochemical cell suicide programme which could explain the perplexing phenomenon of delayed cell death particularly excited Edwards, who brought Huseyin Mehmet, a cell biologist who had worked with Raff and Evan, into his group; there were soon experimental [33,34] and human [35] data to support it.

Amongst the first to try to exploit this new science were Ingmar Kjellmer and Henrik Hagberg in Gothenburg [36,37] and Michael Johnston in Baltimore [38]. There were many potential therapies which might achieve neural rescue and the group of researchers who came together around hypothermia tested several of them. Magnesium was an appealingly simple excitoxin antagonist that protected cells in culture: the Reynolds group tested it without success [39]. Gluckman and Alistair Gunn started by looking unsuccessfully at calcium inhibitors [40]. Edwards picked out nitric oxide inhibition which was also a failure [41]. Gluckman had success with his innovative studies of IGF-1, but could not immediately translate this to clinical practice [42].

## Hypothermic rescue after hypoxia–ischaemia

Many hypothermia researchers cite work published in 1989 from Myron Ginsberg's group as the important catalyst in moving studies of neural rescue towards hypothermia. Ginsberg showed that a short period of hypothermia after hypoxia–ischaemia in adult rats reduced excitotoxin generation [43] and produced significant protection in the hippocampus [44]. Soon Pusanelli's group suggested that at least some of the strong neuroprotective effect of the glutamate antagonist MK-801 was by reducing body temperature [45].

An informal hypothermia interest group was developing. Gluckman visited London; Reynolds and Wyatt went to Oslo; Edwards went to Auckland; and Thoresen contacted Westin, went to Gothenburg and took her boundless enthusiasm for hypothermia to the Reynolds laboratory. Over the next year or so together and separately they produced a series of reports in piglets [46–49], immature rats [50–52] and fetal sheep [53] which showed repeatedly that post-insult hypothermia significantly reduced hypoxic–ischaemic brain damage in the developing brain. They showed that hypothermia specifically reduced apoptosis [64] and interrupted the excitotoxic cascade [65].

This work chimed with an effervescence of experimental work in mature animals [54–61], including evidence of long-term functional benefits [62]. These results also stimulated clinical scientists working with adults whose apparent early success helped sustain a belief in cooling [63].

## From laboratory to cotside

Clinical pilot studies were already being organized, with some trepidation because of the prevailing view that cold was very dangerous for infants. There was disagreement over the relative benefits of selective head against whole body cooling. Gluckman and Gunn tried selective head cooling [66]; Edwards and Azzopardi, after studying the difference between selective head and total body cooling in a computer modelling study [67], started whole body cooling [68]; Thoresen and Andrew Whitelaw, relocated from Oslo to Bristol, tried both methods [69]. Cooling was now a topic of wider discussion in the neonatal community and other groups started to organize further experimental [70] and preliminary clinical studies [71–73] (reviewed in Jacobs *et al*) [74].

However, not everyone was convinced. The highly respected Vannucci laboratory had failed to find any protective effect of post-insult cooling [75] and worse, Ginsberg's group reported that hypothermic protection in mature rats was only temporary [76]. Many clinicians thought that the experiments models were oversimplistic and unrepresentative of the complex clinical situation. Others, perhaps influenced by the important studies of Karen Nelson into the causes of cerebral palsy, thought that infants with encephalopathy had probably had previous insults weeks or months earlier; although a study from Hammersmith dispelled this myth [77].

## Randomized controlled trials

Nevertheless, cooling captured the imagination of one of the most influential figures in neonatal medicine. Jerry Lucey, the editor of *Pediatrics*, had an extraordinarily ability to spot new ideas and he became a strong champion of cooling. He promoted hypothermia tirelessly and in early 1997 made a critical introduction between Olympic Medical, a medium-sized equipment company, and the cooling fraternity. Olympic Medical decided to make a clinical cooling device and provide practical and financial support for the trial. Gluckman and Wyatt would be principal investigators and the scientific committee which developed and ran the trial consisted of the experimentalists supplemented by clinical researchers including Whitelaw, Donna Ferriero, Richard Polin, Roberta Ballard and Charlene Robertson. The new experts were not all convinced baby-coolers – Ferriero, also a distinguished neuroprotection experimentalist,

was sceptical – but they brought a range of new skills essential to taking hypothermia into phase 3 trial. Arguably the most important roles in delivering the trial were taken by Ted Weiler, an indefatigable engineer from Olympic Medical, and Alistair Gunn who became the Scientific Officer.

The CoolCap study tested cooling for 72 hours started within 6 hours of delivery. The protocol was based on the Auckland pilot, but was somewhat arbitrary; the relative merits of different temperatures or lengths of cooling were unclear and the researchers used best estimates based on their animal experiments, cautiously choosing the upper band of the expected therapeutic range. No-one knew with certainty what effect size to predict or even what the best primary outcome was. On the divisive question of selective head versus whole body cooling, in the almost total absence of agreed data they compromised and used rectal temperature to control a head cooling device. CoolCap thus studied the effect of cooling the whole baby to 34.5°C with the expectation (some said hope) that the brain might be a degree or so cooler.

The first infant was enrolled at Columbia Presbyterian Hospital, New York, on July 1, 1999 and all data were collected, audited and prepared for analysis by fall 2003. The result was reported at Lucey's annual Washington DC "Hot Topics in Neonatology" meeting in December 2003 with full publication in the Lancet in 2005. CoolCap did not have quite the definitive result that had been hoped for [78,79], but the researchers remained resolute; as they sat together after the presentation in Washington, Gluckman confided to Edwards that he thought they would never do more important work.

After the CoolCap trial another major study was published by the National Institute for Child Health and Human Development (NICHD) Neonatal Research Network. This network is the best funded and most effective trials grouping in neonatal medicine. The CoolCap researchers had previously had lengthy discussions with the network about collaboration because although the network had little experience of hypothermia it had a strong track record of patient recruitment. However, after detailed discussions around the final CoolCap protocol broke down, the network began a separate trial of whole body cooling led by Seetha Shankaran. Some network members were setting up animal models of hypothermic neural rescue, providing valuable experience for preliminary experiments [70,80]. The NICHD trial found a significant effect of cooling, although the study was criticized in some quarters for temperature instability in the control group [81].

## Uncertainty

The question which now faced the community was: should cooling become standard of care? Opinions were divided. Some observers thought the evidence was sufficient, particularly if the growing number of preliminary studies was considered [82] and in 2006 the Federal Drugs Administration approved the CoolCap device for clinical use. However, others pointed out that the results were at best statistically marginal [83] and urged scepticism. Worryingly, hypothermia trials in adults and older children were failing to show benefit [84,85]. The community held its breath and awaited more data [86].

After a couple of years during which even the original researchers found it difficult always to agree, the last major trial that had grown out of the original experimentalist group was completed. The TOtal Body hYpothermia for neonatal encephalopathy (TOBY) trial, led by Azzopardi and backed by distinguished trials specialist Peter Brocklehurst's National Perinatal Epidemiology Unit, developed from the Hammersmith pilot study of whole body cooling, but collected the data needed to allow meta-analysis with both CoolCap and the NICHD studies. Fortuitously TOBY was delayed by the funding timetable of the UK Medical Research Council, so that it was still in progress when CoolCap and the NICHD trial reported marginal benefits, making it clear that the trial size should be increased. So when TOBY reported it was considerably larger than either previous study. In fact TOBY showed remarkable consistency with both those previous trials; the point estimates for effect were similar and meta-analysis showed unequivocally that cooling increases an infant's chance of surviving without neurological deficits at 18 months, reducing neurodevelopmental impairment in survivors.

The community has been active in pursuing the opportunity of neuroprotection and before there was unequivocal evidence of benefit several groups set up further trials in Europe (neo.Neuro.network), Australia (ICE) and China and reported at least in abstract. While having some differences in design and outcome they are all consistent with a beneficial effect of cooling. Ironically, the relative effects of selective head and whole body cooling seem indistinguishable.

## Acknowledgements

Thanks to Osmund Reynolds, Peter Gluckman, Denis Azzopardi, Alistair Gunn, Marianne Thoresen, Donna Ferriero, Ted Weiler and Andrew Whitelaw: their memories and comments were invaluable.

## References

1. Little WJ. On the influence of abnormal parturition, difficult labours, premature birth and asphyxia neonatorum, on the mental and physical condition of the child, especially in relation to deformities. London: Obstetric Society of London; 1861.

2. Westin B. Hypothermia in the resuscitation of the neonate: a glance in my rear-view mirror. *Acta Paediatr* 2006;**95**:1172–4.

3. Miller JA. Factors in neonatal resistance to anoxia. I. Temperature and survival of newborn Guinea pigs under anoxia. *Science* 1949;**110**:113–4.

4. Enhorning G, Westin B. Experimental studies of the human fetus in prolonged asphyxia. *Acta Physiol Scand* 1954;**31**:359–75.

5. Westin B, Miller JA, Nyberg R, Wedenberg E. Neonatal asphyxia pallida treated with hypothermia alone or with hypothermia and transfusion of oxygenated blood. *Surgery* 1959;**45**:868–79.

6. Auld PA, Nelson NM, Nicolopoulos DA, Helwig F, Smith CA. Physiologic studies on an infant in deep hypothermia. *N Engl J Med* 1962;**267**:1348–51.

7. Silverman WS, Fertig JW, Berger AP. The influence of the thermal environment upon the survival of newly born premature infants. *Pediatrics* 1958;**22**:876–85.

8. Mann TP, Elliott RIK. Neonatal cold injury due to accidental exposure to cold. *Lancet* 1957;**272**:229–34.

9. Brodie HR, Cross KW, Lomer TR. Heat production in new-born infants under normal and hypoxic conditions. *J Physiol* 1957;**138**:156–63.

10. Miller JA Jr, Zakhary R, Miller FS. Hypothermia, asphyxia and cardiac glycogen in guinea pigs. *Science* 1964;**144**:1226–7.

11. Dunn JM, Miller JA Jr. Hypothermia combined with positive pressure ventilation in resuscitation of the asphyxiated neonate. Clinical observations in 28 infants. *Am J Obstet Gynecol* 1969;**104**:58–67.

12. Ehrstrom J, Hirvensalo M, Donner M, Hietalahti J. Hypothermia in the resuscitation of severely asphyctic newborn infants. A follow-up study. *Ann Clin Res* 1969;**1**:40–9.

13. Cordey R, Chiolero R, Miller JA Jr. Resuscitation of neonates by hypothermia: report on 20 cases with

acid-base determination on 10 cases and the long-term development of 33 cases. *Resuscitation* 1973;**2**:169–81.

14. Oates RK, Harvey D. Failure of hypothermia as treatment for asphyxiated newborn rabbits. *Arch Dis Child* 1976;**51**:512–6.

15. Michenfelder JD, Milde JH. Failure of prolonged hypocapnia, hypothermia, or hypertension to favorably alter acute stroke in primates. *Stroke* 1977;**8**:87–91.

16. Kopshev SN. [Craniocerebral hypothermia in the prevention and combined therapy of cerebral pathology in infants with asphyxia neonatorum]. *Akush Ginekol (Mosk)* 1982;56–8.

17. Bohn DJ, Biggar WD, Smith CR, Conn AW, Barker GA. Influence of hypothermia, barbiturate therapy and intracranial pressure monitoring on morbidity and mortality after near-drowning. *Crit Care Med* 1986;**14**:529–34.

18. Delpy DT, Gordon RE, Hope PL, et al. Noninvasive investigation of cerebral ischemia by phosphorus nuclear magnetic resonance. *Pediatrics* 1982;**70**:310–3.

19. Hope PL, Costello AM, Cady EB, et al. Cerebral energy metabolism studied with phosphorus NMR spectroscopy in normal and birth-asphyxiated infants. *Lancet* 1984;**2**:366–70.

20. Kirino T. Delayed neuronal death in the gerbil hippocampus following ischemia. *Brain Res* 1982;**239**:57–69.

21. Pulsinelli WA, Brierley JB, Plum F. Temporal profile of neuronal damage in a model of transient forebrain ischemia. *Ann Neurol* 1982;**11**:491–8.

22. Vannucci RC. Experimental biology of cerebral hypoxia-ischemia: Relation to perinatal brain damage. *Pediatr Res* 1990;**27**:317–26.

23. Lorek A, Takei Y, Cady EB, et al. Delayed ('secondary') cerebral energy failure following acute hypoxia-ischemia in the newborn piglet: continuous 48-hour studies by 31P magnetic resonance spectroscopy. *Pediatr Res* 1994;**36**:699–706.

24. Blumberg RM, Cady EB, Wigglesworth JS, McKenzie JE, Edwards AD. Relation between delayed impairment of cerebral energy metabolism and infarction following transient focal hypoxia ischemia in the developing brain. *Exp Brain Res* 1996;**113**:130–7.

25. Williams CE, Gunn AJ, Mallard C, Gluckman PD. Outcome after ischemia in the developing sheep brain: an electroencephalographic and histological study. *Ann Neurol* 1992;**31**:14–21.

26. Olney JW, Sharpe LG. Brain lesions in an infant rhesus monkey treated with monosodium glutamate. *Science* 1969;**166**:386–8.

27. Olney JW, Ho OL. Brain damage in infant mice following oral intake of glutamate, aspartate or cysteine. *Nature* 1970;**227**:609–11.

28. Simon RP, Swan JH, Griffiths T, Meldrum BS. Blockade of N-methyl-D-aspartate receptors may protect against ischemic damage in the brain. *Science* 1984;**226**:850–2.

29. Kerr JF, Wyllie AH, Currie AR. Apoptosis, a basic biological phenomenon with wide-ranging implications in human tissue kinetics. *Br J Cancer* 1972;**26**:239–57.

30. Ellis HM, Horvitz HR. Genetic control of programmed cell death in the nematode C. elegans. *Cell* 1986;**44**:817–29.

31. Raff MC. Social controls on cell survival and cell death. *Nature* 1992;**356**:397–400.

32. Evan GI, Wyllie AH, Gilbert CS, et al. Induction of apoptosis in fibroblasts by c-myc protein. *Cell* 1992;**69**:119–28.

33. Mehmet H, Yue X, Squier MV, et al. Increased apoptosis in the cingulate sulcus of newborn piglets following transient hypoxia-ischemia is related to the degree of high energy phosphate depletion during the insult. *Neurosci Lett* 1994;**181**:121–5.

34. Beilharz E, Williams CE, Dragunow M, Sirimanne E, Gluckman PD. Mechanisms of cell death following hypoxic-ischemic injury in the immature rat: evidence of apoptosis during selective neuronal loss. *Mol Brain Res* 1995;**29**:1–14.

35. Edwards AD, Yue X, Cox P, et al. Apoptosis in the brains of infants suffering intrauterine cerebral injury. *Pediatr Res* 1997;**42**:684–9.

36. Thiringer K, Hrbek A, Karlsson K, Rosen KG, Kjellmer I. Postasphyxial cerebral survival in newborn sheep after treatment with oxygen free radical scavengers and a calcium antagonist. *Pediatr Res* 1987;**22**:62–6.

37. Hagberg H, Andersson P, Kjellmer I, Thiringer K, Thordstein M. Extracellular overflow of glutamate, aspartate, GABA and taurine in the cortex and basal ganglia of fetal lambs during hypoxia-ischemia. *Neurosci Lett* 1987;**78**:311–7.

38. McDonald JW, Silverstein FS, Johnston MV. MK-801 protects the neonatal brain from hypoxic-ischemic damage. *Eur J Pharmacol* 1987;**140**:359–61.

39. Clemence M, Thornton JS, Penrice J, et al. 31P MRS and quantitative diffusion and T2 MRI show no cerebroprotective effects of intravenous MgSO4 after severe transient hypoxia-ischemia in the neonatal piglet. *MAGMA* 1996;**4**:114.

40. Gunn AJ, Mydlar T, Bennet L, et al. The neuroprotective actions of a calcium channel antagonist, flunarizine, in the infant rat. *Pediatr Res* 1989;**25**:573–6.

41. Marks KA, Mallard C, Roberts I, et al. Nitric oxide synthase inhibition attenuates delayed vasodilation and increases injury following cerebral ischemia in fetal sheep. *Pediatr Res* 1996;**40**:185–91.

42. Gluckman PD, Klempt N, Guan J, et al. A role for IGF-1 in the rescue of CNS neurons following hypoxic-ischemic injury. *Biochem Biophys Res Commun* 1992;**182**:593–9.

43. Busto R, Globus MY, Dietrich WD, et al. Effect of mild hypothermia on ischemia-induced release of neurotransmitters and free fatty acids in rat brain. *Stroke* 1989;**20**:904–10.

44. Busto R, Dietrich WD, Globus MY, Ginsberg MD. Postischemic moderate hypothermia inhibits CA1 hippocampal ischemic neuronal injury. *Neurosci Lett* 1989;**101**:299–304.

45. Buchan A, Pulsinelli WA. Hypothermia but not the N-methyl-D-aspartate antagonist, MK-801, attenuates neuronal damage in gerbils subjected to transient global ischemia. *J Neurosci* 1990;**10**:311–6.

46. Thoresen M, Penrice J, Lorek A, et al. Mild hypothermia following severe transient hypoxia-ischemia ameliorates delayed cerebral energy failure in the newborn piglet. *Pediatr Res* 1995;**37**:667–70.

47. Yue X, Mehmet H, Penrice J, et al. Apoptosis and necrosis in the newborn piglet brain following transient cerebral hypoxia-ischemia. *Neuropathol Appl Neurobiol* 1996;**22**:482–503.

48. Haaland K, Loberg EM, Steen PA, Thoresen M. Posthypoxic hypothermia in newborn piglets. *Pediatr Res* 1997;**41**:505–12.

49. Penrice J, Lorek A, Cady EB, et al. Proton magnetic resonance spectroscopy of the brain during acute hypoxia-ischemia and delayed cerebral energy failure in the newborn piglet. *Pediatr Res* 1997;**41**:795–802.

50. Thoresen M, Bagenholm R, Loberg EM, Apricena F, Kjellmer I. Posthypoxic cooling of neonatal rats provides protection against brain injury. *Arch Dis Child Fetal Neonatal Ed* 1996;**74**:F3–9.

51. Sirimanne E, Blumberg RM, Bossano D, et al. The effect of prolonged modification of cerebral temperature on outcome following hypoxic-ischemic brain injury in the infant rat. *Pediatr Res* 1996;**39**:591–7.

52. Bona E, Loberg E, Bagenholm R, Hagberg H, Thoresen M. Protective effects of moderate hypothermia after hypoxia-ischemia in a neonatal rat model: short and long-term outcome. *J Cereb Blood Flow Metab* 1997;**17**(Suppl 1): S857.

53. Gunn AJ, Gunn TR, De Haan HH, Williams CE, Gluckman PD. Dramatic neuronal rescue with prolonged selective head cooling after ischemia in fetal lambs. *J Clin Invest* 1997;**99**:248–56.

54. Boris-Moller F, Smith M-L, Siesjö BK. Effects of hypothermia on ischemic brain damage: a comparison between preischemic and postischemic cooling. *Neurosci Res Commun* 1989;**5**:87–94.

55. Ikonomidou C, Mosinger JL, Olney JW. Hypothermia enhances protective effect of MK-801 against hypoxic/ischemic brain damage in infant rats. *Brain Res* 1989;**487**:184–7.

56. Minamisawa H, Nordstrom CH, Smith ML, Siesjo BK. The influence of mild body and brain hypothermia on ischemic brain damage. *J Cereb Blood Flow Metab* 1990;**10**:365–74.

57. Cardell M, Boris Moller F, Wieloch T. Hypothermia prevents the ischemia-induced translocation and inhibition of protein kinase C in the rat striatum. *J Neurochem* 1991;**57**:1814–7.

58. Chopp M, Chen H, Dereski MO, Garcia JH. Mild hypothermic intervention after graded ischemic stress in rats. *Stroke* 1991;**22**:37–43.

59. Clifton GL, Jiang JY, Lyeth BG, et al. Marked protection by moderate hypothermia after experimental traumatic brain injury. *J Cereb Blood Flow Metab* 1991;**11**:114–21.

60. Coimbra C, Wieloch T. Hypothermia ameliorates neuronal survival when induced 2 hours after ischemia in the rat. *Acta Physiol Scand* 1992;**146**:543–4.

61. Moyer DJ, Welsh FA, Zager EL. Spontaneous cerebral hypothermia diminishes focal infarction in rat brain. *Stroke* 1992;**23**:1812–6.

62. Colbourne F, Corbett D. Delayed and prolonged post-ischemic hypothermia is neuroprotective in the gerbil. *Brain Res* 1994;**654**:265–72.

63. Marion DW, Penrod LE, Kelsey SF, et al. Treatment of traumatic brain injury with moderate hypothermia. *N Engl J Med* 1997;**336**:540–6.

64. Edwards AD, Yue X, Squier MV, et al. Specific inhibition of apoptosis after cerebral hypoxia-ischemia by moderate post-insult hypothermia. *Biochem Biophys Res Commun* 1995;**217**:1193–9.

65. Thoresen M, Satas S, Puka-Sundvall M, et al. Post-hypoxic hypothermia reduces cerebrocortical release of NO and excitotoxins. *Neuroreport* 1997;**8**:3359–62.

66. Gunn AJ, Gluckman PD, Gunn TR. Selective head cooling in newborn infants following perinatal asphyxia: a safety study. *Pediatrics* 1998;**102**:885–992.

67. Van Leeuwen GMJ, Hand JW, Lagendijk JJW, Azzopardi D, Edwards AD. Numerical modelling of temperature distributions within the neonatal head. *Pediatr Res* 2000;**48**:351–6.

68. Azzopardi D, Robertson NJ, Cowan F, et al. Pilot study of treatment with whole body hypothermia for neonatal encepalopathy. *Pediatrics* 2000;**106**:684–94.

69. Thoresen M, Whitelaw A. Cardiovascular changes during mild therapeutic hypothermia and rewarming in infants with hypoxic-ischemic encephalopathy. *Pediatrics* 2000;**106**:92–9.

70. Laptook AR, Corbett RJ, Sterett R, et al. Modest hypothermia provides partial neuroprotection when used for immediate resuscitation after brain ischemia. *Pediatr Res* 1997;**42**:17–23.

71. Simbruner G, Haberl C, Harrison V, Linley L, Willeitner AE. Induced brain hypothermia in asphyxiated human newborn infants: a retrospective chart analysis of physiological and adverse effects. *Intensive Care Med* 1999;**25**:1111–7.

72. Eicher DJ, Wagner CL, Katikaneni LP, et al. Moderate hypothermia in neonatal encephalopathy: efficacy outcomes. *Pediatr Neurol* 2005;**32**:11–7.

73. Eicher DJ, Wagner CL, Katikaneni LP, et al. Moderate hypothermia in neonatal encephalopathy: safety outcomes. *Pediatr Neurol* 2005;**32**:18–24.

74. Jacobs S, Hunt R, Tarnow-Mordi W, Inder T, Davis P. Cooling for newborns with hypoxic ischemic encephalopathy. *Cochrane.Database Syst Rev* 2007; CD003311.

75. Yager JY, Towfighi J, Vannucci RC. Influence of mild hypothermia on hypoxic ischemic brain damage in the immature rat. *Pediatr Res* 1993;**34**:525–9.

76. Dietrich WD, Busto R, Alonso O, Globus MY, Ginsberg MD. Intraischemic but not postischemic brain hypothermia protects chronically following global forebrain ischemia in rats. *J Cereb Blood Flow Metab* 1993;**13**:541–9.

77. Cowan F, Rutherford M, Groenendaal F, et al. Origin and timing of brain lesions in term infants with neonatal encephalopathy. *Lancet* 2003;**361**:736–42.

78. Gluckman PD, Wyatt JS, Azzopardi D, et al. Selective head cooling with mild systemic hypothermia after neonatal encephalopathy: multicentre randomised trial. *Lancet* 2005;**365**:663–70.

79. Gunn A, Gluckman PD, Wyatt JS, Thoresen C, Edwards AD. Selective head cooling after neonatal encephalopathy. *Lancet* 2005;**365**:1619–20.

80. Shankaran C, Laptook A, Wright LL, et al. Whole-body hypothermia for neonatal encephalopathy: animal observations as a basis for a randomized, controlled pilot study in term infants. *Pediatrics* 2002;**110**:377–85.

81. Shankaran S, Laptook AR, Ehrenkranz RA, et al. Whole-body hypothermia for neonates with hypoxic-ischemic encephalopathy. *N Engl J Med* 2005;**353**:1574–84.

82. Jacobs S, Hunt R, Tarnow-Mordi W, Inder T, Davis P. Cooling for newborns with hypoxic ischemic encephalopathy. *Cochrane Database Syst Rev* 2007; CD003311.

83. Kirpalani H, Barks J, Thorlund K, Guyatt G. Cooling for neonatal hypoxic ischemic encephalopathy: do we have the answer? *Pediatrics* 2007;**120**:1126–30.

84. Hutchison JS, Ward RE, Lacroix J, et al. Hypothermia therapy after traumatic brain injury in children. *N Engl J Med* 2008;**358**:2447–56.

85. Clifton GL, Miller ER, Choi SC, et al. Lack of effect of induction of hypothermia after acute brain injury. *N Engl J Med* 2001;**344**:556–63.

86. Higgins RD, Raju TN, Perlman J, et al. Hypothermia and perinatal asphyxia: executive summary of the National Institute of Child Health and Human Development workshop. *J Pediatr* 2006;**148**:170–5.

87. Robertson NJ, Nakakeeto M, Hagmann C, et al. Therapeutic hypothermia for birth asphyxia in low-resource settings: a pilot randomised controlled trial. *Lancet* 2008;**372**:801–3.

# Clinical trials of hypothermic neural rescue

A. David Edwards and Denis V. Azzopardi

## Introduction

Moderate cooling by 3–4°C is the first successful neural rescue therapy for neonatal encephalopathy. Induced moderate cooling has also been shown to protect the brain in adults following cardiac arrest and has shown promise in other forms of cerebral injury. Although there are several historical reports of induced cooling, the implementation of moderate cooling for neural rescue in newborns with hypoxic–ischaemic brain injury is the culmination of a series of research spanning decades that: proved the potential for neural rescue following perinatal asphyxia [1]; consistently showed benefit in appropriate experimental models [2,3]; examined safety and feasibility in preliminary clinical studies [4,5]; confirmed efficacy by synthesis of the results of several well-conducted randomized clinical trials in newborns [6]; and was followed by rapid implementation into clinical practice and ongoing surveillance [7]. This chapter will examine the findings of the clinical trials of neural rescue therapy with moderate cooling in newborns. The results of these studies led to recommendations by expert groups, specialist advisory committees and regulatory authorities for the rapid implementation into clinical practice of treatment with cooling for neonatal encephalopathy [8–10].

It is interesting to consider why this intervention has succeeded when so many other apparently promising therapies failed to show benefit in clinical trials. The lack of success of neuroprotective interventions in adult stroke led to a series of special meetings of stakeholders, namely neurologists, industry representatives, patient groups and regulatory authorities – the STAIR meetings. These meetings generated recommendations for preclinical evaluation, clinical study design, enhancing trial implementation and completion and, more recently, novel approaches to measuring

outcomes, data analysis and use of new technologies such as telemedicine and electronic databases [11,12]. In many aspects, the development of neural rescue with moderate cooling followed several of the recommendations now being made to facilitate the discovery and evaluation of new neural rescue therapies.

## Preliminary trials

The safety and feasibility of cooling infants with hypoxic ischaemic encephalopathy were investigated in several small preliminary studies before the large randomized controlled trials. One of the first reports was by Gunn who cooled two groups each of six infants to a rectal temperature of 36–36.5°C and 35.5–36°C using a purposely designed cooling cap consisting of coils of silicon tubing filled with circulating water kept at 10°C. The cot overhead radiant warmer was manually adjusted to prevent excessive cooling. No adverse effects due to cooling were observed [4]. Subsequently a commercial device for providing selective head cooling with mild body cooling was developed by Olympic Medical (Olympic Medical Seattle, USA) and used in the first large randomized trial of neural rescue with cooling in infants with perinatal hypoxic ischaemic injury, the Coolcap trial (vide infra) [13].

In other studies the practicality and safety of reducing body temperature by 3–4°C by surface cooling were assessed [5]. Azzopardi and Edwards described the physiological effects of prolonged induced cooling to a rectal temperature of 33.5°C using a commercial air cooling system (Polar Air, Augustine Medical, Eden Prairie, MD) that induces hypothermia by blowing cool air through a translucent perforated paper blanket placed over the infant. The blood pressure rose and heart rate fell linearly with increasing depth of cooling but this was of little clinical significance and no

*Neonatal Neural Rescue*, ed. A. David Edwards, Denis V. Azzopardi and Alistair J. Gunn. Published by Cambridge University Press. © Cambridge University Press 2013.

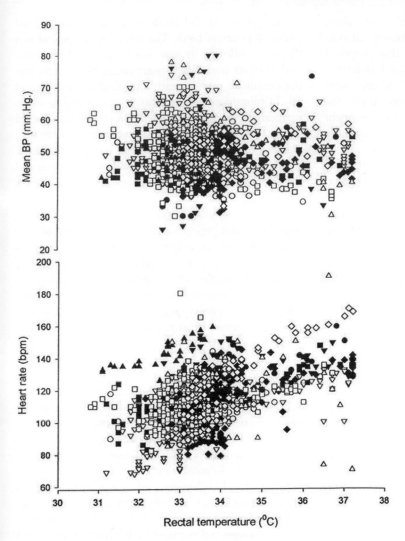

**Figure 4.1.** Relationships among mean blood pressure, heart rate and rectal temperature in cooled infants. Different symbols represent data from individual infants (Reproduced from reference [5] with kind permission from the American Academy of Pediatrics).

arrhythmia or significant hypotension was seen. The relationship between mean blood pressure, heart rate and rectal temperature is shown in Figure 4.1. Whitelaw and Thoresen, using gloves filled with cold water placed around the infant to induce and maintain cooling, reported that inadvertent rapid changes in surface temperature may be associated with hypotension or bradycardia [14]. An observational study using echocardiography in seven infants during cooling and on rewarming found normal tissue perfusion and blood lactate during cooling but cardiac output increased by approximately 30% following rewarming [15].

Safety concerns were raised in Eicher's pilot randomized controlled trial of 65 infants allocated whole body cooling to 33°C for 48 hours or standard care [16]. The group allocated cooling had significantly higher prothrombin times and lower platelet counts and a greater requirement for inotropes and infusions of plasma and platelets. Seizures were also reported to be more frequently observed in the cooled group, compared with the non-cooled infants. These complications were considered to be of mild to moderate severity and easily manageable. These findings may be related to the lower rectal temperature aimed for in this study compared to the other trials (33°C vs. 33.5–34.5°C).

Azzopardi and Edwards investigated a protocol that might be used to enrol infants in prospective randomized controlled trials of neural rescue with hypothermia [5]. The aim was to use objective criteria to select within 6 hours of birth infants with suspected birth asphyxia with a high risk of developing moderate to severe encephalopathy. Because clinical criteria alone were considered poorly predictive of subsequent outcome when applied so soon after birth, they proposed staged entry criteria: first, infants suspected of having suffered perinatal hypoxic–ischaemic injury were defined using clinical criteria and were entered into the study; these infants then underwent objective assessment of their neurological prognosis using amplitude-integrated EEG (aEEG) and those infants with a poor prognosis were selected for treatment with hypothermic neural rescue therapy. Azzopardi and Edwards suggested that this approach increased specificity, which would allow a smaller study size. This method was subsequently used in three large trials of therapeutic cooling in infants with suspected birth asphyxia [13,17,18].

# Clinical trials of neural rescue with cooling

## Outcomes to at least 18 months of age

The initial studies were too small to assess the neuroprotective effect of therapeutic cooling or only reported short-term outcomes. Eicher's pilot randomized study of 65 infants found that cooling was associated with a lower rate of death or severe motor scores up to 12 months of age: 14/27 (52%) in the cooled group compared with 21/25 (84%) in the non-cooled group, $P = 0.019$, but 12 month motor follow-up data were only available in 28/41 survivors [19]. Deaths were similar in the two groups: 10/32 (31%) amongst the infants allocated cooling and 14/33 (42%) in the normothermia group, $P = 0.35$. In this study more than 75% of the infants were born outside the cooling centres but cooling could be initiated during transport. Worryingly, outborn infants were 10 times more likely to die than inborns, but no explanation for this observation could be found.

Six large randomized controlled trials of hypothermic neural rescue therapy in newborns with hypoxic ischaemic encephalopathy with outcomes to at least 18 months were published in the English literature from 2005 to 2011 [13,17,18,20–22]. All six studies had a similar study design, largely based on the Coolcap study, but there were important differences: in two trials the intervention was selective head cooling with mild body cooling [13,21] and three trials used aEEG or EEG for assessment of the severity of encephalopathy and enrolment of infants [13,17,18]. In all six trials infants were full term or near term (up to 36

weeks' gestation) and randomization was completed within 6 hours of birth. The intervention period was 72 hours followed by slow rewarming at 0.5°C/hour and in all six trials the primary outcome measure was the combined rate of death and disability assessed at 18–24 months of age. The target core rectal or oesophageal temperature was 33.5°C in the trials that used whole body cooling. Outcomes were remarkably similar amongst the trials: all showed a reduction in the combined rate of death and disability with cooling and this reached statistical significance in four of the six studies. The rates of death/disability in the control groups were similar in four of the studies (53–66%), suggesting that patient selection and standard of care were likely similar in these trials; the event rate was higher in one study (83%) and lower in another (49%) [18,21]. The studies are summarized in Table 4.1.

The first large trial to be published was the 2005 selective head cooling with mild systemic hypothermia after neonatal encephalopathy trial (the Coolcap trial) [13]. Infants were enrolled if they met the clinical criteria and had a moderately or severely abnormal aEEG or seizures. 116 infants were allocated head cooling for 72 hours and 118 infants allocated conventional care. Follow-up data were available in 218 (93%) infants. There was no difference in the combined rate of death or severe disability at 18 months between the two groups but the odds ratio was reduced with hypothermia after adjustment for the severity of aEEG changes and in a *post hoc* analysis adjusting for clinical severity of encephalopathy [23]. An interaction was present between the severity of aEEG changes and treatment with cooling. No effect of cooling was present in the group with the most severe aEEG abnormalities (severely suppressed aEEG together with seizures), whilst in the remaining infants there was a favourable outcome with cooling. Gluckman has suggested that the combination of seizures and severe suppression of the aEEG before initiation of cooling therapy may indicate the occurrence of irreversible cerebral injury (Peter Gluckman personal communication).

A few months following the Coolcap trial, the National Institute of Child Health and Development, whole body hypothermia for neonates with hypoxic–ischaemic encephalopathy trial (The NICHD trial) reported its results [20]. Of 239 eligible infants, 102 were assigned to whole body cooling to an oesophageal temperature of 33.5°C for 72 hours and 106 infants to normal care. Primary outcome data at 18–22 months

**Table 4.1.** Summary of the main randomized trials of cooling for neonatal encephalopathy with outcome to 18–24 months of age

| Study | Location | Method | Criteria | Rate of death or disability in controls (%) | Rate of death or disability in cooled infants (%) | Risk ratio (RR) | Lower limit of RR | Upper limit of RR |
|---|---|---|---|---|---|---|---|---|
| Coolcap 2005 [13] | USA, New Zealand, UK | Selective head with mild body | Clinical plus aEEG | 73/110 (66.36) | 59/108 (54.62) | 0.82 | 0.66 | 1.02 |
| NICHD 2005 [20] | USA | Whole body | Clinical | 64/106 (60.37) | 45/102 (44.11) | 0.73 | 0.56 | 0.95 |
| TOBY 2009 [17] | UK, Hungary, Ireland, Sweden, Finland, Israel | Whole body | Clinical plus aEEG | 86/162 (53.08) | 74/163 (45.39) | 0.86 | 0.68 | 1.07 |
| Zhou 2010 [21] | China | Selective head with mild body | Clinical | 46/94 (48.93) | 31/100 (31) | 0.63 | 0.44 | 0.91 |
| n.nEURO 2010 [18] | Germany, France, Belgium, Denmark, Italy, South Africa, Singapore | Whole body | Clinical plus aEEG | 48/58 (82.75) | 27/53 (50.94) | 0.62 | 0.46 | 0.82 |
| ICE 2011 [22] | Australia, New Zealand, Canada, USA | Whole body (cool packs) | Clinical | 67/101 (66.34) | 55/107 (51.4) | 0.77 | 0.62 | 0.98 |

of age were available for 205 infants. Death or moderate or severe disability occurred in 45/102 (44%) infants in the cooled group and in 64/103 (62%) infants in the control group: risk ratio (RR) 0.72 95% confidence interval (CI) 0.54–0.95, $P = 0.01$. However, there were no statistical differences between the treated and control groups in the proportion of infants with any of the components of the composite outcome: death, disabling cerebral palsy, the psychomotor and mental developmental indices of the Bayley scales, blindness or impaired hearing. It was not possible to ascertain whether this was due to lack of power of the study or due to lack of effect of therapeutic hypothermia. Therefore, many clinicians remained uncertain of the value of therapeutic hypothermia. There also was no difference in the primary outcome between the

cooled and non-cooled infants grouped according to the clinical severity of encephalopathy. Other differences from the Coolcap study were the absence of aEEG recordings and the inclusion of moderate disability in the composite primary outcome.

The moderate hypothermia to treat perinatal asphyxial encephalopathy trial (the TOBY trial) started enrolment in December 2001 [17]. The investigators planned to enroll 236 infants over 5 years, but this sample size was achieved ahead of schedule and enrollment was continued when the Coolcap and NICHD trial results suggested that a larger sample would be valuable. The enrolment criteria were the same as the Coolcap trial, but trained personnel assessed outborn infants including the aEEG, randomization was carried out and if allocated, cooling was initiated by stopping warming and placing cold gel packs around the baby if necessary during transport to the cooling centre. Of 325 infants enrolled, 163 were assigned to intensive care with cooling and 162 infants to intensive care. Cooling was achieved by a cooling mattress manually adjusted to maintain a rectal temperature of 33.5°C for 72 hours. Sedation was with morphine infusion or chloral hydrate. The reduction in the combined rate of death and severe disability at 18 months of age did not reach statistical significance: In the cooled group, 42 infants died and 32 survived with severe neurodevelopmental disability, whereas in the non-cooled group, 44 infants died and 42 had severe disability (RR for either outcome, 0.86; 95% CI, 0.68 to 1.07; $P = 0.17$). However, infants in the cooled group had an increased rate of survival without neurologic abnormality (RR, 1.57; 95% CI, 1.16 to 2.12; $P = 0.003$) and among survivors, cooling resulted in reduced risks of cerebral palsy (RR, 0.67; 95% CI, 0.47 to 0.96; $P = 0.03$) and improved scores on the Mental Developmental Index and Psychomotor Developmental Index of the Bayley Scales of Infant Development II ($P = 0.03$ for each) and the Gross Motor Function Classification System ($P = 0.01$). Thus the TOBY trial found statistically significant reductions in disabilities with cooling treatment and analysis of MRI images obtained at 8 days of age confirmed a reduction in cerebral abnormalities with cooling [24]. When the results of the TOBY, Coolcap and NICHD trials were synthesized, the improved neurological outcomes with cooling treatment was confirmed [6]. These data together with similar findings in other systematic reviews and meta-analyses led to increasing use of cooling in clinical practice and to early closure of some of the ongoing trials of cooling.

The selective head cooling with mild systemic hypothermia after neonatal hypoxic–ischaemic encephalopathy, a multicentre randomized controlled trial in China by Zhou et al (The Zhou study) was reported in 2010 [21]. Cooling was obtained by a cooling cap around the head servo controlled to attain a nasopharyngeal temperature of 34°C and a servo-controlled radiant body warmer was used to maintain a rectal temperature of 34.5–35°C. Inclusion criteria were evidence of birth asphyxia and presence of encephalopathy on clinical assessment; approximately 20% of enrolled infants had mild encephalopathy only. Randomization was stratified by centre but not severity of encephalopathy, but the degree of encephalopathy was very similar amongst the two treatment groups. The primary endpoint was death

or severe disability at 18 months. Of 235 infants recruited, follow-up data were available for 100 infants in the selective cooling group and 94 controls. Neurodevelopmental assessment was with the Gesell Child Development Scale and severe disability was defined as a developmental quotient <70 or a Gross Motor Function Classification Level 3–5 (i.e., unable to sit without support or worse). The combined rate of death or disability was 31% in the cooling group and 49% in the controls, $P = 0.01$. The proportion of survivors with severe disability was also significantly reduced in the selective cooling group compared with controls (11/80 (14%) vs. 19/67 (28%), $P = 0.03$). The less stringent definition of birth asphyxia and the inclusion of infants with mild encephalopathy probably accounts for the lower event rate observed in this study compared to other studies.

The systemic hypothermia after neonatal encephalopathy trial (the neo.nEURO trial) commenced in 2001 but was terminated in 2006 earlier than planned because of clinical concerns following the positive results of the Coolcap and NICHD trials [18]. The entry criteria were similar to the Coolcap and TOBY trials and required confirmation of encephalopathy by aEEG or EEG. The cooling protocol was the same as that for the TOBY trial. At cessation of enrollment 129 out of a planned 150 infants had been recruited and follow-up data at 18 months of age were available for 111 (86%) infants. The combined rate of death and severe disability was 27/53 (50.9%) in the cooled group and 48/58 (82.8%) in the controls; the odds ratio adjusted for severity of encephalopathy was 0.21, 95% CI 0.09–0.54, $P = 0.001$. The rates of disabling cerebral palsy and of a developmental quotient more than 2 standard deviations below the mean were also significantly reduced with cooling. The high rate of death or disability in both groups was ascribed to a relatively large proportion of outborns (approximately 65%) and of severe encephalopathy. The proportion of infants with severe encephalopathy (defined as the occurrence of a suppressed aEEG/EEG) was approximately 60%, similar to that in the TOBY trial. Unlike the observations of the Coolcap study, the beneficial effect of cooling was maintained in the severe encephalopathy group, probably because of differences in the definition of severe encephalopathy, which required the combination of seizures and a suppressed aEEG in the Coolcap study, but only a suppressed aEEG in the TOBY and neo.nEURO studies. Almost all the infants received regular sedation with morphine or fentanyl and the authors speculated this may have contributed to the improved outcomes observed with cooling, based on the report by Thoresen of a lack of effect of cooling in the absence of sedation in an experimental model of asphyxia [25]. However, the rate of death and disability in the cooled group was no lower in this study than in the other cooling trials.

The final large trial of treatment with cooling for neonatal encephalopathy in well resourced countries was the whole body hypothermia for term and near-term newborns with hypoxic ischaemic encephalopathy trial (The ICE trial) [22]. The study investigators expected the majority of infants to be born outside tertiary centres (outborn) so trained dedicated retrieval teams to identify infants at risk of brain injury and used a simple inexpensive method of systemic cooling that could be used at the birth hospital. Recruitment started in 2001 and terminated in 2007 because of accumulating evidence from the other studies of benefit with cooling, when 221 infants of a planned 300 infants had been enrolled. Cooling was commenced within 6 hours of birth and was achieved by placing cold gel packs around the baby. Similar to the NICHD trial the primary outcome measure was the combined rate of death or moderate or severe disability and was reported at 2 years of age for 208 of 221 (94%) randomized infants and for 139/152 (91.4%) of survivors. The proportion of infants allocated to cooling with the primary outcome was 55/107 (51.7%) and 67/101 (66.3%) in controls, RR 0.77, 95% CI, 0.62–0.98, $P = 0.03$. However, the reduction in death/disability was of borderline significance after adjustment for severity of encephalopathy, $P = 0.05$. Consistent with the results of the TOBY trial, the proportion of infants surviving free of any disability was increased in the cooled group compared with controls: 39.6% vs. 22.7%, RR 1.75, 95% CI, 1.3–2.7, $P = 0.01$. The simple pragmatic methods used in this study for identifying infants at risk of brain injury and for maintaining cooling suggest that therapeutic hypothermia could be used in low-resource countries and further clinical studies are under way to confirm the safety and efficacy of therapeutic cooling in those settings [26].

Two other randomized controlled trials of cooling for neonatal encephalopathy reported outcomes at 18 months of age. Battin reported outcomes for 40 infants that had participated in the preliminary studies of selective head cooling with varying degrees of body cooling, but included 9 infants where treatment allocation was not at random. Amongst children with follow-up data at 18 months of age, there were similar proportions

with death or severe disability among those allocated selective cooling (8/24) and controls (4/13) [27]. In another trial from China with cooling delayed up to 10 hours after birth, the rate of death or disability at 18 months was 7/38 (18.4%) in the hypothermia group and 21/44 (47.7%) in the control group, $P = 0.005$ [28]. In an exploratory analysis the rate of disability amongst survivors did not differ when hypothermia was started before or after 5 hours of age but the numbers in each subgroup were too small to detect a difference. However, these results support the hypothesis that the opportunity for neural rescue therapy in neonatal encephalopathy may extend beyond 6 hours.

# Synthesis of trial data

Although no formal prospective meta-analysis was set up, trial investigators recognized from the outset that meta-analysis of trial data would be required to confirm the safety and efficacy of therapeutic hypothermia for neonatal encephalopathy. Accordingly, the major trials had a similar trial design: clinical enrollment criteria, duration and depth of cooling and outcome measures were similar, albeit different methods of cooling were used. Perhaps for these reasons, synthesis of the trial data shows remarkable consistency with minimal heterogeneity amongst the studies.

The results of a meta-analysis of randomized controlled trials with outcomes to at least 18 months of age and published in the English literature are displayed as typical risk ratios and 95% CI in Figures 4.2–4.7. The meta-analysis was performed with REVMAN V software [29], using a random effects model. These data confirm that prolonged mild cooling, whether provided by a cooling cap or systemically, reduces the rate of death and of severe disability and increases the rate of intact survival at 18 to 24 months of age. The size of the effect (calculated from data from the six large randomized trials with similar entry criteria) is clinically important: for every 7 infants (95% CI 5–11) treated one additional infant is prevented from dying or becoming disabled.

Typical risk ratios for selective head cooling and whole body cooling are similar (Figure 4.7). In view of the simplicity of whole body cooling and the close temperature control achieved with servo-controlled cooling equipment, this is now the most widely practised method of inducing and maintaining cooling therapy in the United Kingdom (data from UK TOBY Cooling Register [30]).

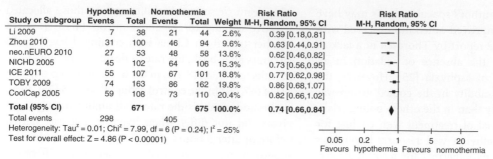

**Figure 4.2.** Forest plot of risk ratios of the combined rates of death and disability in cooled infants and controls at 18–24 months of age.

| Study or Subgroup | Hypothermia Events | Total | Normothermia Events | Total | Weight | Risk Ratio M-H, Random, 95% CI |
|---|---|---|---|---|---|---|
| CoolCap 2005 | 29 | 116 | 20 | 118 | 15.8% | 1.48 [0.89, 2.45] |
| NICHD 2005 | 32 | 102 | 22 | 106 | 18.5% | 1.51 [0.94, 2.45] |
| ICE 2011 | 42 | 106 | 22 | 97 | 21.5% | 1.75 [1.13, 2.70] |
| TOBY 2009 | 71 | 163 | 45 | 162 | 44.3% | 1.57 [1.16, 2.12] |
| **Total (95%CI)** | | **487** | | **483** | **100.0%** | **1.58 [1.29, 1.93]** |
| Total events | 174 | | 109 | | | |

Heterogeneity: Tau² = 0.00; Chi² = 0.31, df = 3 (P = 0.96); I² = 0%
Test for overall effect: Z = 4.43 (P < 0.00001)

**Figure 4.3.** Forest plot of risk ratios of the rate of survival with normal neurological outcome in cooled infants and controls at 18–24 months of age.

Synthesis of trial results grouped by severity of encephalopathy suggests that cooling reduced the rates of death and disability at 18–24 months of age both in the moderate and the severe encephalopathy sub groups (Figure 4.6). However, these data need to be interpreted with caution: clinical assessment of encephalopathy probably differed somewhat between studies because the criteria are imprecise and within each group there is probably a range of severity of encephalopathy. Some studies used the aEEG for assessing encephalopathy, but the aEEG grade is not necessarily equivalent to the clinical grade of encephalopathy. This was evident in the Coolcap study where the combined rate of death and disability in the subgroups differed according to the method of assessment of encephalopathy [13,23]. Furthermore, there was a higher proportion of infants with severe encephalopathy noted in the trials where assessment of encephalopathy was by aEEG, yet the outcomes were broadly similar amongst all the trials. Assessment of severity of encephalopathy by aEEG is less precise during the first 6 hours after birth, since even in the pre cooling era, a proportion of cases with severely suppressed aEEG showed return of cerebral electrical activity over the subsequent few hours and made a full recovery [31]. It remains difficult to determine from clinical and aEEG criteria within 6 hours of birth when cooling is likely to be unnecessary or futile.

## Safety outcomes

Hypothermia has several adverse physiological effects, including immunosuppression, coagulopathy, increased insulin resistance, alterations in electrolyte levels and cardiovascular and haemodynamic effects [32]. These side effects are more likely to occur when core body temperature is less than 30–31°C and are unlikely to cause significant clinical abnormalities at the temperature range used for neural rescue therapy (33–34°C).

Safety outcomes were assessed in several preliminary and randomized controlled trials of moderate cooling for neonatal encephalopathy. Although several short-term adverse events occurred in both cooled and control infants only a low platelet count occurred significantly more frequently in the cooled infants (Figure 4.8). The other adverse events were related to the systemic hypoxic ischaemic injury that accompanied neonatal encephalopathy. The mortality rate at 18 months of age was similar in both treated and controls in most of the trials but was significantly reduced with cooling in the ICE trial and on meta-analysis of trial data (Figure 4.5).

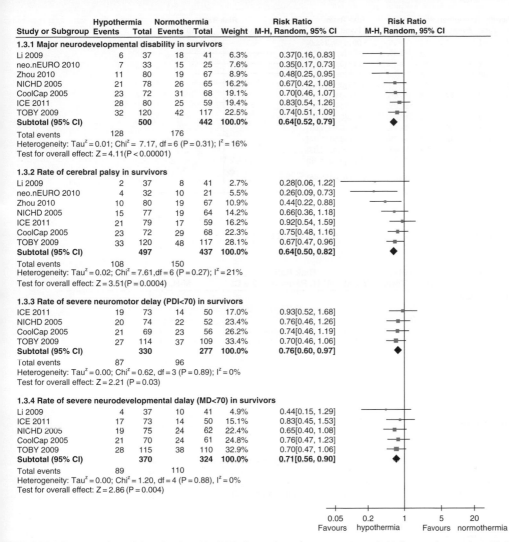

**Figure 4.4.** Forest plots of the risk ratios of individual neurological outcomes in cooled infants and controls at 18–24 months of age.

A mild coagulopathy occurred commonly in both cooled and non-cooled infants and bleeding did not occur more frequently with cooling. In the TOBY trial, mild intracranial haemorrhage on MRI was observed in approximately 30% of cooled and control infants [17,24].

Sinus bradycardia and prolongation of the QT interval in the electrocardiogram are physiological responses to hypothermia and were almost universally observed in the cooled infants [22]. However, clinically significant arrhythmias were very rare and not more frequent with cooling. A severe bradycardia was reported in a few cases in association with lignocaine or phenytoin

administration, irrespective of cooling (data reported by the TOBY trial).

Minor skin changes such as reddening or hardening of the skin were observed in a few infants treated with whole body cooling and similar changes occurred rarely on the scalp with head cooling. Subcutaneous fat necrosis occurred in one infant allocated whole body cooling in the NICHD trial. This complication is notified in approximately 1% of cases registered with the UK Cooling Register and is probably directly related to surface cooling in asphyxiated infants [33].

Neither sepsis nor pneumonia were found to be associated with cooling in the trials. The frequencies

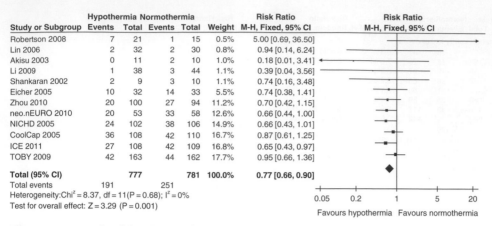

**Figure 4.5.** Forest plot of the risk ratios of mortality rate in cooled infants and controls.

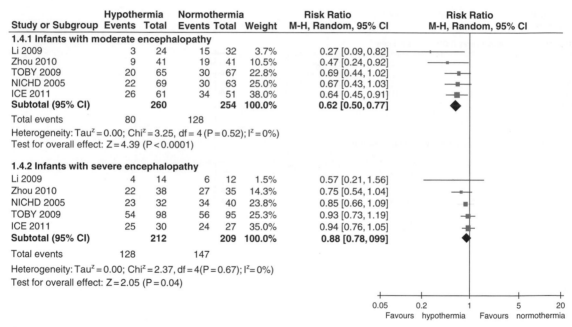

**Figure 4.6.** Forest plot of the risk ratios of the combined rates of death and disability in cooled infants and controls at 18–24 months of age, grouped by the severity of encephalopathy. The severity of encephalopathy was by aEEG grade in the TOBY and n.nEURO studies, by aEEG and clinical grade in the Coolcap study (data from clinical assessment only displayed in forest plot) and by clinical grade only in the other studies.

of other pulmonary complications were similar in cooled and non-cooled infants; the incidence of persistent pulmonary hypertension varied with individual trials, occurring most frequently (approximately 25%) in the NICHD trial.

## Exploratory analysis

*Post hoc* exploratory analyses of data from the randomized trials have been performed to attempt to address some of the clinical uncertainties surrounding therapeutic hypothermia in newborns with encephalopathy, such as the influence of temperature control on outcomes [23,34], effect of cooling on clinical predictors of outcome [35,36], cardiovascular effects of cooling [37] and others [38].

The effect of pyrexia on neurological outcome in infants allocated standard care without cooling was examined in the Coolcap and NICHD trials [23,39]. A rectal or oesophageal temperature of 38 °C or greater on at least one occasion was observed in approximately

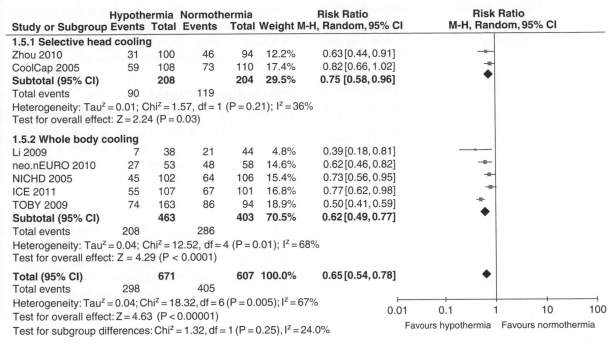

**Figure 4.7.** Forest plot of the risk ratios of the combined rates of death and disability in cooled infants and controls at 18–24 months of age, grouped by the method of cooling.

**Figure 4.8.** Forest plot of the odds ratio of the occurrence of thrombocytopenia in cooled infants and controls. Thrombocytopenia was defined as a platelet count <150,000 cells/μL in the Eicher, TOBY and ICE trials and <100,000 cells/μL in the Coolcap, n.nEURO and Zhou trials. For the NICHD trial, the rates of infants requiring platelet transfusion are shown.

30% of controls and a direct relationship was found between elevated core temperature and subsequent outcome: the odds of death or disability were increased 3-fold in the infants with pyrexia in the Coolcap trial and increased 3.6- to 4-fold with each degree C increase in the highest quartile of oesophageal temperature in the NICHD trial. These observations strongly suggest that pyrexia is injurious following hypoxic ischaemic injury and is consistent with experimental data.

In the clinical trials, excessive cooling commonly occurred in the infants allocated cooling, most often during the induction phase of cooling. An oesophageal temperature of <32°C was observed in approximately 30% of infants allocated cooling in the NICHD trial, despite using servo-controlled cooling equipment. It occurred more frequently in the infants with lower birth weights, but did not cause systemic or cardiovascular complications and was not associated with a worse neurological outcome [34]. Although this is reassuring, there are several case reports of cardiac arrhythmias and other adverse events following accidental hypothermia to <32°C so excessive cooling should be avoided.

In experimental studies, the brain sparing effect of moderate hypothermia is critically affected by the interval between the insult and start of cooling; delay in induction of hypothermia beyond 8 hours is associated with attenuation or loss of neuroprotection [40]. In the cooling trials, cooling was initiated at a median age of approximately 4 hours with little variability amongst the trials. Therefore, it is not surprising that no interaction effect was seen between age at initiation of cooling and outcome. Further information about the effect of delay in starting cooling may be available from a clinical trial of cooling after 6 hours of age currently under way (Evaluation of Systemic Hypothermia Initiated After 6 Hours of Age in Infants with Hypoxic Ischaemic Encephalopathy: A Bayesian Evaluation NCT00614744), as well as from data from the cooling registries. Another trial, Optimizing Hypothermia as Neuroprotection at < 6 Hours of Age for Neonatal Hypoxic Ischaemic Encephalopathy, is also planned by the NICHD to determine the optimal duration of cooling therapy and the depth of cooling.

The ability to predict outcome and the response to cooling treatment soon after birth is vitally important for clinical management of infants with hypoxic ischaemic encephalopathy. This was investigated by the Coolcap and NICHD trial investigators [23,35,41]. In the Coolcap study, following multivariate analysis, treatment with cooling, lower grade of encephalopathy, greater aEEG amplitude, lower birth weight and absence of seizures were associated with a better outcome. The encephalopathy grade at randomization was the strongest predictor of outcome, closely followed by aEEG background amplitude. There was no evidence of interaction between treatment with cooling and these variables. The NICHD investigators used two approaches: (1) a score was developed from the most predictive variables following logistic regression analysis; and (2) prognostic algorithms were developed from classification and regression tree analysis. Prediction of death or death/disability by either method was comparable to or better than the grade of encephalopathy before randomization and was not altered by treatment with cooling; approximately 75% of infants were correctly classified. It is uncertain whether this is sufficiently precise for guiding clinical management. Interestingly, they found that abnormal posture, absence of spontaneous activity and absent suck were the only features of the neurological examination that contributed to the prognosis.

## Concluding remarks

The implementation of therapeutic hypothermia for neonatal encephalopathy is a milestone in neonatal medicine. Neonatal encephalopathy is the largest cause of mortality and serious morbidity affecting children in poorly resourced countries, accounting for over 1 million deaths annually [42]. Preliminary investigation of therapeutic hypothermia in these settings has been carried out and large clinical trials are planned (Therapeutic Hypothermia for Birth Asphyxia in a Low Resource Setting ISRCTN89547571). In well-resourced countries, where the incidence of moderate/severe neonatal encephalopathy is approximately 1–2/1000 births, the societal benefits are likely to be large: treatment with cooling for 72 hours cooling is cost saving by 18 months of age and can be calculated to have major benefits to the health economy in countries where the intervention is applied widely [43]. For example, in the United Kingdom, from the synthesis of trial data and the UK TOBY Cooling Register, we estimated that within 3 years of the introduction of therapeutic hypothermia following the TOBY trial, the total economic benefit, calculated from the increase in numbers of economically active lives and the reduction in the costs of care for disabilities, is in excess of £100 million.

These remarkable benefits need to be put in perspective. It is important to bear in mind that infants with moderate to severe neonatal encephalopathy continue to have a high rate of severe neurological outcome: the rate of death or moderate to severe disability following treatment with cooling was 46% (95% CI 40%-53%) in the six cooling trials with similar enrolment criteria. The success of treatment with moderate cooling has shown that neural rescue therapy for neonatal encephalopathy is achievable. There still is scope and a pressing need for additional therapies to further improve outcomes following this devastating condition.

## References

1. Azzopardi D, Wyatt JS, Cady EB, et al. Prognosis of newborn infants with hypoxic-ischemic brain injury assessed by phosphorus magnetic resonance spectroscopy. *Pediatr Res* 1989;**25**:445–51.

2. Thoresen M, Penrice J, Lorek A, et al. Mild hypothermia after severe transient hypoxia-ischemia ameliorates delayed cerebral energy failure in the newborn piglet. *Pediatr Res* 1995;**37**:667–70.

3. Gunn AJ, Gunn TR, de Haan HH, Williams CE, Gluckman PD. Dramatic neuronal rescue with prolonged selective head cooling after ischemia in fetal lambs. *J Clin Invest* 1997;**99**:248–56.

4. Gunn AJ, Gluckman PD, Gunn TR. Selective head cooling in newborn infants after perinatal asphyxia: a safety study. *Pediatrics* 1998;**102**(Pt 1):885–92.

5. Azzopardi D, Robertson NJ, Cowan FM, et al. Pilot study of treatment with whole body hypothermia for neonatal encephalopathy. *Pediatrics* 2000;**106**:684–94.

6. Edwards AD, Brocklehurst P, Gunn AJ, et al. Neurological outcomes at 18 months of age after moderate hypothermia for perinatal hypoxic ischaemic encephalopathy: synthesis and meta-analysis of trial data. *BMJ* 2010;**340**:c363.

7. Azzopardi D, Strohm B, Edwards AD, et al. Treatment of asphyxiated newborns with moderate hypothermia in routine clinical practice: how cooling is managed in the UK outside a clinical trial. *Arch Dis Child Fetal Neonatal Ed* 2009;**94**:F260–4.

8. Higgins RD, Raju TN, Perlman J, et al. Hypothermia and perinatal asphyxia: executive summary of the National Institute of Child Health and Human Development workshop. *J Pediatr* 2006;**148**:170–5.

9. British Association of Perinatal Medicine. Position statement on therapeutic cooling for neonatal encephalopathy. http://www.bapm.org/publications/documents/guidelines/Position_Statement_Therapeutic_Cooling_Neonatal_Encephalopathy_July%202010.pdf 2010 [cited 2012 May 15]; Available from: http://www.bapm.org

10. National Institute for Health and Clinical Excellence. Therapeutic hypothermia with intracorporeal temperature monitoring for hypoxic perinatal brain injury. http://guidance.nice.org.uk/IPG347 2010 [cited 2012 May 15]; Available from: http://www.nice.org.uk/

11. Fisher M, Hanley DF, Howard G, Jauch EC, Warach S. Recommendations from the STAIR V meeting on acute stroke trials, technology and outcomes. *Stroke* 2007;**38**:245–8.

12. Fisher M, Feuerstein G, Howells DW, et al. Update of the stroke therapy academic industry roundtable preclinical recommendations. *Stroke* 2009;**40**:2244–50.

13. Gluckman PD, Wyatt JS, Azzopardi D, et al. Selective head cooling with mild systemic hypothermia after neonatal encephalopathy: multicentre randomised trial. *Lancet* 2005;**365**:663–70.

14. Thoresen M, Whitelaw A. Cardiovascular changes during mild therapeutic hypothermia and rewarming in infants with hypoxic-ischemic encephalopathy. *Pediatrics* 2000;**106**(Pt 1):92–9.

15. Gebauer CM, Knuepfer M, Robel-Tilling E, Pulzer F, Vogtmann C. Hemodynamics among neonates with hypoxic-ischemic encephalopathy during whole-body hypothermia and passive rewarming. *Pediatrics* 2006;**117**:843–50.

16. Eicher DJ, Wagner CL, Katikaneni LP, et al. Moderate hypothermia in neonatal encephalopathy: safety outcomes. *Pediatr Neurol* 2005;**32**:18–24.

17. Azzopardi DV, Strohm B, Edwards AD, et al. Moderate hypothermia to treat perinatal asphyxial encephalopathy. *N Engl J Med* 2009;**361**:1349–58.

18. Simbruner G, Mittal RA, Rohlmann F, Muche R. Systemic hypothermia after neonatal encephalopathy: outcomes of neo.nEURO.network RCT. *Pediatrics* 2010;**126**:e771–8.

19. Eicher DJ, Wagner CL, Katikaneni LP, et al. Moderate hypothermia in neonatal encephalopathy: efficacy outcomes. *Pediatr Neurol* 2005;**32**:11–7.

20. Shankaran S, Laptook AR, Ehrenkranz RA, et al. Whole-body hypothermia for neonates with hypoxic-ischemic encephalopathy. *N Engl J Med* 2005;**353**:1574–84.

21. Zhou WH, Cheng GQ, Shao XM, et al. Selective head cooling with mild systemic hypothermia after neonatal hypoxic-ischemic encephalopathy: a multicenter randomized controlled trial in China. *J Pediatr* 2010;**157**:367–72.

22. Jacobs SE, Morley CJ, Inder TE, et al. Whole-body hypothermia for term and near-term newborns with hypoxic-ischemic encephalopathy: a randomized controlled trial. *Arch Pediatr Adolesc Med* 2011;**165**:692–700.

23. Wyatt JS, Gluckman PD, Liu PY, et al. Determinants of outcomes after head cooling for neonatal encephalopathy. *Pediatrics* 2007;**119**:912–21.

24. Rutherford M, Ramenghi LA, Edwards AD, et al. Assessment of brain tissue injury after moderate hypothermia in neonates with hypoxic-ischaemic encephalopathy: a nested substudy of a randomised controlled trial. *Lancet Neurol* 2010;**9**:39–45.

25. Thoresen M, Satas S, Loberg EM, et al. Twenty-four hours of mild hypothermia in unsedated newborn pigs starting after a severe global hypoxic-ischemic insult is not neuroprotective. *Pediatr Res* 2001;**50**:405–11.

26. Robertson NJ, Nakakeeto M, Hagmann C, et al. Therapeutic hypothermia for birth asphyxia in low-resource settings: a pilot randomised controlled trial. *Lancet* 2008;**372**:801–3.

27. Battin MR, Dezoete JA, Gunn TR, Gluckman PD, Gunn AJ. Neurodevelopmental outcome of infants treated with head cooling and mild hypothermia after perinatal asphyxia. *Pediatrics* 2001;**107**:480–4.

28. Li T, Xu F, Cheng X, et al. Systemic hypothermia induced within 10 hours after birth improved neurological outcome in newborns with hypoxic-ischemic encephalopathy. *Hosp Pract (Minneap)* 2009;**37**:147–52.

29. Review Manager (RevMan). [computer program]. Version 5 2008.

30. Azzopardi D, Strohm B, Edwards AD, et al. Treatment of asphyxiated newborns with moderate hypothermia in routine clinical practice: how cooling is managed in the UK outside a clinical trial. *Arch Dis Child Fetal Neonatal Ed* 2009;**94**:F260–4.

31. van Rooij LG, Toet MC, Osredkar D, et al. Recovery of amplitude integrated electroencephalographic background patterns within 24 hours of perinatal asphyxia. *Arch Dis Child Fetal Neonatal Ed* 2005;**90**: F245–51.

32. Polderman KH. Mechanisms of action, physiological effects and complications of hypothermia. *Crit Care Med* 2009;**37**(Suppl): S186–202.

33. Strohm B, Hobson A, Brocklehurst P, Edwards AD, Azzopardi D. Subcutaneous fat necrosis after moderate therapeutic hypothermia in neonates. *Pediatrics* 2011;**128**:e450–2.

34. Shankaran S, Pappas A, Laptook AR, et al. Outcomes of safety and effectiveness in a multicenter randomized, controlled trial of whole-body hypothermia for neonatal hypoxic-ischemic encephalopathy. *Pediatrics* 2008;**122**:e791–8.

35. Gunn AJ, Wyatt JS, Whitelaw A, et al. Therapeutic hypothermia changes the prognostic value of clinical evaluation of neonatal encephalopathy. *J Pediatr* 2008;**152**:55–8.

36. Laptook AR, Shankaran S, Ambalavanan N, et al. Outcome of term infants using apgar scores at 10 minutes following hypoxic-ischemic encephalopathy. *Pediatrics* 2009;**124**:1619–26.

37. Battin MR, Thoresen M, Robinson E, et al. Does head cooling with mild systemic hypothermia affect requirement for blood pressure support? *Pediatrics* 2009;**123**:1031–6.

38. Pappas A, Shankaran S, Laptook AR, et al. Hypocarbia and adverse outcome in neonatal hypoxic-ischemic encephalopathy. *J Pediatr* 2011;**158**:752–8.

39. Shankaran S, Laptook AR, McDonald SA, et al. Temperature profile and outcomes of neonates undergoing whole body hypothermia for neonatal hypoxic-ischemic encephalopathy. *Pediatr Crit Care Med* 2012;**13**:53–9.

40. Gunn AJ, Bennet L, Gunning MI, Gluckman PD, Gunn TR. Cerebral hypothermia is not neuroprotective when started after postischemic seizures in fetal sheep. *Pediatr Res* 1999;**46**:274–80.

41. Ambalavanan N, Carlo WA, Shankaran S, et al. Predicting outcomes of neonates diagnosed with hypoxemic-ischemic encephalopathy. *Pediatrics* 2006;**118**:2084–93.

42. Lawn JE, Cousens S, Zupan J. 4 million neonatal deaths: when? Where? Why? *Lancet* 2005;**365**:891–900.

43. Regier DA, Petrou S, Henderson J, et al. Cost-effectiveness of therapeutic hypothermia to treat neonatal encephalopathy. *Value Health* 2010;**13**:695–702.

## Chapter 5

# Economic evaluation of hypothermic neural rescue

Dean A. Regier and Stavros Petrou

## Introduction

Health care economic evaluation is the study of how the inputs of health care activities, such as medicine or physician labour, affect output, where output is a measure of health status. The aim of economic evaluation is to inform decision makers as to the best, i.e., most efficient, allocation of scarce health care resources with a view to optimizing value for money. Implicit in these definitions is the idea of choice: health care resources are scarce and choices between interventions or programmes are necessary because not all desired outputs can be achieved given constrained health care budgets. Economic evaluation does not, therefore, investigate an intervention in isolation; it is a comparative exercise that examines the costs and consequences of possible decisions between multiple courses of action.

The focus of this chapter is to review the methods used and evidence informing the economic costs and consequences of hypothermia for neonatal rescue. The chapter will begin by providing an overview of the study designs, economic methods and approaches to incorporating statistical uncertainty that are available when conducting an economic evaluation where the patient group of interest is young children. This will be followed by a summary and critique of published economic evaluations that have examined resource allocation issues surrounding inducing hypothermia in children with encephalopathy. The final section will highlight significant differences between the identified studies and will critically discuss the effects alternative assumptions have on the study conclusions.

## Economic evaluation

Economic evaluations can be conducted on the basis of several different study designs. The two most common study designs are, first, prospective assessment on the basis of a randomized controlled trial (RCT) and, second, decision-analytic modelling [1]. An economic evaluation conducted prospectively alongside a RCT considers resource allocation issues as adjunct to the RCT by adding economic variables to those data already being collected. These "piggy-back" economic evaluations are typically underpowered [2], even when RCT efficacy endpoints are adequately powered. An economic evaluation conducted prospectively alongside a RCT should include the input of health economists with respect to all aspects of the RCT design, including formal sample size calculations to ensure adequate power to detect joint differences in both costs and consequences. In practice, the conduct of trial-based economic evaluations is often problematic in the perinatal context where RCT sample sizes are typically small. Moreover, a single RCT might not compare all the relevant options available, might not be conducted over a long enough time horizon to capture all the relevant differences in economic outcomes, or might not provide evidence specific to a particular setting or patient group. Under these circumstances, the study design for the conduct of economic evaluation is provided by decision analytic modelling. Decision modelling involves the application of mathematical techniques that synthesize data from multiple sources, including RCTs, but might also draw upon evidence from non-randomized studies if appropriate. Synthesizing data from multiple sources increases the statistical precision of the variables in an economic evaluation and allows the economic evaluation to be more generalizable [3]. For example, decision modelling can extend the time horizon of an economic evaluation beyond that of the available RCTs through the use of cohort data. This is a desirable aspect of

*Neonatal Neural Rescue*, ed. A. David Edwards, Denis V. Azzopardi and Alistair J. Gunn. Published by Cambridge University Press. © Cambridge University Press 2013.

**Table 5.1.** Approaches to economic evaluation by type

| Type of economic evaluation | Unit of measurement: cost | Unit of measurement: outcomes | Tradeoff between cost and consequences |
| --- | --- | --- | --- |
| Cost minimization | Monetary | None | None |
| Cost-effectiveness | Monetary | Clinical effectiveness | Incremental cost per unit of effectiveness |
| Cost utility | Monetary | Preference-based utility value | Incremental cost per increase in utility |
| Cost benefit | Monetary | Monetary | Incremental benefit minus incremental cost |

decision modelling because current published RCTs examining hypothermia for neonatal rescue are restricted to 18 months after birth [4–6], which may underestimate the long-term costs and consequences of the intervention. Next we describe the methodologies that underpin economic evaluation.

Table 5.1 summarizes the four approaches available when conducting an economic evaluation: cost-minimization, cost-effectiveness, cost-utility and cost-benefit. Each approach characterizes the inputs or cost of an intervention in monetary units, where the costs can be estimated from the perspective of the health care payer(s) or from the perspective of society. The health care payer perspective includes direct medical costs arising from the use of resources that the Ministry of Health, health insurance provider or patient incurs directly. The societal perspective is broader in scope and includes all direct and indirect costs related to an intervention, irrespective of whether the costs are borne by the health care payer or by other parties, including families or informal caregivers. Indirect costs include time costs such as lost days from work or the impaired ability to work.

Each of the four approaches or types of economic evaluation differs in terms of how output or consequences are measured. Cost-minimization (CMA) analysis assumes that the strategies under consideration are equal with respect to outcome and that the study design was such that equivalence of outcomes can be statistically tested [7]. By implication, only costs are important in CMA and the best strategy is the least expensive strategy.

Cost-effectiveness analysis (CEA) measures the output of competing interventions or programmes in naturalistic units [1], such as the number of deaths prevented or improvement in neurological function. Effectiveness measures can also incorporate the amount of time spent in a health state. For example, effectiveness metrics such as disability-free life years (DFLY) have been used in economic evaluations examining interventions in young children [8]. The primary outcome in CEA is typically the incremental cost-effectiveness ratio (ICER; $\Delta C/\Delta E$), which has incremental cost ($\Delta C$, where $\Delta$ represents treatment minus control) in the numerator and the incremental effectiveness ($\Delta E$) in the denominator. The ICER is a composite measure that summarizes the tradeoff between cost and effectiveness. CEA can be considered a limited approach because it can solely inform decisions between interventions that have the same unit of naturalistic outcome [1].

Cost-utility analysis (CUA) values the output of the intervention using the concept of utility, which is broadly defined as the relative desirability of being in a particular health state [9]. Valuing utility for use in CUA can be accomplished using preference elicitation methods such as the standard gamble [10] or time tradeoff techniques [11]. The valuation exercise for health states that children may experience has been completed by children as young as 12 [12], or by means of a proxy, such as the parent of a young child [13,14]. Utility weights can be also assigned to the patient using a generic "off-the-shelf" multi-attribute utility instrument such as the EQ-5D [15] or Health Utilities Index (HUI) [16]. These instruments are thought to be appropriate for children as young as age 6 when completed by parents [17], but have also been completed by paediatricians [18] and adolescents [19]. When used as the effectiveness metric, utility weights are scaled such that perfect health is given the (maximum) weight of 1 and death is given a value of 0. A widely accepted measure of benefit for CUA is the quality adjusted life year (QALY) metric [9]. The QALY is calculated by multiplying the utility weight of a health state by the amount of time the patient spends in that state [9]. The primary endpoint in CUA is usually the ICER ($\Delta C/\Delta QALY$). CUA allows resource allocation decisions to be made between disparate clinical areas that use the same approach to inform output.

The final approach to economic evaluation is cost-benefit analysis (CBA). CBA quantifies both costs and consequences in monetary terms [1]. Estimating health value in monetary units can be achieved directly by using methods that ask respondents' willingness to pay for a good; this approach is called contingent valuation. The value of an effectiveness gain can also be monetized by eliciting respondents' preferences for alternative courses of action using a discrete choice experiment; willingness to pay for different interventions or programmes can then be quantified by deriving values of monetary equivalence. Contingent valuation and discrete choice methods have been applied to several perinatal issues and applications concerning children, including antenatal carrier screening for cystic fibrosis [20], prenatal screening for developmental disability[21] and diagnosing genetic causes of developmental disability [22,23]. The primary outcome of CBA is incremental cost subtracted from incremental benefits. The reach of CBA in terms of informing resource allocation is the broadest of the evaluative approaches because it can inform decisions not only between clinical interventions, but also between all sectors of the economy.

Regardless of the approach to economic evaluation used or the perspective taken, it is recommended that costs and consequences be discounted and that uncertainty surrounding the outcomes of the economic evaluation are adequately reported [1,9]. Applying a discount rate to cost and consequences reflects the economic idea of time preference because it acknowledges that it is advantageous to receive health benefits from interventions earlier and to incur the costs of medical interventions later [1,9].

Several different types of uncertainty can arise in economic evaluations. In trial-based economic evaluations, *sampling (or stochastic) uncertainty* is most commonly reported as a confidence interval, depending on variation in both the numerator and the denominator of the ICER. A common method for estimating confidence intervals for the ICER is the non-parametric bootstrap, which re-samples with replacement cost-effect pairs from the trial data under the assumption that the trial population is a valid representation of the underlying population of interest [24]. In modelling-based economic evaluations, parameter uncertainty deals with the statistical precision of model variables, be it the probability of an event, mean resource usage, or the inferred utility weight associated with a health state [25]. Parameter uncertainty can be incorporated into the decision model by assigning each variable an empirical distribution; Monte Carlo simulation techniques are then used to propagate parameter uncertainty throughout the model [25].

Regardless of the methodological framework, the results of economic evaluations should be presented on the cost-effectiveness (CE) plane and decision uncertainty communicated using the cost-effectiveness acceptability curve (CEAC). The CE plane [26] presents the results on a Cartesian coordinate system by plotting the difference in effectiveness per patient against the difference in cost per patient. Specifying the effectiveness difference on the horizontal axis and the cost difference on the vertical axis allows the slope of a line that joins any point on the plane to the origin to be equal to the ICER. Using the four quadrants of the plane, the possible tradeoffs between cost and consequences are depicted. For example, points in the south east quadrant suggest that the new intervention is more effective and less costly, i.e., it is dominant in health economic terms, whilst a point in the northwest quadrant suggests the new treatment is less effective and more costly, i.e., it is dominated. If there is a clear tradeoff between costs and consequences, the points will be in the north east or south west quadrants (see Figure 5.1). The CEAC [27] uses the bootstrapped or Monte Carlo replications to predict the percentage of ICER draws that are cost-effective at a given willingness to pay for an effectiveness or QALY gain. The willingness to pay threshold for an effectiveness gain, commonly denoted as $\lambda$, is often cited as between £20,000 and £30,000 in the United Kingdom [28] and $50,000 in the United States and Canada [29].

## Methods

Economic evaluations of hypothermia for neonatal rescue were identified by performing a systematic

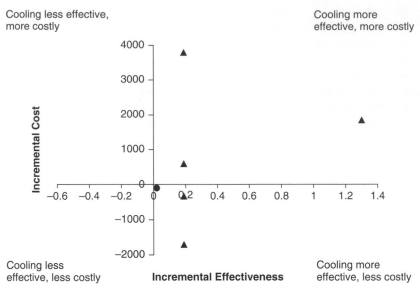

Cooling less effective, more costly

Cooling more effective, more costly

**Figure 5.1.** The cost-effectiveness plane; results from examined studies.

Cooling less effective, less costly

**Incremental Effectiveness**

Cooling more effective, less costly

● denotes mean ICERs published by Gray *et al* [30]
▲ denotes mean ICERs published by Regier *et al* [31]

literature review using MEDLINE and the National Health Services (UK) Economic Evaluation databases. The following medical subject heading (MeSH) terms were used: "infant, newborn", "hypoxia–ischaemia, brain", "hypothermia, induced", "costs and cost analysis" and "cost-benefit analysis". Although all identified studies were reviewed, only those studies published before August 2010 that focused on the evaluation of the economic costs and consequences of therapeutic hypothermia to treat neonatal encephalopathy were included. Manuscripts that were not available in English or simply stated they questioned or endorsed the cost-effectiveness, cost-benefit or cost-utility of the therapeutic hypothermia for neonatal encephalopathy, but did not conduct a quantitative economic evaluation, were excluded.

Studies were reviewed according to the study design used; i.e. whether the cost and consequences were an economic evaluation performed alongside a RCT or a data synthesis study using decision modelling. Descriptive information relating to key aspects of each economic evaluation was extracted and summarized. The results of each study were discussed and the conclusions of each study were compared and evaluated. A discussion of the methodological issues surrounding economic evaluation raised by these studies is also presented.

# Results

Three studies met the initial search criteria [30,31]; one study [32] was excluded because it questioned cost-effectiveness but did not include a quantitative economic evaluation. The details of the included studies according to country of origin, time horizon, study design, the perspective taken on cost and consequences, the metric used to inform consequences, the discount rate and the type of sensitivity analysis and stated conclusions are presented in Table 5.2.

# Study design and evaluative approach

The study by Gray *et al* [30] used hypothetical cohort analysis where discrete event simulation was used to examine the economic consequences of selective head cooling (SHC) plus intensive care versus intensive care alone in the U.S. state of Massachusetts. Several different scenarios informed the cost-effectiveness of SHC. Each scenario differed with respect to the availability of amplitude-integrated electroencephalogram (aEEG) or SHC at different centres. The centres were defined by the level of care they could provide (Levels 1 to 4), which were defined according to guidelines

**Table 5.2.** Characteristics of economic evaluations examining hypothermia for neonatal rescue

| Authors | Country | Comparators | Time horizon | Study design | Viewpoint | Effectiveness measure | Discount rate | Sensitivity analysis | Stated conclusions |
|---|---|---|---|---|---|---|---|---|---|
| Gray et al, 2008 [30] | United States | Selective head cooling vs. intensive care | Life time | Hypothetical cohort via discrete event simulation | Societal | Quality adjust life year | 3% | One way; two way; Monte Carlo | Cooling results in lower costs and increased effectiveness |
| Regier et al, 2010 [31] | United Kingdom | Whole body cooling and head cooling vs. intensive care | 18 months; 18 years | Hypothetical cohort via decision analytic model | Health Care Payer | Disability free life year | 3.5% | One way; structural; Monte Carlo | 19,931 per DFLY over 18 months 1,421 per DFLY over 18 years |

DFLY, disability free adjusted life year.

published by the American Academy of Pediatrics [33]. Data to inform the identification of children with encephalopathy and their subsequent management and clinical outcome were obtained from the CoolCap RCT by Gluckman et al [5]. Information on resource usage, unit costs and long-term mortality rates was obtained from secondary sources. The time horizon of the model was the lifetime of the infant, where it was assumed that a child assessed to have neurodevelopmental impairment continued in that state throughout their life. The primary outcome of the model was $\Delta C/\Delta QALY$. Costs and effects were discounted at 3% per year. Costs were reported in 2006 U.S. dollars. The perspective of the study was societal.

In a UK setting, Regier et al [31] employed decision analytic modelling to synthesize data on mortality and morbidity from the TOBY [4], NICHD [6] and CoolCap [5] trials. The intervention and comparator were respectively intensive care plus cooling and intensive care alone. Resource usage was directly obtained from the TOBY trial [4], which was the sole source of prospectively collected resource usage data for infants with encephalopathy. Regier et al [31] did not, therefore, need to model the ability of a centre to offer aEEG or head cooling because these were informed by means of the TOBY RCT [4]. Three final, mutually exclusive health states were modelled in the baseline analysis: survival without neurological abnormality, survival with neurological abnormality or death. The primary outcome of the economic evaluation was the ICER and the perspective of the analysis was the health care payer perspective. Costs and effects were discounted at a rate of 3.5% per year. Costs were valued at 2006–2007 prices. The time-horizon of the baseline model was the first 18 months after birth, which was the length of the TOBY RCT [4]. In sensitivity analyses, the time horizon was extended to 18 years, where children could transition between health states using transition probabilities reported by Mangham et al [34]. Other sensitivity analyses included patient throughput reflecting the national incidence of neonatal encephalopathy distributed across the current configuration of neonatal services, or, alternatively, excluded the cost of acquiring an aEEG.

## Measurement and valuation of resource usage and costs

Gray et al [30] synthesized resource usage data from published literature and administrative databases.

Information on total length of stay after birth for those in the cooling or standard care strategies was derived from published literature [6,35–37], but the model did not discriminate length of stay by level of care. Transport costs were based on per-mile rates from published sources specific to Massachusetts. Unit costs were assigned to resource usage using cost-to-charge ratios calculated from Medicare and Medicaid Services Hospital Cost reports. The cost of the cooling equipment and aEEG machine was obtained using market prices. It is not apparent that the variable costs associated with head cooling were examined. The cost of the capital outlays were amortized over 5 years using a discount rate of 3% and were distributed evenly across infants who were cooled. Gray et al [30] incorporated the long-term costs associated with developmental impairment by using costs associated with cerebral palsy obtained from the US Centre for Disease Control and Prevention [38]. The costs associated with any productivity lost from premature mortality or inability to work were also included, as were special education costs and out-of-pocket expenses for caregivers.

Regier et al [31] report the health care resource usage collected alongside the TOBY [4]. Included in the analysis was the personnel required during transport to/from a cooling hospital and the personnel required throughout the hospital stay. The average number of days in each level of neonatal care as defined by the British Association of Perinatal Medicine [39] was also reported. Information on hospital readmissions, outpatient hospital visits and the use of other health care services after the infant was discharged was derived from TOBY follow-up questionnaires at 6, 12 and 18 months post-discharge. Unit costs were attached to resource usage using data from the National Health Service Reference Costs database [40] and the British National Formulary [41].

Regier et al [31] used the market costs of the aEEG machine and the Tecotherm total body cooling system. The non-capital variable costs associated with these machines were obtained by means of telephone interviews with the UK suppliers or from UK TOBY centres. The cost of each machine was annuitized over 5 years using a discount rate of 3.5%. The cost of aEEG and total body cooling was calculated by dividing the equivalent annual cost of the machines by the number of infants per year that received total body cooling in each TOBY participating centre.

## Outcome measures

Gray *et al* [30] used the QALY metric in their study using the HUI Mark 3 multi-attribute measure [42] to inform health utilities. Specifically, Gray *et al* [30] used a utility weight of 0.67 for children with neuro-developmental impairment, where impairment was defined by Gluckman *et al* [5]; those without impairment had a utility weight of 1 and death was assigned a weight of 0. Although the QALY metric is recommended for CUA [9], it is unclear how Gray *et al* [30] obtained their weighting because detail regarding who and how many individuals completed the HUI3 was not reported. The 0.67 utility weighting should, therefore, be interpreted with caution.

The effectiveness measure used by Regier *et al* [31] was the disability-free life year (DFLY). The DFLY endpoint is similar to the clinical endpoint of survival without neurological abnormality (defined by Edwards *et al* [43] as Bayley Mental Developmental Index [MDI] score > 84; Bayley Psychomotor Development Index [PDI] > 84; no neuromotor impairment; normal vision). The difference between the approaches is that the DFLY accounts for the duration of time spent in the health state. Children without a neurological abnormality were, therefore, assigned a health state value of 1 for each disability-free year of survival. Children with neuro-developmental abnormalities or who died were assigned a health state value of 0. This approach was limited because children expected to have a neurological abnormality are assigned a weight of 0, which likely underestimates the value of being in that health state.

## Statistical modelling and sensitivity analysis

Gray *et al* [30] conducted probabilistic sensitivity analyses using Monte Carlo simulation techniques for selected inputs. A normal distribution was assigned to the mortality rate of children in the neonatal intensive care unit and a binomial distribution was assigned to children with encephalopathy, neurodevelopmental impairment and for the probabilities surrounding any side effects of treatment. For resource usage, any delay in the initiation and stabilization of a child who was cooled was assigned a triangular distribution. With the exception of length of stay and the life expectancy at birth for those without developmental impairment, the other model variables were varied in deterministic sensitivity analyses. It is not clear why parameter

uncertainty was not incorporated for all variables. The results of the probabilistic sensitivity analysis for one of the scenarios was plotted on the CE plane and although CEACs were not developed in the study, the proportion of Monte Carlo replications above $\lambda = \$50,000$ was reported for the scenario that examined Level 4 centres having access to aEEG and SHC.

Probabilistic sensitivity analysis was conducted for each model variable in each analysis by Regier *et al* [31]. Deterministic sensitivity analysis was conducted to address the concern that local configuration of resources may differ from those encountered in TOBY. Modelling the probabilistic clinical outcomes from the three RCTs was achieved using Bayesian meta-analysis, where the beta distribution was assigned to the prior and likelihood data for transition probabilities based on binomial data, and the Dirichlet distribution was assigned to the prior and likelihood data for probabilities based on multinomial data. The gamma distribution was assumed for all cost variables except the cost per infant of aEEG and total body cooling, which was modelled using non-parametric bootstrapping. Monte Carlo simulation was used to propagate uncertainty throughout the model. The joint uncertainty of cost and effectiveness was represented using the CE plane and a CEAC was presented for each analysis.

## Results and conclusions of the studies

Results from both studies are summarized in Figure 5.1. Relative to usual care, Gray *et al* [30] report that cooling resulted in lower costs and greater effectiveness (by means of utility) in each of the scenarios examined. The degree of cost savings or effectiveness gains differed depending on scenario, but the mean costs savings were generally in the range of $6 to $57, whilst the QALYs gained were between 0.0066 and 0.0088. Confidence intervals generated by the Monte Carlo analysis were not reported for the cost or effectiveness estimates. The authors did report that the percentage of replications that were jointly cost saving and more effective was between 68% and 73%, depending on the scenario selected. The percentage of ICERs that were expected to be below a willingness to pay threshold of $50,000 per QALY ranged between 88% and 92%.

In their deterministic sensitivity analyses, Gray *et al* [30] examined the effects of requiring all Level 3 or Level 2 centres to have an aEEG machine or to have an aEEG machine and the ability to cool children with encephalopathy. These analyses demonstrated increased effectiveness (confidence intervals not reported) and decreased costs (confidence intervals not reported) for all scenarios except the scenario where aEEG was required for all Level 2 centres. In this scenario, the ICER was $84,211. Gray *et al* [30] conclude their study with a statement that aEEG with selective head cooling is "extremely" likely to be a cost-effective intervention.

Regier *et al* [31] were more conservative in their statements regarding the cost-effectiveness of cooling. The study reported that cooling resulted in an incremental cost of £3,787 (95% confidence interval [CI]: -2,516, 12,360) over the first 18 months after birth. The probabilistic sensitivity analysis demonstrated that cooling resulted in expected cost savings in 15% of the replications. Cooling resulted in incremental effectiveness where the mean number of DFLYs gained was 0.19 (95% CI: 0.07, 0.31) over the first 18 months after birth. The reported ICER in the baseline analysis was £19,931 per DFLY gained. The CEAC showed the exact probability of cost-effectiveness was 69% when $\lambda$ = £30,000. If $\lambda$ = £20,000, the probability of cost-effectiveness was 52%.

The deterministic sensitivity analyses demonstrated an improvement in the ICER. For example, when the number of infants per centre per year reflected current data from the UK Cooling Register, cooling was, on average, cost-saving (£-295; 95% CI: -4,555, 5,414) and there was a 92% probability that cooling is cost-effective at $\lambda$ = £20,000. When the time-horizon of the model was extended to 18 years after birth, the incremental effectiveness was 1.30 DFLYs gained (95% CI: 0.51, 2.15) and the incremental cost was £1,847 (95% CI: -4,494, 10,303). The ICER was £1,421 per DFLY gained and there was a 99% probability that cooling is cost-effective when $\lambda$ = £20,000. Regier *et al* [31] state that the cost-effectiveness of therapeutic hypothermia is finely balanced in the first 18 months after birth because the probability that cooling is cost-effective only reached 69% when the willingness to pay threshold was £20,000.

## Discussion

The allocation of scarce health care resources has been hoisted into the spotlight over the past 40 years – as new medicines and technologies have been developed, health care consumers have increasingly demanded cutting-edge health technologies and expenditure on health care has risen dramatically. The phenomenon of increasing heath care costs has resulted in decision-making institutions, such as the National Institute for Health and Clinical Excellence (NICE) and the Canadian Common Drug Review, to incorporate economic evaluations into their recommendation processes. The reality of using economic evaluations as part of a process to inform resource allocation decisions necessitates that economic evaluations of therapeutic neonatal rescue follow established methodological guidelines such as those published by NICE [28].

We found the reviewed studies did employ accepted methodological approaches in their analyses, but used different tools to inform their conclusions. The first difference between the studies was the study design. The strategy pursued by Gray *et al* [30] was to examine a hypothetical cohort of patients by synthesizing data extracted from multiple sources. Costs and consequences were projected beyond CoolCap [5] by using Markov assumptions, where 18 months after birth individuals would continue in a designated state of disability and disutility. This is a limitation as children may transition to different states or levels of disability. Regier *et al* [31] benefited from a piggyback economic evaluation conducted alongside the TOBY RCT [4] and partly used individual level data to inform their analysis. Given the uncertainty in the clinical efficacy endpoint reported in TOBY [4], Regier *et al* [31] pursued a strategy of data synthesis for effectiveness and patient level data for cost. Regier *et al* [31] also projected outcomes beyond 18 months using Markov modelling with patients able to transition between levels of disability.

A second divergence between the studies was the perspective taken in the cost analysis. Gray *et al* [30] used a broader informational base by taking a societal perspective. Although the societal approach is preferred [9], it is often difficult to successfully incorporate into a model. Debate surrounding the merits of incorporating societal costs has led NICE to recommend that societal costs should only be included in sensitivity analysis [28]. Regier *et al* [31] used a narrow informational base by only examining the health care payer perspective.

The third difference between the studies was how effectiveness was measured. Gray *et al* [30] used a HUI3 estimate to inform the QALY metric. The limitation to this approach was that the authors did not report who completed the HUI3 questionnaire; for example, the authors did not report if the respondents were parents of children with neurodevelopmental impairment, or physicians or individuals with neurodevelopmental impairment. Regier *et al* [31] used the DFLY metric and cited that the QALY was not used because of concerns surrounding the use of preference-based measurement in early childhood [30]. The limitation of the DFLY metric is that it does not distinguish between varying levels of disability.

The last significant difference between the studies centred on the approaches to sensitivity analysis. Gray *et al* [30] focused on point estimates of cost and utility differences, making it difficult for the reader to draw any conclusions as to the statistical significance of the reported differences. The authors did present the joint uncertainty of costs and effects on the CE plane. The CE plane revealed a great deal of statistical uncertainty because the simulated ICERs straddled each quadrant of the CE plane. Although the authors did not discuss the proportion of ICERs falling in each quadrant, they do state that 87.5% of the replications fell below a λ of $50,000 per QALY gained. However, this statement is not an adequate substitute for the CEAC. Furthermore, the final conclusion that aEEG and SHC is an "economically desirable" intervention seems overstated given the probability of cost-effectiveness fails to reach a 95% certainty threshold when λ = $50,000. Regier *et al* [31] produced a CE plane for their baseline analysis and also constructed CEACs for each of their sensitivity analyses. The CE plane revealed that ICER bootstrap replicates straddled all four quadrants, but the replicates were concentrated in the NE and SE quadrants. The CEACs revealed significant decision uncertainty.

The evidence surrounding the economic costs and consequences of therapeutic hypothermia for neonatal encephalopathy seems to favour its implementation, but further studies are needed to provide definite recommendations. Regier *et al* [31] state that the cost-effectiveness of hypothermia is finely balanced when the time horizon is 18 months after birth. This conclusion was based on the considerable decision uncertainty surrounding the cost and consequences of therapeutic hypothermia over the short-term. Both Gray *et al* [30] and Regier *et al* [31] concluded that therapeutic hypothermia was likely to be cost-effective over a long-term time horizon. Conclusions surrounding the cost-effectiveness of therapeutic hypothermia over the long-term should, however, be treated with some caution as the data used to project outcomes beyond the published RCTs

[4–6] were not prospectively collected for the purpose of projecting outcomes of hypothermic neural rescue. Prospectively collected data following children who participated in the TOBY RCT [4] to the ages of 6–7 years of age will be available in the next few years and these data will better inform the cost-effectiveness of therapeutic hypothermia over a medium-term time horizon.

# References

1. Drummond MF, Obrien BJ, Stoddart GL, et al. *Methods for the economic evaluation of health care programmes. 3rd edition*. Oxford: Oxford University Press; 2005.

2. Briggs AH, Gray AM. Power and sample size calculations for stochastic cost-effectiveness analysis. *Med Decis Making* 1998;**18**:S81–92.

3. Sculpher MJ, Claxton K, Drummond M, et al. Whither trial-based economic evaluation for health care decision making? *Health Econ* 2006;**15**:677–87.

4. Azzopardi DV, Strohm B, Edwards AD, et al. Moderate hypothermia to treat perinatal asphyxial encephalopathy. *N Engl J Med* 2009;**361**:1349–58.

5. Gluckman PD, Wyatt JS, Azzopardi D, et al. Selective head cooling with mild systemic hypothermia after neonatal encephalopathy: multicentre randomised trial. *Lancet* 2005;**365**:663–70.

6. Shankaran S, Laptook AR, Ehrenkranz RA, et al. Whole-body hypothermia for neonates with hypoxic-ischemic encephalopathy. *N Engl J Med* 2005;**353**:1574–84.

7. Briggs AH, O'Brien BJ. The death of cost-minimization analysis? *Health Econ* 2001;**10**:179–84.

8. Petrou S, Bischof M, Bennett C, et al. Cost-effectiveness of neonatal extracorporeal membrane oxygenation based on 7-year results from the United Kingdom Collaborative ECMO Trial. *Pediatrics* 2006;**117**:1640–9.

9. Gold MR, Siefel JE, Russel LB, et al. *Cost-effectiveness in health and medicine*. New York: Oxford University Press; 1996.

10. Von Neumann J, Morgenstern O. *Theory of games and economic behavior. 3rd edition*. New York: Wiley; 1953.

11. Torrance GW, Thomas WH, Sackett DL. A utility maximization model for evaluation of health care programs. *Health Serv Res* 1972;**7**:118–33.

12. Sung L, Young NL, Greenberg ML, et al. Health-related quality of life (HRQL) scores reported from parents and their children with chronic illness differed depending on utility elicitation method. *J Clin Epidemiol* 2004;**57**:1161–6.

13. Saigal S, Stoskopf BL, Burrows E, et al. Stability of maternal preferences for pediatric health states in the perinatal period and 1 year later. *Arch Pediatr Adolesc Med* 2003;**157**:261–9.

14. Sung L, Greenberg ML, Young NL, et al. Validity of a modified standard gamble elicited from parents of a hospital-based cohort of children. *J Clin Epidemiol* 2003;**56**:848–55.

15. EuroQol – a new facility for the measurement of health-related quality of life. The EuroQol Group. *Health Policy* 1990;**16**:199–208.

16. Torrance GW, Furlong W, Feeny D, et al. Multi-attribute preference functions. Health Utilities Index. *Pharmacoeconomics* 1995;**7**:503–20.

17. Sung L, Petrou S, Ungar W. Measuring health utilities in children and their parents. In: Ungar W, editor. *Economic evaluation in child health*. Oxford: Oxford University Press; 2009:77–90.

18. Oostenbrink R, HA AM, Essink-Bot ML. The EQ-5D and the Health Utilities Index for permanent sequelae after meningitis: a head-to-head comparison. *J Clin Epidemiol* 2002;**55**:791–9.

19. Feeny D, Juniper EF, Ferrie PJ, et al. Why not just ask the kids? Health-related quality of life in children with asthma. In: Drotar D, editor. *Measuring health-related quality of life in children and adolescents*. London: Lawrence Erlbaum Associates; 1998.

20. Donaldson C, Shackley P, Abdalla M, et al. Willingness to pay for antenatal carrier screening for cystic fibrosis. *Health Econ* 1995;**4**:439–52.

21. Ryan M, Diack J, Watson V, et al. Rapid prenatal diagnostic testing for Down syndrome only or longer wait for full karyotype: the views of pregnant women. *Prenat Diagn* 2005;**25**:1206–11.

22. Regier DA, Ryan M, Phimister E, et al. Bayesian and classical estimation of mixed logit: An application to genetic testing. *J Health Econ* 2009;**28**:598–610.

23. Regier DA, Friedman JM, Marra CA. Value for money? Array genomic hybridization for diagnostic testing for genetic causes of intellectual disability. *Am J Hum Genet* 2010;**86**:765–72.

24. Briggs AH, Wonderling DE, Mooney CZ. Pulling cost-effectiveness analysis up by its bootstraps: a non-parametric approach to confidence interval estimation. *Health Econ* 1997;**6**:327–40.

25. Briggs AH, Claxton K, Schulpher M. *Decision modelling for health economic evaluation*. Oxford: Oxford University Press; 2006.

26. Black WC. The CE plane: a graphic representation of cost-effectiveness. *Med Decis Making* 1990;**10**:212–4.

27. van Hout BA, Al MJ, Gordon GS, et al. Costs, effects and C/E-ratios alongside a clinical trial. *Health Econ* 1994;**3**:309–19.

28. National Institute for Clinical Excellence (NICE). *Guide to the methods of technology appraisal*. London: Nice; 2008.

29. Laupacis A, Feeny D, Detsky AS, et al. How attractive does a new technology have to be to warrant adoption and utilization? Tentative guidelines for using clinical and economic evaluations. *CMAJ* 1992;**146**:473–81.

30. Gray J, Geva A, Zheng Z, et al. CoolSim: using industrial modeling techniques to examine the impact of selective head cooling in a model of perinatal regionalization. *Pediatrics* 2008;**121**:28–36.

31. Regier DA, Petrou S, Henderson J, et al. Cost-effectiveness of therapeutic hypothermia to treat neonatal encephalopathy. *Value Health* 2010;**13**:695–702.

32. Horn A, Thompson C, Woods D, et al. Induced hypothermia for infants with hypoxic-ischemic encephalopathy using a servo-controlled fan: an exploratory pilot study. *Pediatrics* 2009;**123**:e1090–8.

33. Stark AR. Levels of neonatal care. *Pediatrics* 2004;**114**:1341–7.

34. Mangham LJ, Petrou S, Doyle LW, et al. The cost of preterm birth throughout childhood in England and Wales. *Pediatrics* 2009;**123**:e312–27.

35. Zupancic JAF. A systematic review of costs associated with preterm birth. In: Behrman R, Sith-Butler A, editors. *Preterm birth: causes, consequences and prevention*. Washington, DC: National Academic Press; 2006.

36. Akisu M, Huseyinov A, Yalaz M, et al. Selective head cooling with hypothermia suppresses the generation of platelet-activating factor in cerebrospinal fluid of newborn infants with perinatal asphyxia. *Prostaglandins Leukot Essent Fatty Acids* 2003;**69**:45–50.

37. Battin MR, Penrice J, Gunn TR, et al. Treatment of term infants with head cooling and mild systemic hypothermia (35.0 degrees C and 34.5 degrees C) after perinatal asphyxia. *Pediatrics* 2003;**111**:244–51.

38. Centers for Disease Control and Prevention. Economic costs associated with mental retardation, cerebral palsy, hearing loss and vision impairment: United States. *MMWR Morb Mortal Wkly Rep* 2004;**53**:57–9.

39. Report of working group of the British Association of Perinatal Medicine and Neonatal Nurses Association on categories of babies requiring neonatal care. *Arch Dis Child* 1992;**67**:868–9.

40. Department of Health. *NHS reference costs 2006–2007*. London: Department of Health; 2008.

41. BNF 56. British Medical Association and Royal Pharmaceutical Society of Great Britain; 2008.

42. Feeny D, Furlong W, Torrance GW, et al. Multi-attribute and single-attribute utility functions for the health utilities index mark 3 system. *Med Care* 2002;**40**:113–28.

43. Edwards AD, Brocklehurst P, Gunn AJ, et al. Neurological outcomes at 18 months of age after moderate hypothermia for perinatal hypoxic ischaemic encephalopathy: synthesis and meta-analysis of trial data. *BMJ* 2010;**340**:c363.

Chapter

6

# Challenges for parents and clinicians discussing neuroprotective treatments

Peter Allmark, Claire Snowdon, Diana Elbourne and Su Mason

## Introduction

Speaking to stressed parents in difficult circumstances about the care and prognosis for their very sick newborn baby is one of the challenges involved in providing neonatal intensive care. The regularity of the task can allow clinicians to develop their personal style and to refine their skills in communication, especially as many discussions have standard features such as explanations of a condition, an environment, a piece of equipment. Highly variable contextual and inter-personal elements can, however, add unpredictable dimensions to the discussions which can be demanding, professionally and personally. When a baby is a candidate for neural rescue, there are several additional issues which can increase these demands on clinicians.

The purpose of this chapter is to help clinicians who are thinking through issues involved with communication in these difficult situations. We draw upon accounts from parents of critically ill babies of their experiences of discussing hypothermic neural rescue with clinicians. These data are taken from our own research; we have conducted two studies of the views and experiences of parents and clinicians involved in studies of hypothermia and neuroprotection. Allmark and Mason carried out a qualitative study which focused on the continuous consent processes used in the TOBY trial [1,2]; data from their TOBY-QUAL study are indicated by [TQ][1]. Snowdon and Elbourne carried out a qualitative study of parent and clinician-researcher views of a pre-trial safety study of hypothermia and ECMO [3]; data from

their Views of Hypothermia and ECMO study are indicated by [VHE][2].

These studies considered the experiences of parents and clinicians in the context of neuroprotective research. Data were collected at a time when hypothermic neural rescue was a promising but unproven intervention. Discussions of treatment options for the parents in these studies were different to those which take place outside of a research context. Parents had to take on board the then experimental nature of cooling and the underlying uncertainty over treatment. They also had to grasp key features of the research aims and processes. In the TOBY trial these were the use of randomization and experimental and control arms and in the Hypothermia Pilot pre-allocated control and intervention groups. They were required to consider the situation carefully to make a decision. Those consenting would formally sign to enrol their baby as a research participant. Now that cooling is the current best treatment for perinatal asphyxia, the emphasis has shifted. Parents are given information about hypothermia as a routine and recommended treatment for which there is no requirement for signed permission. Hypothermia may in fact be under way by the time the subject is raised. Conversations with parents are to inform them about the treatment and to attend to any questions that they might have. The TQ and VHE data discussed below have been selected to illuminate aspects of the parental experience which are of relevance and use to clinicians preparing to discuss neural rescue with parents in research and non-research situations.

---

[1] This study includes the following data: 30 recordings of discussions between the TQ researcher and parents of babies that had entered the trial and 10 interviews with clinician-researchers responsible for the *TOBY* study.

[2] This study includes the following data: 16 recordings of discussions between Hypothermia Pilot Study Research Fellow and parents of eligible babies, 16 subsequent parental interviews and six interviews with CS.

---

*Neonatal Neural Rescue*, ed. A. David Edwards, Denis V. Azzopardi and Alistair J. Gunn. Published by Cambridge University Press. © Cambridge University Press 2013.

## Context

The emotions and anxiety experienced by parents of babies cared for in neonatal intensive care units have been well documented [4–8]. It is clear that the nature and degree of this stress changes over time and not necessarily in a linear manner [9,10]. There can be huge emotional peaks and troughs and these can be experienced differently by men and women [11]. We know that information needs shift and that parents become increasingly familiar with the intensive care environment [12]. The nature and content of discussions change according to where they are on the trajectory of their baby's illness and care [13]. Discussions about asphyxia and neural rescue necessarily take place very early in that trajectory, when parental stress is high and acclimatization to the environment is low. This can shape the content and style of such discussions in several important ways. These are considered below.

## Proximity to difficult experiences

Asphyxia can be an unexpected consequence of the difficult and traumatic delivery of a previously healthy term baby. Neural rescue must be initiated as soon as possible after the injury. If the process of care is to be transparent and inclusive and parents are to be informed, all parties will be propelled into a rapidly moving series of discussions and events. The conversation in which parents learn about the implications of the injury to their baby and the potential benefits of neural rescue typically takes place within a few hours of delivery and close to initiation of intensive care. The timing can be difficult for parents as indicated by a father interviewed for the TQ Study who commented:

> I think because of the panic at the beginning it was such a rush I think we weren't totally clear. [TQ]

The nature of the birth, the condition of the baby and the implications for the family up-end parental expectations of going home with a healthy child shortly after delivery and shape early experiences of neonatal intensive care. Long and complicated labours can leave women exhausted and in pain; rapid labours, especially those which follow dramatic emergencies such as placental abruptions, can be overwhelming in a different way. Delivery is often instrumental or surgical and many women will have had painkilling drugs, an epidural or a general anaesthetic. A mother interviewed for the VHE Study had complications after an emergency caesarean section and was in severe pain. She found transferring hospitals and getting in and out of a wheelchair to go to see her son very hard. She explained how difficult it was to be in the unit and the hospital accommodation as her circumstances were different from those of other parents of sick babies. She said: "I was different. I was sick myself and couldn't get about". Like several women interviewed for the study, the price of being with her sick baby was that her own needs were not fully met. Some women disregarded their needs and pushed for discharge as early as possible, to be with their babies. Several described walking with stitches and paying little attention to a lack of food, rest and pain killers. Physical problems are also emotionally draining and the comments of one mother [TQ] convey something of the experience for parents trying to take on board information in these circumstances.

> I really can't remember anything at the time; I remember we went to see him later on and I was asking him [the doctor] questions and I was smacking myself on the nose to keep myself awake because I was just like this [gestures sleepy] my head was spinning, most of the day is a blur anyway, most of the labour's a blur . . . they give you morphine. [TQ]

Men can be exhausted by accompanying their partner through a long labour, traumatized by the events they have just witnessed and fearful for their baby. One father explained that they had had "a long day" asking his partner: "It was 26 hours or something wasn't it without sleep?" [TQ]. Often men are not allowed to attend an emergency delivery, a decision which may be problematic for some couples [14]. Some fathers are absent throughout labour and birth, especially where events have moved quickly, arriving afterwards to learn of the delivery and its outcome all at the same time. This can be difficult for women who are on their own and for men who have to catch up on complicated events with far-reaching implications.

## Implications of the information about the condition of the baby

Any discussion of the potential value of neural rescue requires a clear acknowledgement of the possibility of brain damage and subsequent disability. The period in which a baby is a candidate for neural rescue is, however, often a time of clinical ambiguity, when the extent of damage is undetermined and the likelihood of survival unclear. While the first thing that some parents will ask is whether their baby has suffered brain damage, for others the introduction of this subject at such an early stage can seem to pile on bad news. In their interviews for TQ and VHE, parents commonly spoke of being overwhelmed. Discussions with parents in the VHE Study make it clear that the acknowledgement that their child may survive but with a degree of impairment is a difficult moment in the conversation; in at least one recording the mother starts to quietly cry at this point. In contrast, the TQ Study showed some evidence of parents not acknowledging the bad news imparted:

FATHER: . . . certain things went in one ear and out the other; certain things you wanted to hear, other bits . . .

MOTHER: yes, you try to hear the best bits. [TQ]

Given the variety of coping styles that exists, clinicians face a difficult balance between conveying information about potential disability in a clear and unambiguous way while avoiding what might seem to parents to be a harsh or brutally pessimistic approach. It is also important that discussion of neural rescue does not raise unrealistic hopes of survival when death is still a possible outcome. Talking to parents about whether or not their child might have problems with walking or co-ordination is necessary but for some could inhibit acceptance and preparation for a possible death.

Finally, there is a more subtle issue which might arise from discussion about potential disability and the value of neural rescue; complicated and occasionally mismanaged labours can be the subject of litigation, primarily for obstetric colleagues rather than for neonatologists [15]. This places the neonatologists who discuss these issues with parents in a potentially delicate situation. Their summary of events and implications for a baby might prove to be important in assuaging or stimulating concerns. Some neonatologists might feel cautious about what they say, wary of the possibility of being drawn into litigious processes.

## Perceptions of hypothermic treatment

When neural rescue involves cooling, this can seem strange from a parent's viewpoint, running counter to a desire to warm and protect the baby. Some parents in the TQ study found this difficult.

MOTHER: How will [it] help my baby . . . people say, wrap up babies. [TQ]

MOTHER: The thought of him going on the frozen mattress was like, oh my God, you know, extreme really. [TQ]

Parents of one baby in the VHE Study were aware of issues around temperature change but described the intervention as warming rather than the possibly counter-intuitive notion of cooling their baby.

Father: There was something about the heating . . . [The doctor] was saying they're trying it out and if we wouldn't mind putting her on the heating before she went on ECMO. . . . It was just to help her warm up or something and [the doctor] was saying it would help her at the early stages. For kids who get learning difficulties [it is] supposed to improve it. [VHE]

For some parents, however, the idea that cooling could be protective was not so strange. For one couple the mother described being "a little bit sceptical" about cooling, but her partner believed that he could see how it might be helpful, adding:

you see the news, people falling in ice and you know they've come out a few hours later and they've been perfectly fine, And I thought well I've heard of that and it might just work, you know it's worth that chance! [VHE]

The idea and the reality of a cool baby can be discomforting, particularly for parents considering the possibility that their baby might die. A TQ father commented: "because we didn't know if he was going to survive at that point, we didn't want his last few hours to be in discomfort". To pre-empt unnecessary concerns and assumptions, it is important that parents are given a clear account of sedation practices, what their baby will and will not experience when cooled, what they will witness themselves and how their baby will feel to them.

## Research and complex information

As suggested above parents of asphyxiated babies new to neonatal intensive care have a range of informational and support needs. They might be baffled that an apparently normal pregnancy has ended so badly. At some point, they will want to know what has happened and what it means for the future. The answers to these questions are complex and will probably require multiple conversations and iterations. They also need to know about the intensive care environment and the treatment plan for their baby. Parents can feel bombarded by the amount and the complexity of information they are given and neural protection adds a further dimension to discussions [16]. If treatment is proposed as part of a randomized trial there is an extra layer of information to give and to absorb.

Parents may have questions that they need answers to straightaway, but in the initial stage some of their questions may not be fully formulated. When parents might be given the bulk of the information is an important consideration. In the VHE Study, ECMO and the Hypothermia Pilot were discussed in one conversation, usually while babies were being prepared for transfer to the ECMO centre. In this research situation the Hypothermia Pilot research fellow was not involved in the transfer and could devote a generous amount of time to discuss the situation with parents. It is clear from the recorded discussions that the information was complex; while some parents were active discussants, in some meetings parents were relatively silent, asking few questions.

Whilst an early conversation with additional time for information and questions seems intuitively a good thing, the variety of information needs and the potential for overwhelming parents is highlighted by one particular case in which it was not possible to have a discussion before transfer. The parents were approached on arrival at the ECMO centre after a long drive from their referring hospital. Parents would often be hungry for information at this point and delays would be frustrating. This couple, however, had a different set of needs. They wanted to compose themselves and to feel prepared and calm at the time of the discussion. Rather than feeling positive about the time made available for immediate discussion, the father explained that they had found being confronted with the information very quickly when they were unprepared to be a difficult experience:

> . . . she hit us soon as we walked in, we were still in a bit of shock, you know what I mean. . . . What I would have preferred . . . is let us come in, we an't even – we'd just walked in, was give us an hour 'cos we hadn't even put us luggage away what we brought up, shown down, walked in, see as she's okay, go upstairs, get settled in, had a shower, come downstairs, nice pot of tea and walked

down, would have been okay, would have been a lot calmer. [VHE]

Although the use of neural rescue requires clinicians to speak to parents as early as possible, information can be given in a staged and ongoing way [17]. A flexible strategy of "continuous consent" was developed for use in the multicentre TOBY trial. The most minimal form of information was a leaflet giving preliminary details of the trial which could be given to parents whilst their baby was being assessed for eligibility. This could be used primarily where babies would need to be transferred to a cooling centre. If the baby was found to be eligible, a second and more comprehensive leaflet was to be given to the parents and the trial discussed with them; written consent was then sought. During the intervention period the consultant neonatologists committed to meeting with the parents to go through the information again and to check that they were still happy for the intervention to continue. This approach was developed in recognition of the difficulties for some parents at the very earliest stage in their experiences. It involves repetition and a gradual increase in detail and offers the opportunity for further discussion and questions. Clinicians were, however, free to take the lead from parents and to give more information whenever it was required and the TOBY QUAL study indicated parents were often given a relatively complete account of the situation and the proposed research in their early discussions.

## Pace of decision-making and freedom to choose

If clinicians wish to speak to parents before commencing neural rescue, or if permission is required for research participation, discussions will be conducted with some sense of urgency. The treatment window is narrow and there is little time for reflection and wider consultation. If babies need to be transferred to a cooling centre this exerts additional time pressures on clinicians and parents. Parents react to this situation in very different ways. When neural rescue is initiated as part of a trial, some can feel pressured to make their decision within the necessarily rigid timeframe:

INTERVIEWER: Did the 2 hours feel, like, short?

MOTHER: It was short!

FATHER: . . . I was thinking maybe we could relax a bit and maybe the following day or the third day we could think about it, but at that precise moment it was difficult... [TQ]

In the same situation others can feel frustration that things do not move even faster.

INTERVIEWER: You had the hour to make up your mind; did you feel like that was enough time?

MOTHER: It was too long.

INTERVIEWER: Too long?

MOTHER: Too long. It don't take long to read the booklet.

INTERVIEWER: You made your mind up very quickly?

FATHER: He was stressing to us that this treatment has to start within 6 hours; he was stressing that to us a lot; so we more or less said well, yes we agree, get on with it, get it started.

INTERVIEWER: You didn't really need the hour?

MOTHER: No, we made our mind up straightaway hadn't we? [TQ]

The decisions that parents made about care and research could have implications for their future well-being and family life and all parents were required to make this choice in what was a relatively contracted time period. In the two settings considered here hypothermia was presented to parents as an unevaluated trial procedure rather than (as now) an evaluated form of care. The formal decision-making process was explicit and parental needs and preferences were brought into focus, as indicated by the TQ parents below.

INTERVIEWER: What made you say yes?

FATHER: Desperation, I suppose, there was no other option and it was worth a shot and that is the truth. [TQ]

Those asked to consider trial participation in emergency or life-threatening situations can feel that they have little option other than to agree [18]. This can be because the scenario that they face is devastating and few alternatives are available and they take any chance they can to improve the situation. The situation in which parents in these studies found themselves when neural protection was raised, rendered the offer compelling; they commonly presented their decision as an obvious choice or no real choice. This feeling can be shared by clinicians as this TQ interviewee suggests.

Neonatologist: ... It's easy for someone to put a gun to your head and say it's your decision. And the gun being that their baby is born and is damaged and is needing a lot of resuscitation and here we are saying, look there's a trial happening and this is the only thing available and there's nothing else available... [TQ]

Where a treatment is part of a trial protocol, the conditions under which a choice is made can be further removed from the standard care situation, as clinician-researchers may be less directive, reluctant to steer parental decision-making in any one direction.

## Value of involvement for the parents

It is clear from several studies that even in very difficult situations, parents want to be involved in decisions about the care of their child; there is very little support for overriding or excluding parents from decisions either in care or research [19–22]. This is endorsed by two TQ parents.

FATHER: Because it's your child and you want to make the decision. You don't want some doctor saying, I'm doing this and I'm doing that, because it's your baby. [TQ]

MOTHER: ... You feel all the time that everyone else is making decisions because, what can you do, you can't look after your own baby. So if you can't even have that decision [about the trial] you then, what are you left with? [TQ]

Even where information is complex and where it is emotionally challenging, parents seem to feel that they would rather shoulder this burden than be excluded from processes and decisions which are fundamental to the care of their child.

MOTHER: I think parents ought to be told all possibilities. ... If I was told after I don't think I would be very happy. I would want to know from the start everything I need to know.

INTERVIEWER: No matter how stressful?

MOTHER: No matter. [VHE]

## The discussion with parents

The circumstances surrounding discussion of perinatal asphyxia are difficult and parents vary tremendously in how much information they wish to have and what they are able to absorb. Personality types, coping strategies and contextual factors such as fatigue and medication may constrain some parents' ability to engage in detailed discussion. For others, however, information and understanding can be important tools for orientation and control and despite difficult circumstances they can be calm and focused with a strong desire for information.

These situations require different approaches and skill sets. For an individual clinician, the task is to pick up cues from parents as to how much information they want and the pace at which they are able to move and then to adapt their practice accordingly. In terms of unit policy, it is important that strategies are encouraged which will give good quality information and which are sufficiently flexible to accommodate the range of parental responses. In addition, both individual and policy approaches involve careful reflection on the interplay between these factors and several overarching practical and ethical considerations.

One example of this interplay relates to the speed at which events unfold for a given family, the pace and style of information-giving and degree of engagement in the decision-making process. In pressured circumstances, the pace may need to be rapid to allow initiation of treatment, or because only basic details may be given when parents indicate that they are unable to assimilate the information in the prescribed timeframe. If a decision is formally required from parents before proceeding to an intervention and they prefer a particularly slow pace, then the clinician faces a difficult situation in which the needs of the parents may differ from those of the baby. A fine line has then to be taken to encourage parents to engage in a focussed and to some extent limited discussion without overwhelming them at a vulnerable time. In these situations a strong commitment to an ongoing process of information giving is important; the concept of consent as a continuous process rather than a single event, whether around formal permission in a trial situation, or for information-giving for standard care, is a key element in the process. Parents aware that continuous consent is being used might then find it easier to make provisional decisions.

These balancing acts are not unusual in neonatal intensive care; they arise in relation to many discussions with parents and occur in a variety of circumstances as well as in discussions of neural rescue. This latter situation can, however, involve additional challenges. Conversations may be highly complex,

involving multiple layers of information as well as practical and ethical considerations. Taking parents through the events surrounding a difficult delivery, the condition of the baby and hypothermic neural rescue (standard care) is already a substantial task. The introduction of neural rescue research into the situation brings additional issues and complications.

Hypothermia is the first neural rescue tool to have been evaluated. The push to further improve the evidence base means that there are likely to be other interventions for evaluation. Some may be assessed in their own right. Others, such as xenon or erythropoietin, are adjuncts trialled in combination with hypothermia. This means that clinicians need to make clear that only one dimension of care is being carried out under research conditions and that the rules that govern this single dimension are different from those governing the rest of the care their baby receives.

Neural rescue is likely to occupy this middle ground, part standard care, part research protocol, for some time yet. It is, therefore, important that clinicians involved in discussing the situation with parents are themselves clear about the different frameworks within which care and research are governed. When care and research are difficult to distinguish, parents may agree to research participation under the assumption that the decisions about treatment are made with the individual's personal need for care at the centre. This has been described as a therapeutic misconception [23]. Whilst it has been argued that clinician-researchers should strive for a clear separation of care and research, in practice the boundary between the two can be somewhat blurred for professionals as well as for patients and their proxies [24].

Research essentially has the aim of contributing to knowledge; treatment has the aim of advancing the best interest of the patient. If parents or clinicians believe that research activity has a therapeutic aim some may argue that their therapeutic intention may blur the clarity of the discussion [25,26]. When participants enrol in research it is important they understand that they (or those they represent) will be exposed to a degree of uncertainty and risk for the sake of future knowledge. Parents should understand also that they can (and must) choose whether to consent to research, whereas established treatment will usually be given anyway. The challenge is to help parents to distinguish that part of the neural rescue treatment which is established from another part which is conducted under research conditions and for which the terms of engagement are different. That there is the potential for an intervention, however promising, to be ineffective, harmful or to save life but with an increase in disability, is a message which should be a foremost consideration for all those who discuss neural rescue research with parents. The extent to which this can be effectively and sensitively communicated to parents is clearly subject to the limiting effects of the contextual factors and individual variations discussed above.

This discussion has so far focussed on issues around giving information and support and where necessary making the distinction between research and care especially clear. It is important to also point out that other strategies for tackling consent problems in neonatal research have been suggested; these relate to deferring or waiving the information given to parents.

One suggestion made by Zelen is for pre-randomized consent, where the baby is randomized before parents are asked for consent [27]. This model has been defended on several grounds; for example, it is said to protect parents of babies randomized to the control arm from the disappointment of not getting a new treatment that has been explained to them [28]. However, in the only study of parents' views that we are aware of, there was not majority support for the design. Importantly, the parents in the control group seemed particularly hostile [22]. The evidence is insufficient to draw a definitive conclusion, but any use of Zelen design would need strong justification backed by evidence from public consultation that it would be acceptable to parents. This design does not lend itself to openness and trust of parents for their babies' carers and as such may not be supported by clinicians either.

The second suggestion is for deferred and waived consent [29] in situations where it is not possible to secure prior consent to an intervention, probably extreme emergency where an intervention has to be given at a time of crisis. Our data suggest that parents appear to want to be involved, even where they know they are limited in their abilities to understand or cope with what's happening and clinicians appear to be keen to try to discuss care and research up front, even in circumstances as constrained and difficult as those encountered in the TOBY trial [30]. Robust data on parents' views are not yet available but it is likely that deferred consent would seem preferable to that which is waived entirely; with deferred consent parents can at least give (or refuse) permission for ongoing treatment or data collection.

## Conclusions

Communication concerning neural rescue between clinicians and parents takes place when all are under stress; it concerns the treatment of very sick infants whose condition is almost always unexpected, the treatment needs to be given quickly, within hours of birth and parents are often still subject to the effects of perhaps traumatic births. If parents are to understand the treatment options or to give meaningful consent to research participation, they need to process a lot of complex and challenging information. This includes information about an often poor prognosis. Nonetheless, parents greatly value involvement in making decisions. The clinicians who help them with this task, therefore, have a demanding role to play.

In this role, treating consent and communication as a continuous process in which information can be reiterated and built upon seems effective, although careful thought needs to be given to which information is held back at first, if any. In the main, parents should know at least what is about to happen. The pace of decision-making is problematic for some parents but not necessarily for all; even in time-pressured research situations some parents will make their mind up quickly and express comfort with their decision [18].

We have considered the distinction between research and treatment now that cooling is an established treatment. There is an important difference insofar as formal parental consent is almost always required for research but not for treatment. In practice, the boundaries are less clear, but we have suggested that as a minimum parents need to know what is being tested and what is established. We do not underestimate the challenges involved in making the distinction clear in this highly charged and pressured situation.

## References

1.  Allmark P, Mason S. Was the continuous consent process used by researchers on the TOBY study successful at getting valid informed consent from parents for their infants to take part in that study? Report to the TOBY trial Steering Committee (unpub). 2005.

2.  Allmark P, Mason S. Improving the quality of consent to randomised controlled trials by using continuous

consent and clinician training in the consent process. *J Med Ethics* 2006;**32**:439–43.

3. Snowdon C, Elbourne D, Garcia J. Preliminary report of the study of parental and professional views of ECMO and hypothermia at Glenfield Hospital. Confidential report to Heartlink (unpub). 2001.

4. Shellabarger S, Thompson T. The critical times: meeting parental communication needs throughout the NICU experience. *Neonatal Netw* 1993;**12**:39–45.

5. Carter J, Mulder R, Bartram A, Darlow B. Infants in a neonatal intensive care unit: parental response. *Arch Dis Child Fetal Neonatal Ed* 2005;**90**:F109–13.

6. Hall E. Being in an alien world: Danish parents' lived experiences when a newborn or small child is critically ill. *Scand J Caring Sci* 2005;**19**:179–85.

7. Cleveland L. Parenting in the neonatal intensive care unit. *J Obstet Gynecol Neonatal Nurs* 2008;**37**:666–91.

8. Vanderbilt D, Bushley T, Young R, Frank D. Acute posttraumatic stress symptoms among urban mothers with newborns in the neonatal intensive care unit: a preliminary study. *J Dev Behav Pediatr* 2009;**30**:50.

9. Wigert H, Johansson R, Berg M, Hellström A. Mothers' experiences of having their newborn child in a neonatal intensive care unit. *Scand J Caring Sci* 2006;**20**:35–41.

10. Mundy C. Assessment of family needs in neonatal intensive care units. *Am J Crit Care* 2010;**19**:156.

11. Pohlman S. Fathering premature infants and the technological imperative of the neonatal intensive care unit: an interpretive inquiry. *Adv Nursing Sci* 2009;**32**:E1–16.

12. Heermann J, Wilson M, Wilhelm P. Mothers in the NICU: outsider to partner. *Pediatr Nursing* 2005;**31**:176–81.

13. De Rouck S, Leys M. Information needs of parents of children admitted to a neonatal intensive care unit: a review of the literature (1990–2008). *Patient Educ Couns* 2009;**76**:159–73.

14. Koppel G, Kaiser D. Fathers at the end of their rope: a brief report on fathers abandoned in the perinatal situation. *J Reprod Infant Psyc* 2001;**19**:249–51.

15. Cowan P. Litigation. *Semin Fetal Neonatal Med* 2005;**10**:11–21.

16. Ward F. Parents and professionals in the NICU: communication within the context of ethical decision making – an integrative review. *Neonatal Netw* 2005;**24**:25–33.

17. Mason S, Megone C. *European neonatal research*. Farnham: Ashgate; 2001.

18. Snowdon C, Elbourne D, Garcia J. "It was a snap decision": parental and professional perspectives on the speed of decisions about participation in perinatal randomised controlled trials. *Soc Sci Med* 2006;**62**:2279–90.

19. Alderson P, Hawthorne J, Killen M. Parents' experiences of sharing neonatal information and decisions: consent, cost and risk. *Soc Sci Med* 2006;**62**:1319–29.

20. Burgess E, Singhal N, Amin H, McMillan D, Devrome H. Consent for clinical research in the neonatal intensive care unit: a retrospective survey and a prospective study. [erratum appears in Arch Dis Child Fetal Neonatal Ed 2004;89:F83]. *Arch Dis Child Fetal Neonatal Ed* 2003;**88**:F280–5; discussion F285–6.

21. Morley C, Lau R, Davis P, Morse C. What do parents think about enrolling their premature babies in several research studies? *Arch Dis Child Fetal Neonatal Ed* 2005;**90**:F225–8.

22. Snowdon C, Elbourne D, Garcia J. Zelen randomization: attitudes of parents participating in a neonatal clinical trial. *Control Clin Trials* 1999;**20**(2):149–71.

23. Appelbaum P, Roth L, Lidz C. The therapeutic misconception: informed consent in psychiatric research. *Int J Law Psychiatry* 1982;**5**:319–29.

24. Snowdon C. Collaboration, participation and nonparticipation: Decisions about involvement in randomised controlled trials for clinicians and parents in two neonatal trials. Ph.D. thesis. London: London School of Hygiene and Tropical Medicine, University of London; 2005.

25. Miller F, Brody H. A critique of clinical equipoise - Therapeutic misconception in the ethics of clinical trials. *Hastings Cent Rep* 2003;**33**:19–28.

26. Lidz C, Appelbaum P, Grisso T, Renaud M. Therapeutic misconception and the appreciation of risks in clinical trials. *Social Sci Med* 2004;**58**:1689–97.

27. Torgerson D. The use of Zelen's design in randomised trials. *BJOG* 2004;**111**:2.

28. Allmark P. Should Zelen pre-randomised consent designs be used in some neonatal trials? *J Med Ethics* 1999;**25**:325–9.

29. Manning D. Presumed consent in emergency neonatal research. *J Med Ethics* 2000;**26**:249–53.

30. Culbert A, Davis D. Parental preferences for neonatal resuscitation research consent: a pilot study. *J Med Ethics* 2005;**31**:721–6.

# The pharmacology of hypothermia

Alistair J. Gunn and Paul P. Drury

## Introduction

The possibility that hypothermia might prevent or lessen asphyxial brain injury is a "dream revisited", first proposed more than 300 years ago by Floyer [1]. Early experimental studies, mainly in precocial animals such as rat pups and kittens, demonstrated that hypothermia during severe hypoxia/asphyxia greatly extended the "time to last gasp" and improved functional recovery [2]. These encouraging data led to uncontrolled studies in the 1950s and 1960s, in which infants who were not breathing spontaneously at 5 minutes after birth were immersed in cold water until respiration resumed and then allowed to slowly spontaneously rewarm [3]. Outcomes after cooling at birth were reported to be better than for historical controls. Although these studies preceded the development of active resuscitation, immersion cooling was able to be combined with positive pressure resuscitation [4]. These provocative studies were not followed up because of the recognition that mild hypothermia was associated with increased oxygen requirements and greater mortality in premature newborns (<1500 g) [5] and disappointing outcomes from a small cohort of children resuscitated from near-drowning [6].

In retrospect, a key conceptual limitation of the early preclinical studies was that they tested cooling *during* severe hypoxia [2], in contrast with the clinical setting where cooling was induced many hours after resuscitation [7]. This chapter reviews the key empirical developments that helped to delineate the experimental parameters that determine whether post-resuscitation cooling is or is not successful and then relates the parameters to potential mechanisms of hypothermic neuroprotection.

## Pathophysiologic phases of cerebral injury

The central concept that enabled successful trials of cooling was the clinical and experimental observation in term fetuses, newborns and adults that injury to the brain is not a single "event" occurring at, or just after, an insult, but rather an evolving process that leads to cell death well after the initial insult [8]. Critically, Azzopardi and colleagues showed that infants with evidence of moderate to severe asphyxia often have normal cerebral oxidative metabolism shortly after birth, measured using magnetic resonance spectroscopy, but many then went on to develop delayed energy failure 6 to 15 hours later [9]. Infants who did not show transient recovery had a very high mortality, while in survivors, the degree of secondary energy failure after 24 to 48 hours was closely associated with impaired neurodevelopmental outcome at 4 years of age [10]. An identical pattern of initial recovery of cerebral oxidative metabolism followed by secondary failure of mitochondrial activity and production of high-energy metabolites has been demonstrated after hypoxia–ischaemia in the piglet, rat pup and fetal sheep and correlated to the severity of neuronal injury [11–15]. It is this delay between insult and injury that raised the tantalizing possibility that asphyxial cell death may be prevented even well after the insult.

These studies suggested that there are distinct phases of evolving injury, as illustrated in Figure 1. The actual period of hypoxia and ischaemia is the *primary* phase of cell injury. During this phase, there is progressive hypoxic depolarization of cells, leading to severe cytotoxic oedema, with extracellular accumulation of excitatory amino acids (*excitotoxins*) related to a combination of depolarization-mediated release

*Neonatal Neural Rescue*, ed. A. David Edwards, Denis V. Azzopardi and Alistair J. Gunn. Published by Cambridge University Press. © Cambridge University Press 2013.

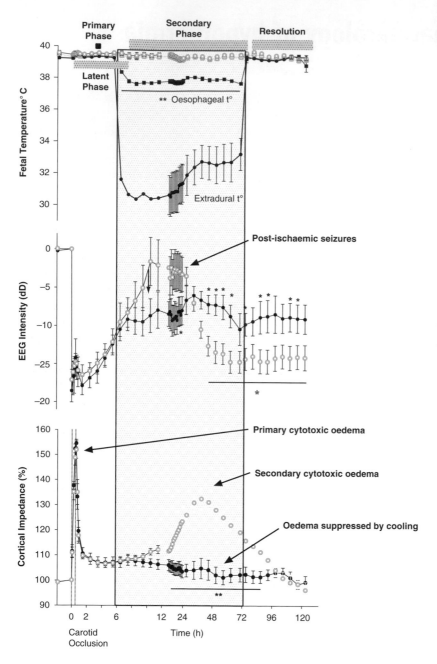

**Figure 7.1.** The effect of hypothermia started 5.5 hours after reperfusion from 30 minutes of cerebral ischaemia in near-term fetal sheep. The period of ischaemia is shown by *dotted lines*, whereas cooling is shown by the *bar*. The *top panel* shows changes in extradural (*solid circles*) and oesophageal (*solid squares*) temperature in the hypothermia group and extradural (*open circles*) and oesophageal (*open squares*) temperature in the sham-cooled group. The *lower two panels* show changes in electroencephalographic (EEG) intensity and cortical impedance (expressed as percentage of baseline) in the hypothermia (*solid circles*) and sham-cooled (*open circles*) groups. Impedance is a measure of cytotoxic oedema (cell swelling). The hypothermia group showed greater recovery of EEG intensity after resolution of delayed seizures and complete suppression of the secondary rise in impedance. Mean ± SEM, *P < .05, **P < .001 hypothermia versus sham-cooled fetuses. Reproduced from reference [43] with kind permission from the American Association of Pediatrics.

and failure of reuptake by astrocytes [16]. Excessive levels of excitatory amino acids promote further channel-specific entry of salt, water and calcium into the cells. After reperfusion during resuscitation from an asphyxial insult, the initial hypoxia-induced cytotoxic oedema may transiently resolve over approximately 30 to 60 minutes, with at least partial recovery of cerebral oxidative metabolism (*latent phase*). This is followed by a secondary phase of deterioration starting many hours later (~6 to 15 hours later) that may extend over many days [10,15]. This so-called *secondary phase* is marked by delayed onset of seizures [17,18], secondary cytotoxic oedema (see Figure 7.1) [19], accumulation of excitotoxins [16], failure of mitochondrial oxidative metabolism [11,15] and ultimately cell death.

The studies discussed in this chapter strongly suggest that it is the early recovery, or latent phase, that represents the key window of opportunity for intervention.

# Factors determining effective neuroprotection with hypothermia

Experimentally, the efficacy of hypothermia is highly dependent on certain factors, including the timing of initiation of cooling, its duration and its depth.

## Cooling during resuscitation and reperfusion

Brief hypothermia, for 1 to 2 hours, appears to be modestly neuroprotective, provided it is initiated immediately after the insult. For example, after 15 minutes of reversible ischaemia in the piglet, mild hypothermia (2–3°C) for 1 to 3 hours significantly improved recovery and reduced neuronal loss 3 days later [20,21]. Critically, protection appears to be lost if the brief interval of hypothermia is delayed by as little as 15 to 45 minutes after the primary insult [22–25]. This extreme sensitivity to delay is consistent in part with the hypothesis that resuscitative hypothermia can suppress damage secondary to oxygen free radical production during reperfusion [26,27]. Alternatively, however, this strategy may merely represent intervention at the end of the primary phase, when cerebrovascular perfusion is being re-established [28], cell function is just starting to recover as shown by delayed resolution of cytotoxic oedema [19] and levels of excitatory amino acids are still high [16].

Even if such immediate cooling during resuscitation were consistently effective, it would be almost impossible to test in practice. It is simply not possible at present to reliably identify the few infants requiring resuscitation who will go on to develop significant encephalopathy until some hours after birth.

## Prolonged cooling

A more recent approach has been to try to suppress the secondary encephalopathic processes by maintaining hypothermia throughout the course of the secondary phase. Such extended periods of cooling of between 5 and 72 hours appear to be consistently effective [29–32]. For example, in a study of reversible middle cerebral artery occlusion in the adult rat,

21 hours, but not 1 hour, of mild hypothermia reduced the area of infarction after 48 hours recovery [33]. After severe global ischaemia in the adult gerbil, 12 hours of mild hypothermia was ineffective, whereas extending the interval to 24 hours was associated with almost complete protection of CA1 neurons in the hippocampus [30].

Newborn studies support these data. In unanaesthetized infant rats subjected to moderate hypoxia–ischaemia, mild hypothermia (2–3°C reduction in brain temperature) for 72 hours from the end of hypoxia prevented cortical infarction, whereas 6 hours of cooling only had intermediate, non-significant results [34]. In the same model greater reduction in body temperature (by 5°C) for 6 hours, starting immediately after the insult, gave significant neuroprotection both after 1 and 6 weeks survival as well as neurobehavioural improvement [35]. Finally, in the anaesthetized piglet exposed either to hypoxia with bilateral carotid ligation or to hypoxia with hypotension, 12 to 48 hours of moderate whole body hypothermia or head cooling with mild systemic hypothermia (started immediately after hypoxia) prevented delayed energy failure [31,32,36], reduced neuronal loss [32,37–39] and suppressed post-hypoxic seizures [38].

## How late is too late? Recent evidence

At present, the window of opportunity for any particular therapy can only be determined empirically. However, some general principles can be discerned. For example, initiation of neuronal degeneration is accelerated by more severe insults. DNA fragmentation in the hippocampus can be detected as early as 10 hours after a 60-minute hypoxic–ischaemic injury in the rat, whereas DNA fragmentation in the hippocampus is only detectable 3 to 5 days after a 15-minute hypoxic–ischaemic injury [40]. However, the appearance of DNA fragmentation and classic ischaemic cell change represent only the terminal events of this cascade and thus are unlikely to be a good guide to determining when cell death may still be reversible. *In vitro* studies have distinguished *latent* and active or *execution* phases during the process of programmed or apoptotic cell death [41]. Whereas the active phase involves downstream factors that could induce DNA fragmentation and chromatin condensation within previously normal nuclei, the preceding latent phase is characterized by caspase activation (a large family of enzymes that mediate and amplify apoptosis) [42] confined to the

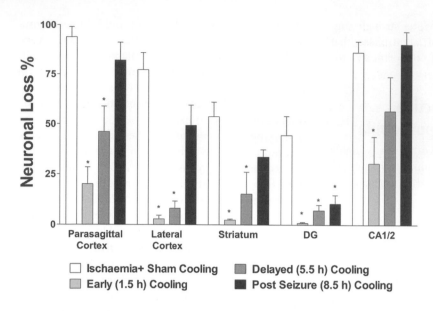

**Figure 7.2.** Comparison of the effect of cerebral cooling in the fetal sheep started at different times after reperfusion and continued until 72 hours on microscopically assessed neuronal loss in the neuronal regions of cortex after 5 days' recovery from 30 minutes of cerebral ischaemia. Compared with the sham-cooled group (n = 13), cooling that was started 90 minutes after reperfusion (n = 7) or just before the end of the latent phase (5.5 hours after reperfusion, n = 11) was protective, whereas there was no significant overall protection with cooling started shortly after the start of the secondary phase (8.5 hours after reperfusion, n = 5), although there was possible improvement within individual regions such as the dentate gyrus (DG) of the hippocampus. Only cooled fetuses in which the extradural temperature was successfully maintained at less than 34°C have been included. CA; Cornu Ammonis. *P < 0.005 compared with sham-cooled (control) fetuses. Data are mean ± SEM [18,43,44].

cytoplasm, without downstream factors. These data suggest that activation of the downstream, intranuclear factors is the critical event that occurs at the transition from the latent to the execution phases of programmed neuronal death. Thus, in principle, it seems far more likely that intervention would be protective if applied during the initial, latent phase of programmed cell death rather than during the execution phase, even though the latter still precedes DNA fragmentation and cell death [41].

Systematic *in vivo* studies support the central role of the latent phase. In the near-term fetal sheep, moderate hypothermia induced 90 minutes after reperfusion from 30 minutes of carotid occlusion (i.e., in the early latent phase) and continued until 72 hours after ischaemia prevented secondary cytotoxic oedema and improved electroencephalographic recovery [18]. There was a concomitant, substantial reduction in parasagittal cortical infarction and improvement in neuronal loss scores in all regions. When the start of hypothermia was delayed in this paradigm until just before the onset of secondary seizures, 5.5 hours after reperfusion, only partial protection was seen (Figure 7.2) [43]. With further delay (until after seizures were established 8.5 hours after reperfusion), there was no electrophysiologic or overall histologic protection with cooling [44]. Similarly, subsequent studies in the anaesthetized newborn piglet have shown that delayed

hypothermia from 2 to 26 hours after hypoxia–ischaemia improved magnetic resonance markers of injury and reduced overall neuronal loss [36,45,46]. In this paradigm, more severe injury was associated with a short latent phase before secondary energy failure, leading to apparently less effective neuroprotection [46].

Data from adult models are consistent with this concept. For example, 5 hours of moderate hypothermia (32.5°C) initiated under anaesthesia in adult rats reduced selective neuronal loss when it was started up to 12 hours after brief global ischaemia, although the degree and extent of neuroprotection markedly declined as the start of cooling was delayed beyond 2 hours [47]. In adult gerbils, when the delay before initiating a 24-hour period of cooling was increased from 1 to 4 hours after ischaemia, neuroprotection in the CA1 field of the hippocampus after 6 months of recovery fell from 70 to 12% [48]. However, this deterioration could be largely overcome by extending the interval of moderate hypothermia (a reduction in body temperature of up to 5°C) to 48 hours or more, even when the start of cooling was delayed until 6 hours after reperfusion [49,50].

## Is neuroprotection maintained long-term?

There have been reports that hypothermia may only delay, rather than prevent, neuronal degeneration after global ischaemia in the adult rat [51–53] and after moderate hypoxia–ischaemia in the 7-day-old rat [54]. The most likely explanation is that the duration or degree of hypothermia may have been inadequate as suggested by the finding that 5°C of cooling for 6 hours [35] or 2 to 3°C for 72 hours in infant rats were associated with long-term improvement after carotid occlusion and hypoxia [34]. Subsequent studies both in the 7-day-old rat and in adult species have confirmed that a sufficiently prolonged phase of moderate cooling can be associated with persistent behavioural and histological protection for many weeks and months [35,49,50,55–58]. Broadly, these studies tend to suggest that the later cooling is started, the more prolonged the treatment needs to be to achieve neuroprotection [59].

An additional issue may have been rebound hyperthermia in the secondary phase. Even short periods of hyperthermia, 24 hours after either global or brief focal ischaemia in the adult rat, exacerbated injury [60,61]. Similarly, in 10-day-old rat pups a 1.5°C increase in brain temperature for several hours during induced seizures after hypoxia–ischaemia was associated with preventable exacerbation of neural injury up to 20 days later [62]. Furthermore, when moderate hypothermia 2 to 9 hours after global ischaemia in the rat was combined with prevention of spontaneous delayed pyrexia with antipyretics, histologic protection was seen after 2 months of recovery [53]. Each intervention alone had essentially short-term benefit only. Whether mild hypothermia could have had additional benefit compared with normothermia in this late interval is, regrettably, unknown. More generally, these findings further support the critical importance of maintaining hypothermia until the encephalopathic processes resolve.

## If some is good, is more better?

There appears to be a critical depth of cerebral hypothermia between 32°C and 34°C required for effective neuronal rescue. In the fetal sheep cooled from 90 minutes after ischaemia, substantial neuroprotection was seen only in fetuses that had a sustained fall of the extradural temperature to less than 34°C (normal temperature in the fetal sheep is 39.5°C), with no substantial improvement below approximately 32–33°C [18]. Similarly, in piglets, during whole body cooling, rectal temperatures of 33 and 35°C were associated with similar improvements in

recovery of oxidative metabolism compared with normothermia (38.5–39°C) [36]. In the adult gerbil, cooling to a rectal temperature of 32°C was associated with greater behavioural and histologic neuroprotection than 34°C [57]. Intriguingly, recent short-term recovery studies in the piglet suggest that the optimal depth of cooling may be greater for the cortex than for the basal ganglia [39]. Supporting this experimental observation, in a recent case series, head cooling but not whole body cooling seemed to be associated with a reduction in the incidence of severe cortical lesions on MRI scans [63].

Overall, these studies suggest that although the "optimal" depth remains unclear and likely varies with region and severity of injury [18,36], there is unlikely to be further neural benefit from cooling to less than 32°C. Supporting this, in the adult dog, deep hypothermia (to a rectal temperature of 15°C) after cardiac arrest was detrimental, whereas mild hypothermia (34 to 36°C), from 10 minutes until 12 hours after cardiac arrest was beneficial [64]. Furthermore, it is reasonable to consider that there is likely to be a tradeoff between the adverse systemic effects of cooling, which in adults increase progressively below a core temperature of approximately 34°C [65] and cerebral benefits.

## Mechanisms of action of hypothermia

The precise mechanisms of hypothermic neuroprotection are still unclear. Although this does not affect its pragmatic clinical use, better understanding is critical to efforts to develop more effective strategies such as combination treatments [66–68]. Broadly, it is now well established that cooling suppresses many of the pathways leading to delayed cell death. As well as reducing cellular metabolic demands [69,70], hypothermia reduces excessive accumulation of cytotoxins such as glutamate and oxygen free radicals, suppresses the post-ischaemic inflammatory reaction and inhibits the intracellular pathways leading to programmed (i.e., apoptosis-like) cell death.

## Cerebral metabolism, excitotoxins and free radicals during the primary and reperfusion phases

The combination of hypoxic depolarization and extracellular excitotoxin accumulation are key factors in the initiation of neuronal injury in the primary phase. Hypothermia produces a graded reduction in cerebral metabolism of approximately 5% for every degree of temperature reduction [69] and, thus, delays the onset of anoxic cell depolarization [71]. However, the protective effects of hypothermia even in this phase are not simply the result of reduced metabolism delaying the onset of anaerobic depolarization, because cooling disproportionately improves outcome even when the absolute duration of depolarization is controlled [72]. Cooling potently reduces post-depolarization release of numerous toxins including excitatory amino acids [73], nitric oxide [74,75] and other free radicals [26,76]. Similarly, cooling begun during reperfusion reduces levels of extracellular excitatory amino acids and nitric oxide production in the piglet [27]. However, these mechanisms are not active during the latent phase and thus cannot readily account for the protective effects of delayed cooling.

## Cooling and cerebral blood flow and metabolism in the latent phase

Following reperfusion, cerebral blood flow typically recovers transiently, followed by secondary hypoperfusion. This is consistently seen during the latent phase; indeed one of the markers of the end of the latent phase is a transition to hyperperfusion [14]. The duration of hypoperfusion in the latent phase is broadly proportional to the severity of the insult [77]. The significance of this apparently low perfusion has been controversial, since prolonged cerebral hypoperfusion after perinatal HI is associated with an adverse clinical outcome [78]. However, there is now increasing evidence that it does not reflect "poor" perfusion, but rather is actively mediated by suppressed cerebral metabolism and is associated with increased not decreased tissue oxygen levels [79].

In fetal sheep, delayed post-ischaemic hypothermia was associated with a marked extension of the phase of secondary hypoperfusion, to nearly 24 hours after the insult [43]. This prolongation of reduced blood flow was associated with improved neural outcome [43]. Hypothermia started at both 1.5 hours [80] and 5.5 hours [43] after ischaemia also prevented the later development of hyperperfusion during the secondary phase. Post-insult hyperperfusion is strongly associated with injury and appears to reflect a true luxury "perfusion", i.e., excess perfusion contrasting with progressive failure of oxidative metabolism in the phase of secondary deterioration [14,15].

Mitochondrial failure is a hallmark of the phase of secondary deterioration [15]. Clearly, maintaining mitochondrial function is crucial in promoting survival after HI. Post-ischaemic hypothermia maintains mitochondrial respiratory activity after 2 hours' reperfusion in the adult gerbil [81]. Hypothermia suppressed reactive oxygen species-mediated mitochondrial damage and preserved mitochondrial membrane potential in cultured myocytes [82]. To date, there are no data directly evaluating mitochondrial function in vivo during therapeutic hypothermia following hypoxia–ischaemia. However, prolonged cooling in the piglet and in rodents preserves cerebral high-energy metabolite production, strongly suggesting that mitochondrial function was preserved by hypothermia [13,31].

Interestingly, despite these effects on cerebral metabolism and perfusion and the reduction in neuronal loss, post-insult hypothermia did not significantly reduce the rate of electrographic seizures [43,80]. In contrast with the lack of effect on total numbers of events, in at least one study in preterm fetal sheep cooling markedly reduced mean post-asphyxial seizure amplitude [80]. It is likely that cooling may have ameliorated in part the excessive local metabolic demand associated with seizure activity, which in turn has been linked with local neuronal death in some settings [83,84]. Nevertheless, a prolonged period of hypothermia delayed until just before the onset of post-ischaemic seizures was not associated with a significant reduction in neuronal loss [44]. Furthermore, strikingly, hypothermia delayed until this point, 8.5 hours after reperfusion, was able to abolish secondary cytotoxic oedema; a major feature of delayed energy failure, despite not affecting neuronal loss. Consistent with this finding, infusion of MK-801, a highly potent, selective glutamate antagonist, between 6 and 24 hours prevented delayed post-ischaemic seizures and completely suppressed the fetal EEG. Despite this finding, there was no improvement in parasagittal neuronal loss scores, although there was a small reduction in less severely affected regions [85]. These data suggest that alterations of delayed overt electrographic seizure activity in isolation are unlikely to be a major therapeutic target in infants with HIE and cannot be critical to hypothermic neuroprotection.

## Intracellular pathways in the latent phase

The effects of hypothermia on pathways distal to cell membrane ion channels are likely to be more important for post-insult neuroprotection than preventing release of toxic factors. For example, intra-insult hypothermia did not prevent intracellular accumulation of calcium during cardiac arrest *in vivo* [86]. or during glutamate exposure *in vitro* [87]. Indeed, there is evidence in the adult rat that the apparent neuroprotective effect of NBQX, a glutamate antagonist, administered from 1 hour after mild ischaemia, was actually mediated by mild hypothermia [52]. In contrast, *in vitro* neuronal degeneration was prevented by cooling initiated *after* the excitotoxins had been washed out [87]. Thus, the ability of hypothermia to reduce release of excitotoxins does not appear to be central to its post-insult neuroprotective effects; rather, these data suggest that the critical effect of hypothermia is to block the intracellular consequences of depolarization and excitotoxin exposure.

## Does hypothermia specifically prevent or suppress apoptosis (programmed cell death)?

There is increasing evidence that hypothermia may have a particular role in suppressing the evolution of programmed cell death. Recent clinical studies have shown that apoptosis is a major contributor to post-asphyxial cell death in the developing brain [88,89]. Studies using morphological criteria have had mixed outcomes. In the piglet, hypothermia started after severe hypoxia–ischaemia was reported to reduce apoptotic cell death, but not necrotic cell death [37], with similar results reported after injury in rats [90,91]. However, in the adult rat, delayed post-ischaemic cell death prevented by hypothermia had a necrotic appearance on detailed electron microscopic criteria [92], consistent with findings of a maturity related reduction in caspase-3 expression after hypoxia–ischaemia in the rat [93]. Nonetheless, it is now clear that apoptotic mechanisms can be involved even in "necrotic" cell death [94]. Although multiple pathways are likely to be involved in such post-ischaemic apoptosis, caspase-3 is reported to play a crucial role as the final "executioner" caspase [94].

The delayed toxicity of hypoxia and excitotoxin exposure is mediated by a massive influx of calcium into the cell, which activates a wide range of enzyme systems and proteases, such as calpain. Activated calpain cleaves structural and regulatory proteins, including cell membrane spectins [95]. Moreover, mitochondrial calcium overload induces cytochrome C release and caspase activation [96]. Caspase inhibition may be neuroprotective for up to 6 hours after reversible stroke in the adult rat [97]. Hypothermia is highly likely to inhibit the activity of such enzymes. Although no specific studies of this pathway have been reported to date, protection with post-ischaemic hypothermia in the near-term fetal sheep was closely linked with suppression of activated caspase-3 [98], with a similar suppression with delayed head-cooling after severe asphyxia in preterm fetal sheep [99]. These data are consistent with *in vitro* studies of hypothermia after severe hypoxia in developing rat neurons. Strikingly, in that model hypoxic preconditioning activated a programme that stimulated the expression of anti-apoptotic proteins such as Bcl-2 and HSP-70, whereas hypothermia did not trigger these active processes, but rather depressed cell activity and abolished hypoxia-associated protein synthesis, thus suppressing apoptotic pathways [100].

## Suppression of inflammatory second messengers

Brain injury leads to induction of the inflammatory cascade with increased release of cytokines and interleukins [101]. These compounds are believed to exacerbate delayed injury, whether by direct neurotoxicity and induction of apoptosis through the so-called extrinsic pathways linked to cell death receptors [102] or by promoting leukocyte diapedesis into the ischaemic brain. Experimentally, cooling potently suppresses multiple aspects of the inflammatory reaction [103]. For example, *in vitro*, hypothermia inhibits proliferation, superoxide and nitric oxide (NO) production by cultured microglia [104] and in adult rats, hypothermia suppresses the post-traumatic release of interleukin-1$\beta$ [105] and accumulation of polymorphonuclear leukocytes [106]. Similarly, post-ischaemic hypothermia can suppress microglial activation following transient ischaemia in the fetal sheep [98]. This broad reduction in inflammatory signalling may offer significant mitochondrial protection. Cytokine mediated iNOS expression increases NO levels, which compete with molecular oxygen at its binding site on cytochrome oxidase [107], potently suppressing oxidative metabolism and thus reducing ATP levels [108]. TNF-$\alpha$ also has this effect by inhibiting complex-I of the electron transport chain [109]. Furthermore, TNF-$\alpha$ and interferon-$\gamma$ mediated iNOS expression was associated with mitochondrial DNA damage and apoptosis in cultured oligodendrocytes [110].

Intriguingly, despite the potent suppression of microglia by hypothermia, it has little effect on astrocytic proliferation *in vitro* [104]. Thus, these data suggest that the hypothermic protection against post-ischaemic neuronal damage may be, in part, the result of differential effects on glia, with suppression of microglial activation but relative sparing of potentially pro-survival astrocytic reactions.

## Conclusions

There is now overwhelming experimental evidence that mild to moderate post-asphyxial cerebral cooling can be associated with long-term neuroprotection. The key requirements are that hypothermia be initiated as soon as possible in the latent phase, within the first 6 hours, before secondary deterioration and that it be continued for a sufficient period in relation to the evolution of delayed encephalopathic processes, typically 48 hours or more. These findings are now supported by large randomized trials of both head cooling combined with mild systemic hypothermia and whole body cooling that found that cooling is safe, at least in the intensive care environment, and associated with a significant reduction in the incidence of both death and severe disability following asphyxia [111]. However, it is critical to appreciate that although hypothermia is an important advance, as currently applied, it is not a "silver bullet" and many infants die or survive with disability despite hypothermia.

Suppression of cerebral metabolism has historically been regarded as the primary mechanism of protection. It is now clear that the mechanisms underlying hypothermic neuroprotection are multifactorial. Key potential mechanisms in the latent phase that have been shown to be suppressed by hypothermia include programmed cell death ("apoptosis"), inflammation and the extrinsic cell death pathway and abnormal receptor activity. It is likely that it is the intracytoplasmic, "downstream" effects of these phenomena that are critical to protection. Further elucidation of the contribution of each of these pathways in the latent phase and at what level the cascades become irreversible by hypothermia will be critical to further improving perinatal neuroprotection.

## Acknowledgements

The authors' work reported in this chapter was supported by the Health Research Council of New Zealand, Lottery Health Board of New Zealand, the Auckland Medical Research Foundation and the March of Dimes Birth Defects Foundation. P. Drury is supported by the New Zealand Neurological Foundation W – B Miller Doctoral Scholarship.

## References

1. Floyer J. *An essay to restore the dipping of infants in their baptism; with a dialogue betwixt a curate and a practitioner, concerning the manner of immersion.* London: Holland; 1722.

2. Westin B, Miller JA Jr, Boles A. Hypothermia induced during asphyxiation: its effects on survival rate, learning and maintenance of the conditioned response in rats. *Acta Paediatr* 1963;**52**:49–60.

3. Cordey R, Chiolero R, Miller JA Jr. Resuscitation of neonates by hypothermia: report on 20 cases with acid-base determination on 10 cases and the long-term development of 33 cases. *Resuscitation* 1973;**2**:169–81.

4. Dunn JM, Miller JA Jr. Hypothermia combined with positive pressure ventilation in resuscitation of the asphyxiated neonate. Clinical observations in 28 infants. *Am J Obstet Gynecol* 1969;**104**:58–67.

5. Silverman WA, Fertig JW, Berger AP. The influence of the thermal environment upon the survival of newly born premature infants. *Pediatrics* 1958;**22**:876–86.

6. Bohn DJ, Biggar WD, Smith CR, Conn AW, Barker GA. Influence of hypothermia, barbiturate therapy and intracranial pressure monitoring on morbidity and mortality after near-drowning. *Crit Care Med* 1986;**14**:529–34.

7. Nurse S, Corbett D. Direct measurement of brain temperature during and after intraischemic hypothermia: correlation with behavioral, physiological and histological endpoints. *J Neurosci* 1994;**14**:7726–34.

8. Higgins RD, Raju TN, Perlman J, et al. Hypothermia and perinatal asphyxia: executive summary of the NICHD workshop. *J Pediatr* 2006;**148**:170–5.

9. Azzopardi D, Wyatt JS, Cady EB, et al. Prognosis of newborn infants with hypoxic-ischemic brain injury assessed by phosphorus magnetic resonance spectroscopy. *Pediatr Res* 1989;**25**:445–51.

10. Roth SC, Baudin J, Cady E, et al. Relation of deranged neonatal cerebral oxidative metabolism with neurodevelopmental outcome and head circumference at 4 years. *Dev Med Child Neurol* 1997;**39**:718–25.

11. Lorek A, Takei Y, Cady EB, et al. Delayed ("secondary") cerebral energy failure after acute hypoxia-ischemia in the newborn piglet: continuous 48-hour studies by phosphorus magnetic resonance spectroscopy. *Pediatr Res* 1994;**36**:699–706.

12. Mehmet H, Yue X, Penrice J, et al. Relation of impaired energy metabolism to apoptosis and necrosis following transient cerebral hypoxia-ischaemia. *Cell Death Differ* 1998;**5**:321–9.

13. Blumberg RM, Cady EB, Wigglesworth JS, McKenzie JE, Edwards AD. Relation between delayed impairment of cerebral energy metabolism and infarction following transient focal hypoxia-ischaemia in the developing brain. *Exp Brain Res* 1997;**113**:130–7.

14. Marks KA, Mallard EC, Roberts I, et al. Delayed vasodilation and altered oxygenation after cerebral ischemia in fetal sheep. *Pediatr Res* 1996;**39**:48–54.

15. Bennet L, Roelfsema V, Pathipati P, Quaedackers J, Gunn AJ. Relationship between evolving epileptiform activity and delayed loss of mitochondrial activity after asphyxia measured by near-infrared spectroscopy in preterm fetal sheep. *J Physiol* 2006;**572**:141–54.

16. Tan WK, Williams CE, During MJ, et al. Accumulation of cytotoxins during the development of seizures and edema after hypoxic-ischemic injury in late gestation fetal sheep. *Pediatr Res* 1996;**39**:791–7.

17. Gunn AJ, Parer JT, Mallard EC, Williams CE, Gluckman PD. Cerebral histologic and electrocorticographic changes after asphyxia in fetal sheep. *Pediatr Res* 1992;**31**:486–91.

18. Gunn AJ, Gunn TR, de Haan HH, Williams CE, Gluckman PD. Dramatic neuronal rescue with prolonged selective head cooling after ischemia in fetal lambs. *J Clin Invest* 1997;**99**:248–56.

19. Williams CE, Gunn A, Gluckman PD. Time course of intracellular edema and epileptiform activity following prenatal cerebral ischemia in sheep. *Stroke* 1991;**22**:516–21.

20. Laptook AR, Corbett RJ, Sterett R, et al. Modest hypothermia provides partial neuroprotection when used for immediate resuscitation after brain ischemia. *Pediatr Res* 1997;**42**:17–23.

21. Haaland K, Loberg EM, Steen PA, Thoresen M. Posthypoxic hypothermia in newborn piglets. *Pediatr Res* 1997;**41**:505–12.

22. Laptook AR, Corbett RJ, Burns DK, Sterett R. A limited interval of delayed modest hypothermia for ischemic brain resuscitation is not beneficial in neonatal swine. *Pediatr Res* 1999;**46**:383–9.

23. Shuaib A, Trulove D, Ijaz MS, Kanthan R, Kalra J. The effect of post-ischemic hypothermia following repetitive cerebral ischemia in gerbils. *Neurosci Lett* 1995;**186**:165–8.

24. Busto R, Dietrich WD, Globus MY, Ginsberg MD. Postischemic moderate hypothermia inhibits CA1 hippocampal ischemic neuronal injury. *Neurosci Lett* 1989;**101**:299–304.

25. Kuboyama K, Safar P, Radovsky A, et al. Delay in cooling negates the beneficial effect of mild resuscitative cerebral hypothermia after cardiac arrest in dogs: a prospective, randomized study. *Crit Care Med* 1993;**21**:1348–58.

26. Zhao W, Richardson JS, Mombourquette MJ, et al. Neuroprotective effects of hypothermia and U-78517F in cerebral ischemia are due to reducing oxygen-based free radicals: an electron paramagnetic resonance study with gerbils. *J Neurosci Res* 1996;**45**:282–8.

27. Thoresen M, Satas S, Puka-Sundvall M, et al. Post-hypoxic hypothermia reduces cerebrocortical release of NO and excitotoxins. *Neuroreport* 1997;**8**:3359–62.

28. Bennet L, Roelfsema V, Dean J, et al. Regulation of cytochrome oxidase redox state during umbilical cord occlusion in preterm fetal sheep. *Am J Physiol Regul Integr Comp Physiol* 2007;**292**:R1569–76.

29. Carroll M, Beek O. Protection against hippocampal CA1 cell loss by post-ischemic hypothermia is dependent on delay of initiation and duration. *Metab Brain Dis* 1992;**7**:45–50.

30. Colbourne F, Corbett D. Delayed and prolonged post-ischemic hypothermia is neuroprotective in the gerbil. *Brain Res* 1994;**654**:265–72.

31. Thoresen M, Penrice J, Lorek A, et al. Mild hypothermia after severe transient hypoxia-ischemia ameliorates delayed cerebral energy failure in the newborn piglet. *Pediatr Res* 1995;**37**:667–70.

32. Chakkarapani E, Dingley J, Liu X, et al. Xenon enhances hypothermic neuroprotection in asphyxiated newborn pigs. *Ann Neurol* 2010;**68**:330–41.

33. Yanamoto H, Hong SC, Soleau S, Kassell NF, Lee KS. Mild postischemic hypothermia limits cerebral injury following transient focal ischemia in rat neocortex. *Brain Res* 1996;**718**:207–11.

34. Sirimanne ES, Blumberg RM, Bossano D, et al. The effect of prolonged modification of cerebral temperature on outcome after hypoxic-ischemic brain injury in the infant rat. *Pediatr Res* 1996;**39**:591–7.

35. Bona E, Hagberg H, Loberg EM, Bagenholm R, Thoresen M. Protective effects of moderate hypothermia after neonatal hypoxia-ischemia: short- and long-term outcome. *Pediatr Res* 1998;**43**:738–45.

36. O'Brien FE, Iwata O, Thornton JS, et al. Delayed whole-body cooling to 33 or 35 degrees C and the development of impaired energy generation consequential to transient cerebral hypoxia-ischemia in the newborn piglet. *Pediatrics* 2006;**117**:1549–59.

37. Edwards AD, Yue X, Squier MV, et al. Specific inhibition of apoptosis after cerebral hypoxia-ischaemia by moderate post-insult hypothermia. *Biochem Biophys Res Commun* 1995;**217**:1193–9.

38. Tooley JR, Satas S, Porter H, Silver IA, Thoresen M. Head cooling with mild systemic hypothermia in anesthetized piglets is neuroprotective. *Ann Neurol* 2003;**53**:65–72.

39. Iwata O, Thornton JS, Sellwood MW, et al. Depth of delayed cooling alters neuroprotection pattern after hypoxia-ischemia. *Ann Neurol* 2005;**58**:75–87.

40. Beilharz EJ, Williams CE, Dragunow M, Sirimanne ES, Gluckman PD. Mechanisms of delayed cell death following hypoxic-ischemic injury in the immature rat: evidence for apoptosis during selective neuronal loss. *Mol Brain Res* 1995;**29**:1–14.

41. Samejima K, Tone S, Kottke TJ, et al. Transition from caspase-dependent to caspase-independent mechanisms at the onset of apoptotic execution. *J Cell Biol* 1998;**143**:225–39.

42. Stefanis L. Caspase-dependent and -independent neuronal death: two distinct pathways to neuronal injury. *Neuroscientist* 2005;**11**:50–62.

43. Gunn AJ, Gunn TR, Gunning MI, Williams CE, Gluckman PD. Neuroprotection with prolonged head cooling started before postischemic seizures in fetal sheep. *Pediatrics* 1998;**102**:1098–106.

44. Gunn AJ, Bennet L, Gunning MI, Gluckman PD, Gunn TR. Cerebral hypothermia is not neuroprotective when started after postischemic seizures in fetal sheep. *Pediatr Res* 1999;**46**:274–80.

45. Faulkner S, Bainbridge A, Kato T, et al. Xenon augmented hypothermia reduces early lactate/N-acetylaspartate and cell death in perinatal asphyxia. *Ann Neurol* 2011;**70**:133–50.

46. Iwata O, Iwata S, Thornton JS, et al. "Therapeutic time window" duration decreases with increasing severity of cerebral hypoxia-ischaemia under normothermia and delayed hypothermia in newborn piglets. *Brain Res* 2007;**1154**:173–80.

47. Coimbra C, Wieloch T. Moderate hypothermia mitigates neuronal damage in the rat brain when initiated several hours following transient cerebral ischemia. *Acta Neuropathol (Berl)* 1994;**87**:325–31.

48. Colbourne F, Corbett D. Delayed postischemic hypothermia: a six month survival study using behavioral and histological assessments of neuroprotection. *J Neurosci* 1995;**15**:7250–60.

49. Colbourne F, Li H, Buchan AM. Indefatigable CA1 sector neuroprotection with mild hypothermia induced 6 hours after severe forebrain ischemia in rats. *J Cereb Blood Flow Metab* 1999;**19**:742–9.

50. Colbourne F, Corbett D, Zhao Z, Yang J, Buchan AM. Prolonged but delayed postischemic hypothermia: a long-term outcome study in the rat middle cerebral artery occlusion model. *J Cereb Blood Flow Metab* 2000;**20**:1702–8.

51. Dietrich WD, Busto R, Alonso O, Globus MY, Ginsberg MD. Intraischemic but not postischemic brain hypothermia protects chronically following global forebrain ischemia in rats. *J Cereb Blood Flow Metab* 1993;**13**:541–9.

52. Nurse S, Corbett D. Neuroprotection after several days of mild, drug-induced hypothermia. *J Cereb Blood Flow Metab* 1996;**16**:474–80.

53. Coimbra C, Drake M, Boris-Moller F, Wieloch T. Long-lasting neuroprotective effect of postischemic hypothermia and treatment with an anti-inflammatory/antipyretic drug. Evidence for chronic encephalopathic processes following ischemia. *Stroke* 1996;**27**:1578–85.

54. Trescher WH, Ishiwa S, Johnston MV. Brief post-hypoxic-ischemic hypothermia markedly delays neonatal brain injury. *Brain Dev* 1997;**19**:326–38.

55. Nedelcu J, Klein MA, Aguzzi A, Martin E. Resuscitative hypothermia protects the neonatal rat brain from hypoxic–ischemic injury. *Brain Pathol* 2000;**10**:61–71.

56. Wagner BP, Nedelcu J, Martin E. Delayed postischemic hypothermia improves long-term behavioral outcome after cerebral hypoxia-ischemia in neonatal rats. *Pediatr Res* 2002;**51**:354–60.

57. Colbourne F, Auer RN, Sutherland GR. Characterization of postischemic behavioral deficits in gerbils with and without hypothermic neuroprotection. *Brain Res* 1998;**803**:69–78.

58. Corbett D, Hamilton M, Colbourne F. Persistent neuroprotection with prolonged postischemic hypothermia in adult rats subjected to transient middle cerebral artery occlusion. *Exp Neurol* 2000;**163**:200–6.

59. Colbourne F, Sutherland G, Corbett D. Postischemic hypothermia. A critical appraisal with implications for clinical treatment. *Mol Neurobiol* 1997;**14**:171–201.

60. Baena RC, Busto R, Dietrich WD, Globus MY, Ginsberg MD. Hyperthermia delayed by 24 hours aggravates neuronal damage in rat hippocampus following global ischemia. *Neurology* 1997;**48**:768–73.

61. Kim Y, Busto R, Dietrich WD, Kraydieh S, Ginsberg MD. Delayed postischemic hyperthermia in awake rats worsens the histopathological outcome of transient focal cerebral ischemia. *Stroke* 1996;**27**:2274–80.

62. Yager JY, Armstrong EA, Jaharus C, Saucier DM, Wirrell EC. Preventing hyperthermia decreases brain damage following neonatal hypoxic-ischemic seizures. *Brain Res* 2004;**1011**:48–57.

63. Rutherford MA, Azzopardi D, Whitelaw A, et al. Mild hypothermia and the distribution of cerebral lesions in

neonates with hypoxic-ischemic encephalopathy. *Pediatrics* 2005;**116**:1001–6.

64. Weinrauch V, Safar P, Tisherman S, Kuboyama K, Radovsky A. Beneficial effect of mild hypothermia and detrimental effect of deep hypothermia after cardiac arrest in dogs. *Stroke* 1992;**23**:1454–62.

65. Schubert A. Side effects of mild hypothermia. *J Neurosurg Anesthesiol* 1995;**7**:139–47.

66. Ma D, Hossain M, Chow A, et al. Xenon and hypothermia combine to provide neuroprotection from neonatal asphyxia. *Ann Neurol* 2005;**58**:182–93.

67. Liu Y, Barks JD, Xu G, Silverstein FS. Topiramate extends the therapeutic window for hypothermia-mediated neuroprotection after stroke in neonatal rats. *Stroke* 2004;**35**:1460–5.

68. George SA, Bennet L, Weaver-Mikaere L, et al. White matter protection with insulin like-growth factor 1 (IGF-1) and hypothermia is not additive after severe reversible cerebral ischemia in term fetal sheep. *Dev Neurosci* 2011 [Epub ahead of print].

69. Laptook AR, Corbett RJ, Sterett R, Garcia D, Tollefsbol G. Quantitative relationship between brain temperature and energy utilization rate measured in vivo using 31P and 1H magnetic resonance spectroscopy. *Pediatr Res* 1995;**38**:919–25.

70. Erecinska M, Thoresen M, Silver IA. Effects of hypothermia on energy metabolism in mammalian central nervous system. *J Cereb Blood Flow Metab* 2003;**23**:513–30.

71. Nakashima K, Todd MM, Warner DS. The relation between cerebral metabolic rate and ischemic depolarization. A comparison of the effects of hypothermia, pentobarbital and isoflurane. *Anesthesiology* 1995;**82**:1199–208.

72. Bart RD, Takaoka S, Pearlstein RD, Dexter F, Warner DS. Interactions between hypothermia and the latency to ischemic depolarization: implications for neuroprotection. *Anesthesiology* 1998;**88**:1266–73.

73. Nakashima K, Todd MM. Effects of hypothermia on the rate of excitatory amino acid release after ischemic depolarization. *Stroke* 1996;**27**:913–8.

74. Kader A, Brisman MH, Maraire N, Huh JT, Solomon RA. The effect of mild hypothermia on permanent focal ischemia in the rat. *Neurosurgery* 1992;**31**:1056–60.

75. Loidl CF, de Vente J, van Ittersum MM, et al. Hypothermia during or after severe perinatal asphyxia prevents increase in cyclic GMP-related nitric oxide levels in the newborn rat striatum. *Brain Res* 1998;**791**:303–7.

76. Lei B, Adachi N, Arai T. The effect of hypothermia on H2O2 production during ischemia and reperfusion: a microdialysis study in the gerbil hippocampus. *Neurosci Lett* 1997;**222**:91–4.

77. Karlsson BR, Grogaard B, Gerdin B, Steen PA. The severity of postischemic hypoperfusion increases with duration of cerebral ischemia in rats. *Acta Anaesthesiol Scand* 1994;**38**:248–53.

78. Perlman JM. White matter injury in the preterm infant: an important determination of abnormal neurodevelopment outcome. *Early Hum Dev* 1998;**53**:99–120.

79. Jensen EC, Bennet L, Hunter CJ, Power GG, Gunn AJ. Post-hypoxic hypoperfusion is associated with suppression of cerebral metabolism and increased tissue oxygenation in near-term fetal sheep. *J Physiol* 2006;**572**:131–9.

80. Bennet L, Dean JM, Wassink G, Gunn AJ. Differential effects of hypothermia on early and late epileptiform events after severe hypoxia in preterm fetal sheep. *J Neurophysiol* 2007;**97**:572–8.

81. Canevari L, Console A, Tendi EA, Clark JB, Bates TE. Effect of postischaemic hypothermia on the mitochondrial damage induced by ischaemia and reperfusion in the gerbil. *Brain Res* 1999;**817**:241–5.

82. Huang CH, Chen HW, Tsai MS, et al. Antiapoptotic cardioprotective effect of hypothermia treatment against oxidative stress injuries. *Acad Emerg Med* 2009;**16**:872–80.

83. Pereira de Vasconcelos A, Ferrandon A, Nehlig A. Local cerebral blood flow during lithium-pilocarpine seizures in the developing and adult rat: role of coupling between blood flow and metabolism in the genesis of neuronal damage. *J Cereb Blood Flow Metab* 2002;**22**:196–205.

84. Ingvar M. Cerebral blood flow and metabolic rate during seizures. Relationship to epileptic brain damage. *Ann N Y Acad Sci* 1986;**462**:194–206.

85. Tan WK, Williams CE, Gunn AJ, Mallard CE, Gluckman PD. Suppression of postischemic epileptiform activity with MK-801 improves neural outcome in fetal sheep. *Ann Neurol* 1992;**32**:677–82.

86. Kristian T, Katsura K, Siesjo BK. The influence of moderate hypothermia on cellular calcium uptake in complete ischaemia: implications for the excitotoxic hypothesis. *Acta Physiol Scand* 1992;**146**:531–2.

87. Bruno VM, Goldberg MP, Dugan LL, Giffard RG, Choi DW. Neuroprotective effect of hypothermia in cortical cultures exposed to oxygen-glucose deprivation or excitatory amino acids. *J Neurochem* 1994;**63**:1398–406.

88. Edwards AD, Yue X, Cox P, et al. Apoptosis in the brains of infants suffering intrauterine cerebral injury. *Pediatr Res* 1997;**42**:684–9.

89. Scott RJ, Hegyi L. Cell death in perinatal hypoxic-ischaemic brain injury. *Neuropathol Appl Neurobiol* 1997;**23**:307–14.

90. Xu RX, Nakamura T, Nagao S, et al. Specific inhibition of apoptosis after cold-induced brain injury by moderate postinjury hypothermia. *Neurosurgery* 1998;**43**:107–14.

91. Inamasu J, Suga S, Sato S, et al. Postischemic hypothermia attenuates apoptotic cell death in transient focal ischemia in rats. *Acta Neurochir Suppl* 2000;**76**:525–7.

92. Colbourne F, Sutherland GR, Auer RN. Electron microscopic evidence against apoptosis as the mechanism of neuronal death in global ischemia. *J Neurosci* 1999;**19**:4200–10.

93. Hu BR, Liu CL, Ouyang Y, Blomgren K, Siesjo BK. Involvement of caspase-3 in cell death after hypoxia-ischemia declines during brain maturation. *J Cereb Blood Flow Metab* 2000;**20**:1294–300.

94. Benchoua A, Guegan C, Couriaud C, et al. Specific caspase pathways are activated in the two stages of cerebral infarction. *J Neurosci* 2001;**21**:7127–34.

95. Li S, Jiang Q, Stys PK. Important role of reverse Na(+)-Ca(2+) exchange in spinal cord white matter injury at physiological temperature. *J Neurophysiol* 2000;**84**:1116–9.

96. Schild L, Keilhoff G, Augustin W, Reiser G, Striggow F. Distinct Ca2+ thresholds determine cytochrome c release or permeability transition pore opening in brain mitochondria. *FASEB J* 2001;**15**:565–7.

97. Endres M, Namura S, Shimizu-Sasamata M, et al. Attenuation of delayed neuronal death after mild focal ischemia in mice by inhibition of the caspase family. *J Cereb Blood Flow Metab* 1998;**18**:238–47.

98. Roelfsema V, Bennet L, George S, et al. The window of opportunity for cerebral hypothermia and white matter injury after cerebral ischemia in near-term fetal sheep. *J Cereb Blood Flow Metab* 2004;**24**:877–86.

99. Bennet L, Roelfsema V, George S, et al. The effect of cerebral hypothermia on white and grey matter injury induced by severe hypoxia in preterm fetal sheep. *J Physiol* 2007;**578**:491–506.

100. Bossenmeyer-Pourie C, Koziel V, Daval JL. Effects of hypothermia on hypoxia-induced apoptosis in cultured neurons from developing rat forebrain: comparison with preconditioning. *Pediatr Res* 2000;**47**:385–91.

101. Hagberg H, Mallard C, Jacobsson B. Role of cytokines in preterm labour and brain injury. *BJOG* 2005;**112**(Suppl 1): 16–8.

102. Graham EM, Sheldon RA, Flock DL, et al. Neonatal mice lacking functional Fas death receptors are resistant to hypoxic-ischemic brain injury. *Neurobiol Dis* 2004;**17**:89–98.

103. Gunn AJ, Thoresen M. Hypothermic neuroprotection. *NeuroRx* 2006;**3**:154–69.

104. Si QS, Nakamura Y, Kataoka K. Hypothermic suppression of microglial activation in culture: inhibition of cell proliferation and production of nitric oxide and superoxide. *Neuroscience* 1997;**81**:223–9.

105. Goss JR, Styren SD, Miller PD, et al. Hypothermia attenuates the normal increase in interleukin 1 beta RNA and nerve growth factor following traumatic brain injury in the rat. *J Neurotrauma* 1995;**12**:159–67.

106. Chatzipanteli K, Alonso OF, Kraydieh S, Dietrich WD. Importance of posttraumatic hypothermia and hyperthermia on the inflammatory response after fluid percussion brain injury: biochemical and immunocytochemical studies. *J Cereb Blood Flow Metab* 2000;**20**:531–42.

107. Brown GC. Nitric oxide inhibition of cytochrome oxidase and mitochondrial respiration: implications for inflammatory, neurodegenerative and ischaemic pathologies. *Mol Cell Biochem* 1997;**174**:189–92.

108. Tatsumi T, Matoba S, Kawahara A, et al. Cytokine-induced nitric oxide production inhibits mitochondrial energy production and impairs contractile function in rat cardiac myocytes. *J Am Coll Cardiol* 2000;**35**:1338–46.

109. Samavati L, Lee I, Mathes I, Lottspeich F, Huttemann M. Tumor necrosis factor alpha inhibits oxidative phosphorylation through tyrosine phosphorylation at subunit I of cytochrome c oxidase. *J Biol Chem* 2008;**283**:21134–44.

110. Druzhyna NM, Musiyenko SI, Wilson GL, LeDoux SP. Cytokines induce nitric oxide-mediated mtDNA damage and apoptosis in oligodendrocytes. Protective role of targeting 8-oxoguanine glycosylase to mitochondria. *J Biol Chem* 2005;**280**:21673–9.

111. Edwards AD, Brocklehurst P, Gunn AJ, et al. Neurological outcomes at 18 months of age after moderate hypothermia for perinatal hypoxic ischaemic encephalopathy: synthesis and meta-analysis of trial data. *BMJ* 2010;**340**:c363.

# Selection of infants for hypothermic neural rescue

Ericalyn Kasdorf and Jeffrey M. Perlman

## Introduction

The overwhelming majority of term infants are born without labour and delivery complications and have a benign neonatal course with a favourable outcome. Those infants who do experience some transient interruption in placental blood flow are frequently able to adapt through several mechanisms which will be discussed later in this chapter, and also have a favourable outcome. The incidence of brain injury secondary to interruption of placental blood flow significant enough to result in intrapartum hypoxia–ischaemia is exceedingly uncommon with estimates that range from 1 to 2 per 1000 live term births in the developed world [1]. The ability to identify the high-risk infant in a timely manner is critical for several reasons. First, any novel intervention, including hypothermia, has the potential for significant side effects. Thus, targeting the appropriate population where the benefits outweigh the risks is critical. Second, for an intervention to be potentially neuroprotective it must be administered in a timely manner following a presumed insult, within the so-called "therapeutic window" to minimize or prevent ongoing reperfusion injury. Experimental data indicate that the therapeutic window is short at approximately 6 hours [2–5]. In this chapter, we shall review the perinatal indicators that have been shown to identify the high-risk infant who is likely to derive the most benefit from hypothermic neural rescue.

## Pathophysiology

Severe and prolonged interruption of placental blood flow will ultimately lead to fetal asphyxia, characterized biochemically by progressive hypoxia, hypercarbia and acidosis [6]. Although the degree of acidemia with risk for brain injury may vary amongst infants, a cord umbilical arterial pH < 7.00 reflects a severity whereby the risk is increased [7,8]. Some obstetric complications which may be associated with asphyxia include fetal heart rate abnormalities ± meconium-stained amniotic fluid, placental abruption, uterine rupture and cord prolapse [9,10]. A major consequence of asphyxia is impaired cerebral blood flow (CBF), thought to be the causal mechanism for most of the neuropathology associated with hypoxic–ischaemic encephalopathy (HIE) [11]. Neuronal cell death occurs through two principal mechanisms comprised of necrosis and/or apoptosis. The pathway of cell death is in part determined by the intensity of the initial insult, with severe injury leading to necrosis and more mild injury resulting in apoptosis, although it is not uncommon to see histologic evidence of both processes [1,11].

## Circulatory and non-circulatory responses to interruption of placental blood flow

The fetus responds to interruption of placental blood flow with a redistribution of cardiac output. The initial response is to redirect a larger proportion directly to the brain, resulting in a subsequent increase in CBF as well as increasing blood flow to the myocardium and adrenal gland. To accomplish this, blood flow is decreased to other organs, including kidneys, intestine and skin [6]. This adaptive response has been demonstrated experimentally in the hypoxic fetal lamb model [12,13]. Thus with initial arterial hypoxaemia, fetal cerebral vascular resistance can decrease by at least 50% to maintain CBF with minimal decrease in oxygen delivery [14]. Critical to this adaptation is a normal or elevated blood pressure. However, with persistent hypoxaemia and eventual hypotension, cerebral

---

*Neonatal Neural Rescue*, ed. A. David Edwards, Denis V. Azzopardi and Alistair J. Gunn. Published by Cambridge University Press. © Cambridge University Press 2013.

vascular resistance cannot decrease further, resulting in a marked reduction in CBF [15]. Usually CBF is maintained over a wide range of changes in systemic mean arterial blood pressure, a term referred to as autoregulation. However, this critical response may be impaired by acidosis, hypoxia or changes in carbon dioxide status as seen with asphyxia [14]. When autoregulation is disrupted, CBF becomes dependent on systemic blood pressure (BP) changes, a state known as pressure passive cerebral circulation. Under such circumstances, a moderate decrease in systemic BP puts the infant at increased risk for ischaemic brain injury [16]. As noted above, in the setting of ongoing asphyxia, there is a decline in cardiac output secondary to myocardial pump-failure and hypoxia-induced bradycardia. This leads to hypotension and ultimately a decrease in CBF [17]. The relationship of cardiac output with CBF was demonstrated in chronically catheterized fetal lambs. In this study, CBF was found to have a closer correlation to cardiac output than to BP [18]. In addition to the circulatory responses described above, other factors considered potentially important in preserving neuronal integrity with asphyxia include biologic alterations that accompany maturation. These alterations include a slower depletion of high-energy compounds during hypoxia–ischaemia in the fetus compared to the term infant or adult, the neonatal brain's capacity to use lactate and ketone bodies for energy production and the relative resistance of the fetal myocardium to hypoxia–ischaemia [19,20]. Regarding the latter, in a study evaluating myocardial mitochondria from 14 fetal and 15 newborn lambs as compared with 26 adult sheep, increased respiratory rate and, thus, increased aerobic capacity was demonstrated in the non-adult heart mitochondria [20].

To summarize, the adaptive mechanisms briefly described above allow the fetus to maintain CBF and oxygen even under most clinical states where the risk for a reduction might seem unavoidable. These adaptations likely account for the relatively low occurrence of perinatal hypoxic–ischaemic brain injury.

# Selection of infants for hypothermic neural rescue

## Patient population

The multicentre studies for selective head cooling, as well as whole body hypothermia, have enrolled infants ≥35 weeks' gestation [21–24]. This is in part based on the observation that, although the preterm brain is at increased risk for haemorrhagic–ischaemic injury, the developing brain may be relatively resistant to hypoxia–ischaemia. Thus in a study of infants of 31–36 weeks gestation with an umbilical arterial cord pH <7.00, only increasing gestation was a significant predictor for abnormal neonatal neurologic outcome. With each 1-week increase in gestation, the odds ratio for an abnormal outcome increased by 3.6 [25]. Moreover, the premature infant is more vulnerable to hypothermia, which has been associated with increased mortality and morbidity.

## Initiation of hypothermia

After the initial insult, experimental evidence suggests that cerebral energy metabolism is re-established over 30 minutes, followed by a latent phase in which the patient has near-normal oxidative metabolism. This may progress to secondary energy failure with seizures and cytotoxic swelling, as well as oxidative metabolism failure and cell death evolving from 6 to 15 hours following the initial insult [26]. Therapy is targeted at this phase of secondary energy failure. The importance of time to initiation of hypothermia on the extent of subsequent brain injury was shown in a series of experiments in the fetal lamb [2–4]. Thus, cooling initiated within 30 minutes of ischaemia in fetal lambs significantly reduced cytotoxic oedema and the extent of neuronal loss [2]. In a subsequent study wherein hypothermia was delayed until 5.5 hours after the primary insult and before the onset of seizures, partial neuroprotection was still demonstrated. However, less uniform effect was seen, particularly within the hippocampus. Cytotoxic oedema as measured by cortical impedance was also decreased, yet there was no prevention of delayed seizures [3]. Finally, when cooling was initiated at 8.5 hours after the onset of post-asphyxial seizures no neuroprotection was observed. This series of observations emphasizes the need to begin treatment early during the latent phase, before the onset of secondary injury [4].

## Early identification of high-risk infants

### Assessment during labour

The goal is to identify those high-risk infants who have been subjected to an intrapartum insult sufficient enough to interrupt placental blood flow with subsequent compromise to CBF and oxygen delivery. Thus, the first step in the process of early identification is to have evidence of a significant event during labour such as placental abruption, cord prolapse and/or significant fetal heart rate abnormalities. Regarding the latter, there is now a near four-decade experience with intensive fetal heart rate monitoring. While it was initially postulated that monitoring would reduce brain injury, and indeed the incidence of neonatal seizures was reduced in a large randomized study, the impact on subsequent neurologic and cognitive outcome has been minimal [27,28]. Similarly, while meconium-stained liquor occurs in approximately one out of seven pregnancies [29] and particularly when thick is considered to reflect *in utero* stress, it is rarely associated with subsequent neonatal brain injury. This should not be surprising since neither marker provides insight into the duration of the insult and/or the fetal adaptive abilities to maintain CBF and oxygen delivery. However, when associated with subsequent cardio-respiratory depression in the delivery room, the potential risk for subsequent brain injury is increased [30,31].

### Acid–base status in the delivery room

The fetus produces two types of acids, carbonic and non-carbonic acid. Carbonic acid is formed by the oxidative metabolism of carbon dioxide by hydration which is rapidly cleared by the placenta. This elimination is related to placental blood flow. Non-carbonic acid, such as lactate and ketone bodies, results primarily from anaerobic metabolism as occurs after hypoxia–ischaemia. This type of acid tends to increase at a slower rate causing a sustained decrease in pH, and, therefore, becomes more clinically relevant as it reflects the duration of a prior asphyxial insult [32]. Experimental data from Dawes *et al* demonstrated that, upon dividing the umbilical cord, when the arterial pH was >7.17, asphyxiated fetal rhesus monkeys were able to initially maintain rhythmic respirations followed by apnoea and gasping respirations. By contrast, when the arterial pH was <7.14, there was not an onset of rhythmic respiration, rather the monkey progressed directly to gasping and was only able to do so for a significantly shorter period of time before taking a last gasp [33]. These data suggest that acidaemic infants have less ability to adapt during labour and/or in the delivery room. Translating these observations to the neonate, fetal acidaemia had originally been defined as an umbilical arterial pH < 7.2. However, the majority of infants in this group were unaffected at birth, without obvious

sequelae. Goldaber *et al* suggested a cut-off of an umbilical arterial pH <7.00 to be more predictive of adverse outcome. Such infants were noted to have low Apgar scores, defined as <3 at 1 and 5 minutes, as well as increased occurrence of death and unexplained seizures [7]. The American College of Obstetricians and Gynecologists Task Force on Neonatal Encephalopathy and Cerebral Palsy, in collaboration with the American Academy of Pediatrics, considers a pH < 7.00 as reflective of pathologic or severe fetal acidaemia [8]. This concept is supported by a study in which 20/47 acidaemic infants, defined as umbilical arterial pH < 7.00, required oxygen administration, or bag-mask ventilation in the delivery room and 22/47 required intubation and ventilation. Only 5/47 did not require any intervention [10]. Importantly, a small number of infants (n = 8) developed encephalopathy including seizures. These infants were 234 times more likely to require cardiopulmonary resuscitation in the delivery room as opposed to those infants with severe fetal acidaemia without seizures. This is consistent with a maladaptive response to asphyxia as seen in the Dawes model [33]. Clearly, the presence of severe fetal acidaemia, while a distinctive marker of stress, in and of itself does not provide insight with regard to the fetal adaptive ability to maintain cerebral perfusion. The coupling of severe fetal acidosis, with subsequent intensive delivery room resuscitation, provides early objective evidence of a severe intrapartum insult with compromise to cerebral perfusion and oxygen delivery.

### Postnatal acid–base status

There is increasing evidence that early postnatal metabolic acidosis is associated with an increased risk for neurodevelopmental deficits at long-term follow-up. Thus, in a retrospective review of 35 term infants with HIE, an initial base deficit ≥20 mmol/L obtained within 30 minutes of life before correction with sodium bicarbonate had a predictive value of 94% for death or severe disability at 18 months [34]. Moreover, in a secondary analysis of data from the multicentre whole body cooling study, one of the most influential predictor variables for death/disability was a base deficit >22 mmol/L in the first postnatal gas [35]. Finally, in a recent report of infants treated with selective head cooling, those infants with the more severe deficits could be distinguished from infants with a normal outcome by the presence of a severe metabolic acidosis, i.e., pH < 7.00, observed within the first hour following delivery [36].

## Cardiopulmonary resuscitation

Several studies have also demonstrated an increased risk of adverse outcome with a longer need for resuscitation. Thus, in a study of 178 infants with post-asphyxial HIE, there was an increased risk of severe adverse outcome, defined as death or major neurosensory impairment, with delayed onset of breathing. The risk was 42% for infants with first breath at 1–9 minutes, 56% at 10–19 minutes and 88% at >20 minutes [30]. In addition, the need for chest compressions was one of three most important variables predicting adverse outcome, along with seizures at <4 hours and delayed onset of breathing [30]. In another study from the same investigators of 375 infants with post-asphyxial HIE, the three most significant predictors of outcome were need for chest compressions >1 minute, onset of respiration >30 minutes and base deficit >16 meq/L [31]. The rate for severe adverse outcome was 46% without any predictors, 64% with one predictor, 76% with two predictors and 93% with all three predictors. Administration of chest compressions >1 minute produced an odds ratio of 3.24 (95% confidence interval [CI]: 1.44–7.32) and epinephrine an odds ratio (OR) of 2.64 (95% CI: 1.03–6.75) [31]. The placement of an endotracheal tube and the administration of positive pressure ventilation has been demonstrated to be a significant predictor of outcome. When assessed in combination with other high-risk markers, i.e., low cord pH and/or low 5-minute Apgar score, the need for intubation produced the highest odds ratios for subsequent encephalopathy and seizures [9]. This increased risk for adverse outcome with intubation was again demonstrated in a study assessing short-term neurologic outcomes, such as death due to severe encephalopathy, or evidence of moderate to severe encephalopathy with or without seizures, in a group of term acidaemic infants (umbilical arterial pH < 7.00). The need for intubation with or without cardiopulmonary resuscitation (CPR) provided an OR of 4.7 (95% CI: 4.7–17.9) for adverse outcomes [37].

## Apgar scores

In many studies, the Apgar score has been used as a major criterion for the diagnosis of birth asphyxia; however, its use as an isolated criterion to define this state is inappropriate [38]. The Task Force on Neonatal Encephalopathy and Cerebral Palsy supports ACOG in defining an Apgar score of 0–3 *beyond*

5 minutes to be a potential marker of intrapartum asphyxia [8]. In a retrospective cohort, the value of the Apgar scores and umbilical arterial pH as the best predictor of neonatal death was assessed [39]. A mortality rate of 244 per 1000 in term infants with a 5-minute Apgar of 0–3 was noted, whereas it was 0.2 per 1000 for infants with 5-minute score of 7–10. The risk of neonatal death was higher in infants with an umbilical artery pH <7.0 and Apgar of 0–3 at 5 minutes [39]. A persistently low Apgar score at 5, 10, or 20 minutes despite resuscitation is associated with increasing mortality and morbidity [40]. In a recent secondary analysis of infants enrolled in a multi-centre hypothermia trial, a 10-minute Apgar score was found to be useful in determining risk of death or disability at 18–22 months. Thus, 65% of infants with an Apgar score ≤4 suffered this outcome as compared with 30% for those with a higher score. This remained significant both with and without adjustment for treatment with hypothermia. Each point decrease in the Apgar score was associated with a 45% increase in the odds of death or disability [41].

## Combination of peripartum markers

The cumulative above data clearly indicate that a combination of markers is critical to the early identification, i.e. within the first postnatal hour, of infants who are at highest risk for progression to moderate to severe encephalopathy. These markers have become integral to the enrollment criteria for candidate infants for hypothermia.

# Postnatal markers

### Role of amplitude-integrated electroencephalogram (aEEG)

Since the 1980s, the cerebral function monitor (CFM), a simplified EEG also known as the aEEG, has come into more widespread use. Its ease of application, even by clinicians caring for the patient, allows availability at any time [42]. The aEEG is a single-channel EEG generated from two biparietal electrodes. Frequencies <2 Hz and >15 Hz are filtered, rectified, smoothed and amplitude integrated before tracing at paper speed of 6 cm/hr [43,44]. The aEEG can then be categorized as normal amplitude (upper margin of aEEG activity >10 µV and lower margin >5 µV), moderately abnormal (upper margin >10 µV and lower margin ≤5 µV) and finally suppressed (upper margin <10 µV and lower margin <5 μV) [44]. The aEEG has been especially useful in predicting neurodevelopmental outcome [43–48]. Early studies have demonstrated a good correlation between initial cerebral function monitoring (CFM) recording and EEG in infants with severe asphyxia [45]. In an initial study of 47 infants meeting criteria for birth asphyxia within 6 hours of life, the prognostic efficiency of amplitude EEG was found to be higher in the first 6 hours as compared to the initial 3 hours. Additionally, repetitive seizures within the first 6 hours were significantly associated with poor outcome. Importantly, 86% of infants with an abnormal background at 6 hours had a poor outcome and continuous normal voltage at 6 hours was almost always a good prognostic indicator [43]. This finding has been supported in another study of 73 term asphyxiated infants where an abnormal background at 3 hours after birth had a positive predictive value (PPV) of 78% and a negative predictive value (NPV) of 84% in those who progressed to an abnormal outcome. At 6 hours, the PPV increased to 86% and NPV to 91% [47]. In another study the presence of burst suppression, continuous low voltage, epileptic activity, status epilepticus or a flat tracing from 0 to 6 hours had a likelihood ratio of 2.7 for adverse outcome [48]. Similarly, in a study of 56 infants >35 weeks with neonatal encephalopathy, no infant with a suppressed EEG had a normal outcome. The sensitivity and specificity for poor outcome in infants with an abnormal aEEG was 93% and 70% respectively [44]. Cerebral function monitoring has been compared to other modalities, including cranial ultrasound, resistance index (RI) by Doppler ultrasound of the middle cerebral artery, somatosensory evoked potentials (SEPs) and visual evoked potentials (VEPs) obtained within 6 hours of birth. The CFM has been shown to have the highest positive predictive value (84.2%) and negative predictive value (91.7%) compared with these other techniques in predicting development of encephalopathy and subsequent neurologic sequelae [46]. In a study comparing an early neurologic examination with an abnormal aEEG tracing in predicting short-term neurologic outcome, defined as persistence of moderate/severe encephalopathy beyond 5 days of age, or death in the first week of life attributable to hypoxic–ischaemic cerebral injury, the aEEG was found to be more specific with a greater PPV compared to the neurologic examination. The aEEG coupled with an early neurologic examination produced the highest specificity (94%) and PPV (85%) [49]. This finding emphasizes the importance of combining the two methods rather than using either the aEEG or the clinical examination in isolation. The more recent versions of the aEEG monitor provide a window to visualize a single or dual raw EEG tracing. This has become important given that in a recent report it has been shown that artefact, i.e., motion or electrical interference, may contribute to an indeterminate or a potentially incorrect interpretation of the integrated tracing [50,51] (Figure 8.1). Under such circumstances the clinical examination may become the preferred or only method for enrollment.

## Hypothermia trials and the aEEG

The aEEG was used for entry criteria in the CoolCap trial of selective head cooling with mild systemic hypothermia, as well as a marker of outcome [21]. Selective head cooling was found to decrease the risk of death or severe neurodevelopmental disability at 18 months in infants with moderately suppressed background (upper margin >10 μV and lower <5 μV). However, infants with a severely suppressed background (upper margin <10 μV) and/or who exhibited aEEG seizures upon enrollment did not derive consistent benefit from cooling [21]. The Total Body Hypothermia for Neonatal Encephalopathy (TOBY) trial revealed similar findings. Thus more infants with a severely abnormal aEEG died or had a severe disability compared to those with a moderately abnormal aEEG [23].

### Clinical examination

The Sarnat staging has been the preferred method of assessing encephalopathy. This staging of encephalopathy, initially described by Sarnat and Sarnat in 1976, indicated that infants with evolving Stage 2 or Stage 3 encephalopathy over the first days of life were at increased risk for neurologic impairment or death. Stage 2 encephalopathy was characterized by obtundation, hypotonia, strong distal flexion and multifocal seizures and Stage 3 by stupor, flaccidity and suppression of brainstem and autonomic function [52]. The usefulness of Sarnat staging in predicting outcome was demonstrated in a study of 49 infants with HIE. Thus all infants with Stage 1 encephalopathy were normal when followed up at 27 months, approximately 25% of those infants with stage 2 encephalopathy exhibited mild or moderate handicap and the one infant with stage 3 encephalopathy suffered from a moderate

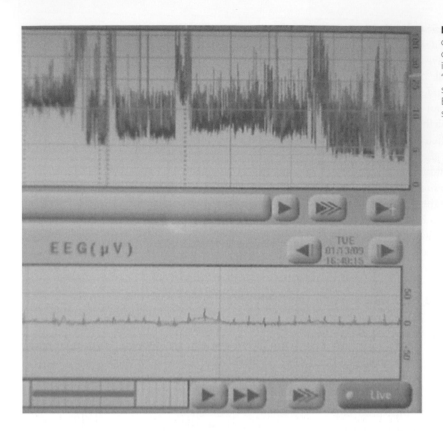

**Figure 8.1.** aEEG tracing obtained from occipito-parietal elctrodes from a comatose unresponsive infant. Note the initial part of the tracing would fall in the "normal range". The narrow band suggest some interference. The corresponding raw EEG tracing shows an EKG signal. Please see plate section for colour version.

handicap [53]. Infants in Sarnat stage 2 or 3 encephalopathy within the first 6 hours of life are considered candidates for treatment with therapeutic hypothermia. Importantly, this assessment of moderate or severe encephalopathy so early in the course of treatment is strongly suggestive of a more severe insult than described in the Sarnats' original report and represents the group of infants who are most likely to benefit from therapeutic hypothermia. The clinical examination as a postnatal marker for eligibility was used in the NICHD trial of whole body hypothermia [22]. Infants were considered candidates if moderate or severe encephalopathy or seizures were present. Moderate or severe encephalopathy was defined as one or more abnormalities in at least three of six categories, including level of consciousness, spontaneous activity, posture, tone, primitive reflexes and autonomic system changes. Death or moderate–severe disability at 18–22 months of age occurred in 44% in the hypothermia group and 62% in the control group. The increase in survival in the cooled group was not accompanied by an increased risk of moderate–severe disability at 18–22 months in infants treated with hypothermia. This addresses the concern for decreasing mortality of infants at high risk for death and disability [22]. The TOBY trial used both the degree of encephalopathy and aEEG abnormalities for enrolment criteria. Infants had to demonstrate evidence of moderate–severe encephalopathy as well as abnormal aEEG background of 30 minutes duration or seizures. Primary outcome of this study was death or severe disability at 18 months. Infants in the cooled group had an increased rate of survival without neurologic disability and a decreased rate of cerebral palsy [23].

## Summary of the selection criteria of infants utilized in the hypothermia studies

Hypothermia ought to be considered in any infant ≥35 weeks' gestation within the first postnatal hour with at least two or more of the following: (1) history of a sentinel event during labour; (2) Apgar score ≤5 at 10 minutes as reflected by a continued need for resuscitation at this time; (3) acidosis defined as cord arterial pH < 7.00 or a postnatal arterial blood gas obtained within the first hour of life with pH < 7.00; (4) base

≥ 36 weeks and two or more of the following

- Sentinel event during labour
- Apgar score ≤5 at 10 minutes reflected by continued need for resuscitation
- Acidosis with umbilical cord arterial pH<7.00 *or* any arterial pH<7.00 within 60 minutes of birth
- Base deficit ≥ – 16 mmol/L in umbilical cord sample *or* any sample obtained within 60 minutes of birth (arterial or venous)

Amplitude EEG with moderate to severe encephalopathy or seizures

Sarnat Stage 2 or 3 encephalopathy

- Stage 2: obtundation, hypotonia, strong distal flexion, and multifocal seizures
- Stage 3: stupor, flaccidity, and suppression of brainstem and autonomic function

**Figure 8.2.** Suggested selection criteria for therapeutic hypothermia: must be initiated within 6 hours of life.

deficit ≥ –16 mmol/L in umbilical cord blood sample or a postnatal sample obtained within 1 hour of life (arterial or venous). An aEEG should demonstrate evidence of moderate to severe encephalopathy or seizures [43–48]. Clinical examination should also be used to guide the decision to cool infants in Sarnat stage 2 or 3 encephalopathy [52,53]. Amplitude EEG and clinical examination used together are a powerful guide in the decision tree to cool [49]. Cooling must be initiated within 6 hours of life (Figure 8.2).

## Gaps in knowledge

In all of the large studies, including our own experience, hypothermia is usually initiated late at approximately 4.5 hours of age [21–24,51]. It remains unclear why there is a relatively protracted period between delivery and time to initiation of therapeutic hypothermia given that high-risk infants often can be initially identified as early as in the delivery room. Survival from cardiac arrest in adults depends on a series of critical interventions termed the "Chain of Survival" [54]. This educational metaphor emphasizes the time-sensitive, sequential actions of early activation of emergency medical services. These actions, including early cardiopulmonary resuscitation and early post-resuscitation advanced life support, have increased intact neurologic survival in adults from 6% to 16% in one population-based study even in the absence of post-resuscitation hypothermia [55]. Because in the neonate it is not survival, but rather early neuroprotection that may improve outcome,

we suggest the modified term "Chain of Brain Preservation" be applied to the delivery room setting so as to improve upon the time-sensitive response in neonates at high risk for evolving brain injury [36]. Since many infants are outborn, educational programmes need to emphasize having skilled providers in the delivery room capable of initiating effective ventilation and intensive resuscitation as indicated (Chain 1). For those depressed babies requiring resuscitation, early activation of a centre capable of providing advanced post-resuscitation care including hypothermia should be undertaken as early as in the delivery room (Chain 2). It is also essential to assess for additional risk factors that may exacerbate ongoing brain injury following hypoxia–ischaemia even before the initiation of cooling including hypoglycaemia, hyperthermia or severe postnatal acidosis. Thus, in a group of infants with severe fetal acidaemia (cord pH <7.00) who received intensive resuscitation including CPR, a blood glucose ≤40 was the strongest predictor of abnormal outcome by multivariate analysis [37]. Additionally, an elevated temperature may exacerbate brain injury in the setting of neonatal hypoxia–ischaemia. In the rat pup model assessing damage following hypoxic–ischaemic seizures, prevention of hyperthermia caused a significant decrease in neuronal damage compared to controls [56]. Indeed in two of the multicentre studies, an elevated temperature before enrollment was an independent risk factor for adverse outcome, with pyrexia defined as ≥38°C in one study [57,58]. This may have practical relevance to the delivery room where infants are initially managed under a radiant warmer. In the context of infants with early profound postnatal metabolic acidosis and in particular those infants with severe encephalopathy, future studies should examine the potential benefit of not actively warming such infants pending arrival of a transport team, as well as initiating hypothermia during transport (Chain 3).

## Conclusion

Selection of the infant appropriate for cooling must be an efficient and thoughtful process. Utilizing a combination of markers has become a powerful determinant of those infants at highest risk for subsequent ongoing cerebral damage. The amplitude EEG is an important tool in assessing cerebral function; however, it must be interpreted with caution in the presence of artefact. Under such circumstances, the clinical examination may be the preferred method of assessing encephalopathy. Early initiation of hypothermia, particularly in those infants with severe encephalopathy, coupled with novel interventions may open up additional avenues of opportunity to reduce long-term morbidity still further in the subgroup of already high-risk infants.

## References

1. Perlman JM. Summary proceedings from the neurology group on hypoxic-ischemic encephalopathy. *Pediatrics* 2006;**117**(Pt 2):S28–33.

2. Gunn AJ, Gunn TR, de Haan HH, Williams CE, Gluckman PD. Dramatic neuronal rescue with prolonged selective head cooling after ischemia in fetal lambs. *J Clin Invest* 1997;**99**:248–56.

3. Gunn AJ, Gunn TR, Gunning MI, Williams CE, Gluckman PD. Neuroprotection with prolonged head cooling started before postischemic seizures in fetal sheep. *Pediatrics* 1998;**102**:1098–106.

4. Gunn AJ, Bennet L, Gunning MI, Gluckman PD, Gunn TR. Cerebral hypothermia is not neuroprotective when started after postischemic seizures in fetal sheep. *Pediatr Res* 1999;**46**:274–80.

5. Karlsson M, Tooley JR, Satas S, et al. Delayed hypothermia as selective head cooling or whole body cooling does not protect brain or body in newborn pig subjected to hypoxia-ischemia. *Pediatr Res* 2008;**64**:74–8.

6. Stola A, Perlman J. Post-resuscitation strategies to avoid ongoing injury following intrapartum hypoxia-ischemia. *Semin Fetal Neonatal Med* 2008;**13**(6):424–31.

7. Goldaber KG, Gilstrap LC III, Leveno KJ, Dax JS, McIntire DD. Pathologic fetal acidemia. *Obstet Gynecol* 1991;**78**:1103–7.

8. American Academy of Pediatrics ACoOaG, editor. *Neonatal encephalopathy and cerebral palsy: defining the pathogenesis and pathophysiology*. Elk Grove Village, IL: AAP; Washington, DC: ACOG2003.

9. Perlman JM, Risser R. Can asphyxiated infants at risk for neonatal seizures be rapidly identified by current high-risk markers? *Pediatrics* 1996;**97**:456–62.

10. Perlman JM, Risser R. Severe fetal acidemia: neonatal neurologic features and short-term outcome. *Pediatr Neurol* 1993;**9**:277–82.

11. Perlman JM. Brain injury in the term infant. *Semin Perinatol* 2004;**28**:415–24.

12. Peeters LL, Sheldon RE, Jones MD, et al. Blood flow to fetal organs as a function of arterial oxygen content. *Am J Obstet Gynecol* 1979;**135**:637–46.

13. Rurak DW, Richardson BS, Patrick JE, Carmichael L, Homan J. Blood flow and oxygen delivery to fetal organs and tissues during sustained hypoxemia. *Am J Physiol* 1990;**258**(Pt 2):R1116–22.

14. Perlman JM. Intrapartum hypoxic-ischemic cerebral injury and subsequent cerebral palsy: medicolegal issues. *Pediatrics* 1997;**99**:851–9.

15. Johnson GN, Palahniuk RJ, Tweed WA, Jones MV, Wade JG. Regional cerebral blood flow changes during severe fetal asphyxia produced by slow partial umbilical cord compression. *Am J Obstet Gynecol* 1979;**135**:48–52.

16. Volpe JJ. *Neurology of the newborn.* 5th edition. Philadelphia: Saunders/Elsevier; 2008. p. 449.

17. Volpe JJ. *Neurology of the newborn.* 5th edition. Philadelphia: Saunders/Elsevier; 2008. p. 296.

18. Ashwal S, Dale PS, Longo LD. Regional cerebral blood flow: studies in the fetal lamb during hypoxia, hypercapnia, acidosis and hypotension. *Pediatr Res* 1984;**18**:1309–16.

19. Volpe JJ. *Neurology of the newborn.* 5th edition. Philadelphia: Saunders/Elsevier; 2008. p. 596.

20. Wells RJ, Friedman WF, Sobel BE. Increased oxidative metabolism in the fetal and newborn lamb heart. *Am J Physiol* 1972;**222**:1488–93.

21. Gluckman PD, Wyatt JS, Azzopardi D, et al. Selective head cooling with mild systemic hypothermia after neonatal encephalopathy: multicentre randomised trial. *Lancet* 2005;**365**:663–70.

22. Shankaran S, Laptook AR, Ehrenkranz RA, et al. Whole-body hypothermia for neonates with hypoxic-ischemic encephalopathy. *N Engl J Med* 2005;**353**:1574–84.

23. Azzopardi DV, Strohm B, Edwards AD, et al. Moderate hypothermia to treat perinatal asphyxial encephalopathy. *N Engl J Med* 2009;**361**:1349–58.

24. Jacobs SE, Morley CJ, Inder TE, et al. Infant Cooling Evaluation Collaboration. Whole-body hypothermia for term and near-term newborns with hypoxic-ischemic encephalopathy: a randomized controlled trial. *Arch Pediatr Adolesc Med* 2011;**165**:692–700.

25. Salhab WA, Perlman JM. Severe fetal acidemia and subsequent neonatal encephalopathy in the larger premature infant. *Pediatr Neurol* 2005;**32**:25–9.

26. Gunn AJ. Cerebral hypothermia for prevention of brain injury following perinatal asphyxia. *Curr Opin Pediatr* 2000;**12**:111–5.

27. Grant A, O'Brien N, Joy MT, Hennessy E, MacDonald D. Cerebral palsy among children born during the Dublin randomised trial of intrapartum monitoring. *Lancet* 1989;**2**:1233–6.

28. Painter MJ, Scott M, Hirsch RP, O'Donoghue P, Depp R. Fetal heart rate patterns during labor: neurologic and cognitive development at six to nine years of age. *Am J Obstet Gynecol* 1988;**159**:854–8.

29. van Ierland Y, de Boer M, de Beaufort AJ. Meconium-stained amniotic fluid: discharge vigorous newborns. *Arch Dis Child Fetal Neonatal Ed* 2010;**95**:F69–71.

30. Ekert P, Perlman M, Steinlin M, Hao Y. Predicting the outcome of postasphyxial hypoxic-ischemic encephalopathy within 4 hours of birth. *J Pediatr* 1997;**131**:613–7.

31. Shah PS, Beyene J, To T, Ohlsson A, Perlman M. Postasphyxial hypoxic-ischemic encephalopathy in neonates: outcome prediction rule within 4 hours of birth. *Arch Pediatr Adolesc Med* 2006;**160**:729–36.

32. Volpe JJ. *Neurology of the newborn*. 5th edition. Philadelphia: Saunders/Elsevier; 2008. p. 337.

33. Dawes GS, Jacobson HN, Mott JC, Shelley HJ, Stafford A. The treatment of asphyxiated, mature foetal lambs and Rhesus monkeys with intravenous glucose and sodium carbonate. *J Physiol* 1963;**169**:167–84.

34. Toh VC. Early predictors of adverse outcome in term infants with post-asphyxial hypoxic ischaemic encephalopathy. *Acta Paediatr* 2000;**89**:343–7.

35. Ambalavanan N, Carlo WA, Shankaran S, et al. Predicting outcomes of neonates diagnosed with hypoxemic-ischemic encephalopathy. *Pediatrics* 2006;**118**:2084–93.

36. Takenouchi T CM, Ross G, Engel M, Perlman JM. Chain of brain preservation-a concept to facilitate early identification and initiation of hypothermia to infants at high risk for brain injury. *Resuscitation* 2010;**81**:1637–41.

37. Salhab WA, Wyckoff MH, Laptook AR, Perlman JM. Initial hypoglycemia and neonatal brain injury in term infants with severe fetal acidemia. *Pediatrics* 2004;**114**:361–6.

38. American Academy of Pediatrics Committee. Fetus and newborn: use and abuse of the Apgar score. *Pediatrics* 1986;**78**:1148–9.

39. Casey BM, McIntire DD, Leveno KJ. The continuing value of the Apgar score for the assessment of newborn infants. *N Engl J Med* 2001;**344**:467–71.

40. Nelson KB, Ellenberg JH. Apgar scores as predictors of chronic neurologic disability. *Pediatrics* 1981;**68**:36–44.

41. Laptook AR, Shankaran S, Ambalavanan N, et al. Outcome of term infants using Apgar scores at 10 minutes following hypoxic-ischemic encephalopathy. *Pediatrics* 2009;**124**:1619–26.

42. Groenendaal F, de Vries LS. Selection of babies for intervention after birth asphyxia. *Semin Neonatol* 2000;**5**:17–32.

43. Hellstrom-Westas L, Rosen I, Svenningsen NW. Predictive value of early continuous amplitude integrated EEG recordings on outcome after severe birth asphyxia in full term infants. *Arch Dis Child Fetal Neonatal Ed* 1995;**72**:F34–8.

44. al Naqeeb N, Edwards AD, Cowan FM, Azzopardi D. Assessment of neonatal encephalopathy by amplitude-integrated electroencephalography. *Pediatrics* 1999;**103**(Pt 1): 1263–71.

45. Bjerre I, Hellstrom-Westas L, Rosen I, Svenningsen N. Monitoring of cerebral function after severe asphyxia in infancy. *Arch Dis Child* 1983;**58**:997–1002.

46. Eken P, Toet MC, Groenendaal F, de Vries LS. Predictive value of early neuroimaging, pulsed Doppler and neurophysiology in full term infants with hypoxic-ischaemic encephalopathy. *Arch Dis Child Fetal Neonatal Ed* 1995;**73**:F75–80.

47. Toet MC, Hellstrom-Westas L, Groenendaal F, Eken P, de Vries LS. Amplitude integrated EEG 3 and 6 hours after birth in full term neonates with hypoxic-ischaemic encephalopathy. *Arch Dis Child Fetal Neonatal Ed* 1999;**81**:F19–23.

48. ter Horst HJ, Sommer C, Bergman KA, et al. Prognostic significance of amplitude-integrated EEG during the first 72 hours after birth in severely asphyxiated neonates. *Pediatr Res* 2004;**55**:1026–33.

49. Shalak LF, Laptook AR, Velaphi SC, Perlman JM. Amplitude-integrated electroencephalography coupled with an early neurologic examination

enhances prediction of term infants at risk for persistent encephalopathy. *Pediatrics* 2003;**111**:351–7.

50. Suk D, Krauss AN, Engel M, Perlman JM. Amplitude-integrated electroencephalography in the NICU: frequent artifacts in premature infants may limit its utility as a monitoring device. *Pediatrics* 2009;**123**:e328–32.

51. Yap V, Engel M, Takenouchi T, Perlman JM. Seizures are common in term infants undergoing head cooling. *Pediatr Neurol* 2009;**41**:327–31.

52. Sarnat HB, Sarnat MS. Neonatal encephalopathy following fetal distress. A clinical and electroencephalographic study. *Arch Neurol* 1976;**33**:696–705.

53. Finer NN, Robertson CM, Peters KL, Coward JH. Factors affecting outcome in hypoxic-ischemic encephalopathy in term infants. *Am J Dis Child* 1983;**137**:21–5.

54. Guidelines 2000 for Cardiopulmonary Resuscitation and Emergency Cardiovascular Care. Part 12: from science to survival: strengthening the chain of survival in every community. The American Heart Association in collaboration with the International Liaison Committee on Resuscitation. *Circulation* 2000;**102**(Suppl):I358–70.

55. Iwami T, Nichol G, Hiraide A, et al. Continuous improvements in "chain of survival" increased survival after out-of-hospital cardiac arrests: a large-scale population-based study. *Circulation* 2009;**119**:728–34.

56. Yager JY, Armstrong EA, Jaharus C, Saucier DM, Wirrell EC. Preventing hyperthermia decreases brain damage following neonatal hypoxic-ischemic seizures. *Brain Res* 2004;**1011**:48–57.

57. Laptook A, Tyson J, Shankaran S, et al. Elevated temperature after hypoxic-ischemic encephalopathy: risk factor for adverse outcomes. *Pediatrics* 2008;**122**:491–9.

58. Wyatt JS, Gluckman PD, Liu PY, et al. Determinants of outcomes after head cooling for neonatal encephalopathy. *Pediatrics* 2007;**119**:912–21.

# Hypothermia during patient transport

Susan E. Jacobs

## Introduction

Therapeutic hypothermia is part of standard care for term and near-term newborn infants with moderate-to-severe hypoxic–ischaemic encephalopathy (HIE) in neonatal intensive care units (NICU) with the expertise, equipment, education, training and protocols to provide this treatment (cooling treatment centres) [1–5]. The safe implementation of hypothermia treatment is being monitored and supported by data from international newborn encephalopathy registries [6–8].

For maximal neuroprotective benefit, therapeutic hypothermia must commence as soon as possible after the hypoxic-ischaemic insult and within the 6-hour "window of opportunity", before the onset of seizures and secondary neuronal injury [9,10]. Neuroprotective effect rapidly declines with delayed initiation of hypothermia treatment [9,11].

Randomized controlled trials (RCT) in term newborn infants with HIE assumed that the insult occurred at the time of birth and initiated hypothermia by 6 hours of age [6,12–17]. Standard thermoregulatory management was maintained until infants were assessed for eligibility, informed parental consent was obtained and randomization occurred; consequently hypothermia treatment was delayed until 4 to 5 hours postnatal age.

Most term infants with moderate-to-severe HIE are born unexpectedly in community, non-tertiary settings, or in NICUs without expertise in therapeutic hypothermia. Following resuscitation and pre-transport stabilization, they are transferred by dedicated neonatal transport teams to the regional cooling treatment centre for ongoing management. Many of these infants will not arrive at the NICU until after 6 hours of age [18], highlighting the need to start hypothermia therapy at the referring hospital before and during transport to the cooling treatment centre [14,19,20].

Regionalized perinatal care is resource efficient, inexpensive and integral to the commencement of hypothermia treatment at referring hospitals and during transport to cooling treatment centres [21]. This includes multidisciplinary collaboration with the regional cooling treatment centre to develop evidence-based referring hospital and transport hypothermia protocols, to ensure equipment availability and with ongoing outreach and transport team support, education and training [22,23]. Whole body therapeutic hypothermia can be initiated during transport as much as 3 to 4.6 hours earlier than if delayed until arrival at the cooling treatment centre [7,20,24].

## Approaches to cooling during transport (methods and techniques)

Target core (rectal or oesophageal) temperature can be reached and maintained with manually adjusted hypothermia devices, passive cooling techniques and servo-controlled systems during therapeutic hypothermia. Individual infant response to hypothermia is variable, related to birth weight, severity of encephalopathy and seizures, anticonvulsant, sedative and muscle relaxant medications and the environment, including incubator or open cot [25–28].

Hypothermia is a normal adaptive response following a perinatal hypoxic–ischaemic insult. The rectal temperature of asphyxiated newborn infants, without any respiratory effort for the first 3 minutes, decreases to around 34.5°C within 2 hours of birth and is at least 1.5°C lower than healthy infants for the first 20 hours of life [29,30]. Dried and wrapped healthy term newborns' rectal temperature decreases from 37.5°C to 36.0°C within 30 minutes of birth [31]. These observations form the basis of a controlled passive, physiological

*Neonatal Neural Rescue*, ed. A. David Edwards, Denis V. Azzopardi and Alistair J. Gunn. Published by Cambridge University Press. © Cambridge University Press 2013.

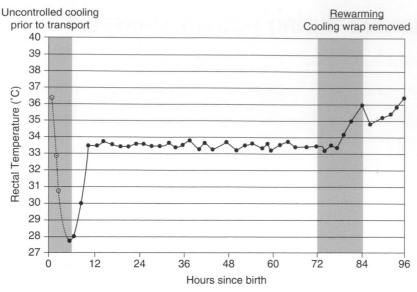

**Figure 9.1.** Overcooling of a term newborn to 27.7°C during passive cooling without rectal temperature monitoring until arrival at cooling treatment centre. Open symbols represent axillary temperature. GA, gestational age; HR, heart rate; Hb, haemoglobin. Reproduced, with permission, from Thoresen [27].

42 wk GA, Apgar 0,0,0,4, HR by 16 min, lactate 24 at birth, cord pH 6.84 meconium aspirated, Hb 9.0, antepartum haemorrhage. 100% $O_2$, $N_2O$ during transport. Low $PCO_2$

approach to induce hypothermia in term and near-term newborns with HIE.

Passive hypothermia allows the baby to cool naturally at ambient environmental temperature by removing all external heat sources (undressed with the overhead radiant warmer or incubator turned off) to facilitate radiant, convective and evaporative heat losses. However, the variable responses to cooling can result in overshoot below the target temperature, particularly during induction of hypothermia, further exacerbated if passive cooling is either unlimited [26] or uncontrolled by continuous core temperature monitoring, shown in Figure 9.1 [7,23,24,27].

Controlled passive cooling is adjusted according to the target core temperature monitored continuously, with the addition of low-technology devices, such as refrigerated [14] or frozen [23,32,33] gel packs and fans [7,34,35], to "actively" lower the infant's core temperature to and maintain it within the target range.

All manually adjusted cooling techniques and devices, including the controlled passive techniques listed above or commercially available water mattresses, are nursing intensive. They require 1:1 care to observe the temperature and to make frequent adjustments to either the thermostat or to apply the gel packs. Variability in individual responses to cooling and response lags to these adjustments result in

frequent overshoot below the therapeutic target in manually adjusted cooling devices and techniques, most evident during induction of hypothermia. Temperature variability is less with servo-controlled systems, which are less demanding on nursing care [8,36]. During the 1- to 5-hour induction phase, the mean (95% CI) of the averaged rectal temperature was 33.4°C (32.5 to 34.3°C) if manually adjusted, compared with much tighter limits of 33.5°C (33.4 to 33.7°C) if servo-controlled [8]. Similarly, the rectal temperature was within 0.5°C of the target for 97% of the time in infants cooled with the CritiCool (MTRE, Charter Kontron, Milton Keynes, UK) servo-controlled system, compared with 81% with the Tecotherm (Tecotherm, TSMed 200M, Tec-Com, Luebeck, Germany) manually adjusted total body cooling system, 76% with the CoolCap selective head cooling with mild systemic hypothermia (Olympic Medical Cool Care System, Olympic medical, Seattle, WA, USA) system and 74% in infants cooled with water-filled gloves [36]. Improved temperature control with servo-controlled devices has been demonstrated in a small number of neonatal transports [37–39].

Other lower technology cooling devices that have been trialled in low-resource settings to induce whole body cooling are water bottles and a phase changing material mattress (PCM) with a 32°C melting point [30,40,41]. The water-bottle technique requires constant tap water temperature of 25°C together with a similar, stable environmental temperature, neither of which is available in transport [20]. The PCM was used in a pilot RCT in south India, with a median (IQR) hypothermia induction time of 35 [10,80] minutes in 10 randomized infants with HIE [41]. This technology has not been assessed during transport.

Therefore, the ideal cooling system would rapidly induce hypothermia to the core target temperature, without overshoot and with minimal fluctuation during the maintenance phase of cooling. It would be automated, servo-controlled, with appropriate safety features and easy to use, thereby minimizing the nursing input required [7,36]. Neonatal retrieval and transport also demands that the device be light, mobile and transferrable both physically and with respect to power requirements between different transport platforms and referring hospitals, and able to be adequately and safely secured in each of these platforms in transport. Whilst the vast majority of transports in the United Kingdom and United States are by road, this is not the case in Australia, New Zealand and Canada. For example, of the 1149 primary retrievals performed in 2009 in Australia by the Victorian Newborn Emergency Transport Service, 141 (12%) were by fixed-wing, 72 (6%) by rotary-wing and 936 (82%) by road (personal communication Dr M. Stewart, Director NETS Victoria). Whilst some transport services have adapted the Criticool servo-control system (weighing 35 kg, without 1–4 litres of water) [37–39], no such purpose-built cooling device is currently available for use during neonatal retrieval and transport.

# Transport data from major randomized controlled trials

Between 45% and 79% of term and near-term newborns with moderate-to-severe HIE enrolled in RCTs of therapeutic hypothermia were outborn in non-participating centres [12,14–17]. However, many limited the commencement of cooling until after admission to the participating NICU [13,15–17]. In some, the transport team started hypothermia treatment at the referring hospital of birth and continued it during transport to the NICU [6,14,32].

Predominantly outborn infants transported to participating NICUs were enrolled in Eicher's pilot RCT [49/65 (75%)] [12,32]. Whole body hypothermia was induced with plastic bags filled with ice wrapped in a washcloth applied to the head in those allocated to hypothermia. In the 26 outborn infants randomized to hypothermia treatment, the transport team initiated cooling at the referring hospital. There was no significant difference in the median (range) time to reach the target rectal temperature of 33 ± 0.5°C between outborn and inborn infants [80 (30–300) vs. 142 (49–300) minutes, $P = 0.2$]. However, mortality was significantly higher in outborn infants with HIE than in those inborn in a participating NICU [22/49 (45%) vs. 1/14 (7%), $P = 0.007$; odds ratio 10.7; 95% confidence intervals 1.3, 90, $P = 0.03$].

Recruitment of infants with HIE born outside participating NICUs in the Total Body Hypothermia for Neonatal Encephalopathy (TOBY) trial occurred in one of two ways [42,43]. If infants could be transferred to the participating NICU within 3 hours of birth, then standard rectal temperature (37 ± 0.2°C) was maintained during the transfer, with infants assessed for eligibility and randomized after admission to the participating NICU. If this was not possible, then trained transport teams assessed infants for eligibility at the referring hospital, including amplitude-integrated electroencephalography (aEEG), obtained parental consent, randomized the infants and then commenced the allocated intervention. Before transfer, infants assigned to cooling were nursed with the overhead radiant warmer turned off. During transport, the transport incubator heater was adjusted and "cooled" gel packs applied around the infant as needed to maintain the rectal temperature between 33.0 and 34.0°C. The method of cooling and temperature of the gel packs is not described. Further information regarding the outborn infants transport in the TOBY trial has not been reported.

The pragmatic Infant Cooling Evaluation (ICE) trial initiated a simple, inexpensive method of whole body hypothermia to 33.5°C for 72 hours at the referring hospital of birth and before 6 hours of age [14]. A secondary aim of the ICE trial was to determine the safety of dedicated retrieval teams initiating therapeutic hypothermia during retrieval and transport for outborn infants. Potentially eligible outborn infants were identified at the time of referral to the participating centre or regional neonatal transport service. Trained retrieval teams then assessed the infant for eligibility at the referring hospital, where they obtained parental consent, randomized the infant and commenced the assigned treatment and monitoring which was continued during transport to the participating NICU.

Treatment and monitoring were exactly the same for inborn and outborn infants in the ICE trial. All infants had their core temperature measured continuously by a disposable thermistor inserted at least 5 cm into the rectum. Controlled whole body hypothermia to the target core temperature of 33.5°C (range, 33–34°C) was achieved by turning the overhead radiant warmer (or transport incubator) off and exposing the infant to the ambient environmental temperature. Two covered refrigerated gel packs at around 10°C were applied across the chest and/or under the head and shoulders if the temperature was above 35.5°C at induction of hypothermia and sequentially removed when the core temperature fell below 35°C and then 34.5°C. The radiant warmer heater output (or transport incubator) was manually adjusted every 15–30 minutes if the core temperature fell below 33.5°C.

One hundred and thirty-four (60%) infants enrolled in the ICE trial were outborn, with 42 inborn and 68 outborn infants assigned to hypothermia treatment. Eighty-five percent of infants allocated to hypothermia were treated with gel packs during the 6-hour induction phase of hypothermia, without any significant difference in core temperature between inborn and outborn infants, shown in Figure 9.2. However, temperature overshoot below 33.0°C was frequent, occurring in 56% of cooled infants, similar to the other trials that used manually adjusted cooling devices during transport [6] and in the NICU [6,15].

There were no significant interactions between therapeutic hypothermia and outborn status ($P = 0.85$), or between hypothermia and age at randomization ($P = 0.22$). Adverse effects of hypothermia were minimal and did not differ significantly between the inborn and outborn cooled infants.

The ICE methodology has been used to develop guidelines for regional referring hospitals whilst awaiting retrieval and transport to the hypothermia treatment centre and for the transport services [44].

# Experience of commencing hypothermia during transport following clinical trials

There are nine implementation reports of commencement of cooling at the birth hospital and during transport to the tertiary NICU [7,20,23–26,37–39].

Anderson et al reported commencing passive cooling by referring hospital staff under guidance of the transport team consultant in two infants with peripartum hypoxia–ischaemia considered at risk of encephalopathy [25]. Referring staff decreased the control point on the radiant warmer to 35°C in one infant, with a fall in temperature to 36.6°C at 2 hours of age; the transport team then turned off the radiant warmer and the infant's temperature was 33.4°C on arrival at the NICU at 4.75 hours of age. The radiant warmer was turned off when the second infant was 30 minutes old, with a reduction in temperature to

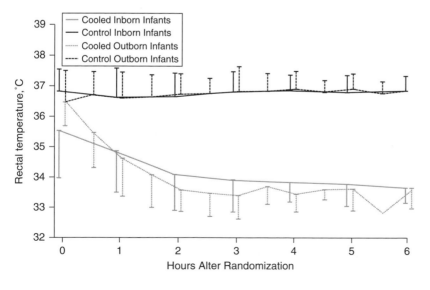

**Figure 9.2.** Temperature (°C) during transport and the 6 hour initiation of intervention period by birth hospital status [14]. Inborn infants were managed in participating neonatal intensive care units (NICUs) and outborn infants were born in non-tertiary settings and transported to participating NICUs. The error bars indicate 1 SD. Reproduced, with permission, from Jacobs [14].

34.3°C at 2 hours of age; the infant's temperature did not reach the target range during transport, but did with active cooling in the NICU.

Safety of initiating cooling at the referring hospital of birth and during transport was explored in a regional cohort of 34 infants who met the Swedish national guidelines for hypothermia treatment following perinatal asphyxia born between December 2006 and April 2008 [26]. At the tertiary hypothermia centres, cooling was initiated and maintained in all infants (inborn and outborn) by the Tecotherm mattress. Referring staff at the birth hospital were advised to passively cool the 18 (53%) outborn infants by stopping all active warming, not limited by the reduction in the infants' temperature. Eight (44%) were normothermic (rectal temperature 35.0–36.9°C), four (22%) were therapeutic (33.0–34.9°C) and six (33%) were sub-therapeutic (below 33.0°C) when the transport team arrived at the referring hospital. The earlier after birth that passive cooling started, the more severe the encephalopathy, ventilation (without humidification and warming), and the lower the birth weight, the more likely the temperature was to be below 33.0°C; outside temperature at transport and infants' rectal admission temperatures were not associated with overcooling. Three of the four deaths were in outborn infants.

Between March 2005 and February 2009, 40 (80%) of 50 newborns with HIE treated with hypothermia at the University of Virginia regional hypothermia NICU were outborn [22–24]. Referring clinicians were trained to not warm infants of 36 weeks' gestation or more with suspected moderate-to-severe HIE by turning off the radiant warmer, to measure rectal temperature every 15 minutes and to consult the on-call neonatologist early. The referring NICU or transport team then commenced continuous rectal temperature monitoring and active cooling with wrapped disposable gel packs around 10°C placed next to the infant's trunk and head until the rectal temperature was below 34.0°C, with the target rectal temperature of 33.0–34.0°C reached within 1 hour. Infants were transferred in a room temperature transport incubator, increasing the air temperature if the infant's temperature was below 33.0°C with a blanket applied. Cool gel packs were reapplied if the rectal temperature was above 34.0°C and warm gel packs if below 31.0°C during transport.

Of the 50 infants treated with hypothermia at the University of Virginia, 10 inborn infants and 5

transported infants were assessed and commenced hypothermia in the NICU. Twenty-five outborn infants had passive cooling alone and 10 infants in outlying NICUs had both passive and active cooling initiated by referring clinicians, such that 35 of the 40 outborn infants were cooled during transport. The transport team arrived at the referring hospital at mean (± SD) 2.9 ± 1.4 hours of age, with the 10 actively cooled infants' mean (± SD) temperature 33.9 ± 2.1°C, the 25 passively cooled infants 34.4 ± 1.9°C and the 5 not cooled 36.6 ± 0.3°C. The 10 inborn infants' rectal temperature was below 34°C at 2.6 ± 1.8 hours postnatal age, the 35 cooled during transport 3.9 ± 1.6 hours and the 5 outborns cooled after transfer to University of Virginia 9.8 ± 6.2 hours of age. Overcooling below 32°C occurred in 12 (34%) transported cooled infants, with 5 (14%) infants having at least one temperature below 30°C and 7 (20%) between 30 and 32°C. Overcooling was related to intermittent, rather than continuous rectal temperature monitoring, the use of frozen rather than refrigerated gel packs and more severe encephalopathy. With experience and education as shown in Figure 9.3, the mean admission temperature increased over time, with two-thirds of transported infants' admission temperatures between 33.0 and 34.0°C in 2008.

The London Neonatal Transfer Service reported their experience with passive cooling before and during transport in 39 infants with HIE referred between January and October 2009 [7]. The protocol was

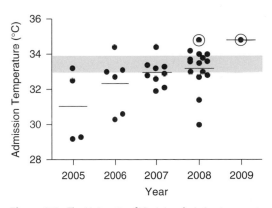

**Figure 9.3.** The University of Virginia admission temperature for 35 outborn infants cooled during transport. The rectal temperature of 35 outborn infants cooled during transport, recorded on admission to the University of Virginia NICU. Grey-shaded area represents target rectal temperature (33 to 34°C). Two patients with only passive cooling during transport (indicated with open circle) had admission temperatures of 34.4 and 34.8°C. All others were transported with active cooling. Reproduced, with permission, from Fairchild et al [24].

A

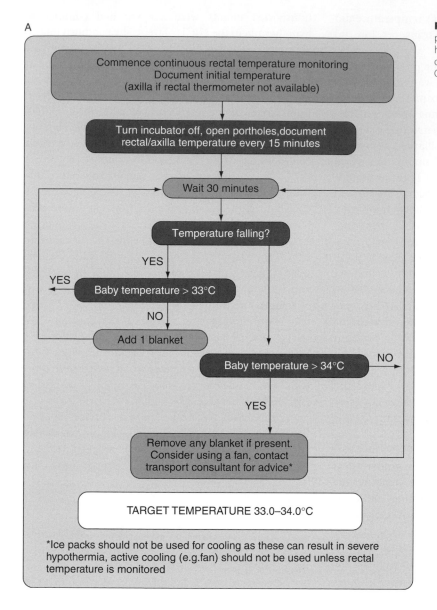

**Figure 9.4.** TOBY register guideline for passive cooling during retrieval. A. Referring hospital. B. Transport incubator. www.npeu.ox.ac.uk/tobyregister/transport, Version 1, October 16, 2009.

Commence continuous rectal temperature monitoring
Document initial temperature
(axilla if rectal thermometer not available)

Turn incubator off, open portholes,document rectal/axilla temperature every 15 minutes

Wait 30 minutes

Temperature falling?

YES

Baby temperature > 33°C    YES

NO

Add 1 blanket

Baby temperature > 34°C    NO

YES

Remove any blanket if present. Consider using a fan, contact transport consultant for advice*

TARGET TEMPERATURE 33.0–34.0°C

*Ice packs should not be used for cooling as these can result in severe hypothermia, active cooling (e.g.fan) should not be used unless rectal temperature is monitored

developed by London centres with expertise in therapeutic hypothermia and transport teams in London, Kent and Cambridge and forms the basis for the TOBY register guideline for cooling on retrieval shown in Figure 9.4 [35].

Referring hospitals of hypothermia eligible infants by TOBY registry criteria [35] were advised to commence passive cooling by turning off the radiant warmer or incubator, opening the incubator portholes, nursing the infant undressed and monitoring the temperature by intermittent rectal and continuous skin temperature measurements. The transport team

commenced continuous rectal temperature monitoring and set the transport incubator temperature at 25°C to minimize fluctuations in ambient temperature during transfer.

Passive cooling (mean ± SD) was initiated at 2.68 ± 1.52 hours of age at the 18 referring hospitals for all 39 infants and continued during transport to the eight hypothermia centres at 7.24 ± 2.19 hours of age, i.e., cooling commenced 4.6 ± 1.8 hours earlier than if delayed until admission to the cooling treatment centre. Passive cooling to the target rectal temperature of 33.0–34.0°C took 2.67 ± 1.00 hours in 33 (85%)

**Figure 9.4.** (cont.)

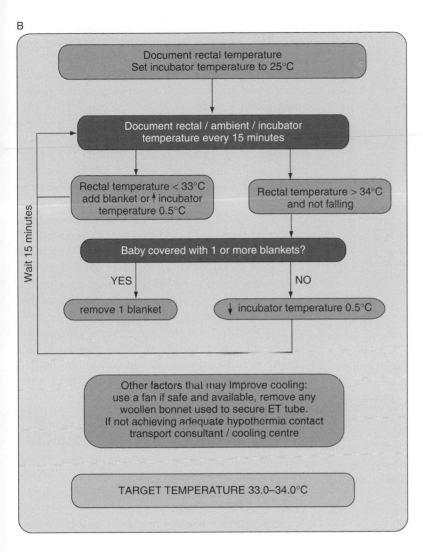

of infants. Referring hospitals did not measure rectal temperature; axilla and core rectal temperature were correlated (mean difference 0.1°C, 95% limits of agreement –1.1, 1.3°C), but not skin and core temperature (skin temperature monitoring has since been removed from the protocol). Two infants, actively cooled by the referring hospitals with a fan without continuous rectal temperature monitoring, were overcooled to below 32.5°C when the transport team arrived. Four infants were actively cooled in consultation with the transport consultant. Figure 9.5 demonstrates that 67% of infants' rectal temperatures were within the 33.0–34.0°C target range on admission to the hypothermia centre.

The correlation between core rectal and axillary temperature was confirmed in a larger single-centre retrospective audit, but large variability between axillary and rectal temperature was reported during both the induction and maintenance phases of whole body hypothermia treatment (95% prediction limits for the difference between rectal and axillary temperatures exceeded 1°C) [45]. Therefore, continuous skin [7] or intermittent axillary [45] temperature measurements can not be recommended as surrogates for continuous core temperature monitoring during whole body therapeutic hypothermia.

The Scottish Neonatal Transport Service reported their experience of cooling nine infants with the servo-controlled Criticool system that was secured in a dedicated ambulance during road transport [38]. The target temperature was rapidly attained with the

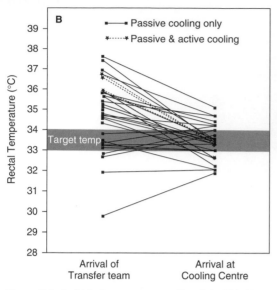

**Figure 9.5.** Individual temperature profiles of the 39 babies during retrieval and transport. Adapted, with permission, from Kendall *et al* [7].

servo-controlled system [median (25th, 75th centiles): time to temperature below 34°C was 45 [30,55] minutes] and the median (range) temperature on arrival at the tertiary cooling centre was 33.5°C (33.4–33.8°C). Similarly, another retrospective audit reported rapid induction and maintenance of temperature within the 33–34°C target range in 19 infants cooled with the servo-controlled system, compared with uncontrolled passive cooling in 10 infants and cooling with manually adjusted low-technology devices in 17 infants [39].

Three case studies described the same servo-controlled Criticool system used in road, rotary and fixed-wing transports [37]. The system was secured and only used when the infant was in the transport platform, with passive cooling in the referring hospitals and between transport platform and NICU; for the two air transports, passive cooling was also used in the road transfers between referring hospital and air platform and between air platform and tertiary cooling centre. Limitations of the servo-controlled Criticool system included the lack of battery backup, the 35 kg weight, the water-filled tubing and the fixation of the device all impeding safe movement from one platform to another.

## Advice on formulating clinical evidence-based protocols

Implementation of any new therapy into neonatal care, including therapeutic hypothermia during neonatal retrieval and transport, requires time, planning and a coordinated multidisciplinary regionalized approach [46]. The risk of overcooling to below 32°C during initiation of hypothermia treatment before and during transport means that "clear and validated" whole body cooling protocols (controlled manually, adjusted passive and/or device servo-controlled) are needed for pre-transport stabilization, for both referring hospitals and the transport team, as well as a transfer protocol for the transport team. These should be developed collaboratively and by the selected regional cooling treatment centres with the expertise and practical experience in hypothermia treatment [21], the referring hospitals and transport service [46]. Once the protocols have been developed, they need to be published to ensure medical and nursing accessibility, exemplified by the Web-based access to the TOBY Cooling Register guideline for passive cooling during retrieval [35,43]. Training in the use of the cooling equipment, the cooling technique and process for consultation with and guidance by the cooling treatment centre or transport service are mandatory, both before implementation to reduce delays in initiating hypothermia treatment and on a continuing basis to maintain familiarity with the protocols and equipment.

## Pre-transport stabilization cooling protocol in referring hospitals

Appropriate resuscitation and stabilization of the infant must be emphasized, with attention to airway, breathing and circulation before considering therapeutic hypothermia [44].

Hypothermia treatment should not be undertaken in referring hospitals without the protocols, training or ability to measure core temperature. In these situations, consideration is given to delaying initiation of hypothermia until the transport team arrives or admission to the cooling treatment centre. Such infants with suspected HIE should be referred to the regional transport service as early as practicable during or after resuscitation, with priority given to maintaining the temperature below 37°C and avoiding hyperthermia.

The referring hospital pre-transport cooling protocol and guidance needs to be detailed enough for infrequent use; some referring hospitals may stabilize and transfer only one infant with HIE requiring hypothermia treatment every 1–2 years. The only equipment required is disposable temperature thermistors and a compliant reusable temperature cable.

**Table 9.1.** Checklist for eligibility for hypothermia treatment

1. Evidence of peripartum hypoxia–ischaemia (asphyxia) – at least two of:
   - Apgar score of 5 or less at 10 minutes
   - Ongoing resuscitation or ventilation (endotracheal tube or mask) at 10 minutes
   - Cord pH < 7.0, or if cord pH not available:
   - Arterial pH < 7.0 or base deficit of 12 or more within 60 minutes of birth
2. Moderate or severe encephalopathy, or seizures (see checklist in Table 9.2)
3. No overt bleeding (including subgaleal haemorrhage)
4. No recognizable major congenital abnormality
5. Less than 6 hours of age

**Table 9.2.** Checklist to assist diagnosis of moderate and severe encephalopathy

| Parameter | Moderate encephalopathy | Severe encephalopathy |
|---|---|---|
| Level of consciousness | Reduced response to stimulation (lethargic) | Absent response to stimulation (obtunded) |
| Spontaneous activity | Decreased activity | No activity |
| Posture | Distal flexion, complete extension | Arms and legs extended (decerebrate) |
| Tone | Hypotonia (focal or general) | Flaccid |
| *Primitive reflexes* | | |
| Suck | Weak | Absent |
| Moro | Incomplete | Absent |
| *Autonomic system* | | |
| Pupils | Constricted | Variable (deviated, non-reactive) |
| Heart rate | Bradycardia | Variable |
| Respiration | Periodic breathing | Apnoea |

Moderate-to-severe encephalopathy defined as seizures or the presence of signs in 3 of the 6 categories (above). Based on modified Sarnat criteria (50,51) and adapted from the TOBY cooling register clinician's handbook (http://www.npeu.ox.ac.uk/tobyregister/docs).

One of the most crucial components of the protocol is early recognition and consultation in infants of 35 weeks' gestation or more with peripartum hypoxia–ischaemia and moderate-to-severe encephalopathy who may benefit from hypothermia treatment. Identification should be based on clinical criteria together with a cord or arterial blood gas, if possible. Checklists used in common by both the referring clinicians and transport personnel should be formulated to assist with telephone evaluation of cooling eligibility (Tables 9.1 and 9.2).

Consent for hypothermia treatment is not necessary as it is a proven therapy, but written information regarding encephalopathy and hypothermia treatment for families is optimal [35,44].

Controlled passive whole body cooling is initiated by discontinuing external heating under guidance of the transport consultant, independent of the ongoing method (whole body or selective head cooling with mild systemic hypothermia) at the cooling treatment centre. The infant is undressed and the radiant warmer or incubator turned off. Rectal temperature measurement is recommended, even if not usual referring hospital practice; if possible continuously by thermistor inserted at least 5 cm into the rectum and secured by tape, or else intermittently. The variability of axillary and skin temperature means that neither should be used. Temperature should be documented every 15 minutes and if it decreases to 34°C whilst awaiting the transport team, then the radiant warmer heater output should be turned on to minimal output and increased every 15–30 minutes to maintain the temperature within the target range of 33.0–34.0°C.

Active cooling with fans or refrigerated gel packs soon after birth, without continuous rectal temperature monitoring, will result in overcooling. Active techniques should only be commenced after 1 hour of controlled passive cooling and after further discussion with the transport consultant. Frozen gel packs should not be used and never be in contact with an infant.

Further treatment and management is according to referring hospital practice guided by the transport team, including the treatment of seizures with anticonvulsants, sedation and fluid management [27]. Sinus bradycardia below 100 beats per minute is expected, with a mean 14 beat per minute reduction in heart rate per 1°C drop in body temperature [47,48].

# Pre-transport stabilization and transfer cooling protocol for transport team

The transport team will require disposable temperature thermistors and a compliant reusable temperature cable for continuous rectal temperature monitoring. Refrigerated gel packs are transported to the referring hospital in a portable cooler and covers for the packs are also needed, and/or a servo-controlled device.

The aEEG is not requisite for the transport team to confirm eligibility for cooling, as both pattern and amplitude are unchanged until core temperature is below 30°C and unaffected at core temperatures of 33.0–34.0°C [27]. The aEEG monitor is applied at the cooling treatment centre and if normal, discontinuation of hypothermia considered [5,35].

Following referring clinician handover and transport team assessment, priority is given to insertion of a thermistor 5 cm into the rectum, with continuous core temperature monitoring and documentation every 15 minutes during stabilization and transfer. If the controlled passive technique is used, two covered refrigerated gel packs are applied across the chest and/or under the head and shoulders when the rectal temperature is above 35.0°C, with sequential removal when the temperature falls below 34.5°C and then 34.0°C. At the referring hospital, the radiant warmer heater output is manually adjusted every 15–30 minutes if the temperature falls below 33.5°C. A wrap or blanket may be applied at this stage, although this may obstruct clinicians' direct and continuous observation of the infant.

The transport incubator may be either turned off [14] or set at minimum temperature [7,35] in infants undergoing active cooling with gel packs during transfer. If the rectal temperature is below 33.5°C, then the transport incubator temperature is manually increased every 15–30 minutes.

Most infants being cooled will be ventilated during transport, with standard warming and humidification of inspired gases recommended. Blood gases may be adjusted for core temperature [49], in accordance with the cooling treatment centre practice. Infants with respiratory failure or pulmonary hypertension in 100% oxygen may be treated with hypothermia.

Clinical seizures, hypotension and fluids should be managed according to transport guidelines. Investigations assessing multi-organ impairment from HIE and effects of hypothermia are deferred until admission to the cooling treatment centre, unless clinically indicated.

In conclusion, therapeutic hypothermia can be commenced in term and near-term newborns with moderate-to-severe HIE at referring hospitals and continued during transport to the regional cooling treatment centre. Protocols, developed with the approach outlined in this chapter, guide this practice that is then overseen by the cooling treatment centre and transport team.

# References

1. Blackmon LR, Stark AR and the Committee on Fetus and Newborn AAP. Hypothermia: a neuroprotective therapy for neonatal hypoxic-ischemic encephalopathy. *Pediatrics* 2006;**117**:942–8.

2. British Association of Perinatal Medicine. Position statement on therapeutic cooling for neonatal encephalopathy, British Association of Perinatal Medicine. 2010. Statement on Therapeutic Cooling for Neonatal Encephalopathy July 2010.pdf [cited August 2010] Available from: http://www.bapm.org/media/documents/publications/Position Statement on Therapeutic Cooling for Neonatal Encephalopathy July 2010.pdf.

3. Higgins RD, Raju T, Edwards AD, et al. Hypothermia and other treatment options for neonatal encephalopathy: an executive summary of the Eunice Kennedy Shriver NICHD workshop. *J Pediatr* 2011;**159**:851–8 e1.

4. Hoehn T, Hansmann G, Bührer C, et al. Therapeutic hypothermia in neonates. Review of current clinical data, ILCOR recommendations and suggestions for implementation in neonatal intensive care units. *Resuscitation* 2008;**78**:7–12.

5. National Health Service. Therapeutic hypothermia with intracorporeal temperature monitoring for hypoxic perinatal brain injury. National Institute for Health and Clinical Excellence, Interventional Procedure Guidance 347. [May 26 2010] Available from: http://www.nice.org.uk/nicemedia/live/11315/48809/48809.pdf.

6. Azzopardi DV, Strohm B, Edwards AD, et al. Moderate hypothermia to treat perinatal asphyxial encephalopathy. *N Engl J Med* 2009;**361**:1349–58.

7. Kendall GS, Kapetanakis A, Ratnavel N, et al. Passive cooling for initiation of therapeutic hypothermia in neonatal encephalopathy. *Arch Dis Child* 2010;**95**:F408–12.

8. Strohm B, Azzopardi D. Temperature control during therapeutic moderate whole-body hypothermia for neonatal encephalopathy. *Arch Disease Child Fetal Neonatal Ed* 2010;**95**:F373–5.

9. Gunn AJ. Cerebral hypothermia for prevention of brain injury following perinatal asphyxia. *Curr Opin Pediatr* 2000;**12**:111–5.

10. Haaland K, Loberg EM, Steen PA, Thoresen M. Posthypoxic hypothermia in newborn piglets. *Pediatr Res* 1997;**41**:505–12.

11. Iwata O, Iwata S, Thornton JS, et al. "Therapeutic time window" duration decreases with increasing severity of cerebral hypoxia-ischaemia under normothermia and delayed hypothermia in newborn piglets. *Brain Res* 2007;**1154**:173–80.

12. Eicher DJ, Wagner CL, Katikaneni LP, et al. Moderate hypothermia in neonatal encephalopathy: safety outcomes. *Pediatr Neurol* 2005;**32**:18–24.

13. Gluckman PD, Wyatt JS, Azzopardi D, et al. Selective head cooling with mild systemic hypothermia after neonatal encephalopathy: multicentre randomised trial. *Lancet* 2005;**365**:663–70.

14. Jacobs SE, Morley CJ, Inder TE, et al. Whole-body hypothermia for term and near-term newborns with hypoxic-ischemic encephalopathy: a randomized controlled trial. *Arch Pediatr Adolesc Med* 2011;**165**: 692–700.

15. Shankaran S, Laptook AR, Ehrenkranz RA, et al. Whole-body hypothermia for neonates with hypoxic-ischemic encephalopathy. *N Engl J Med* 2005;**353**: 1574–84.

16. Simbruner G, Mittal R, Rohlmann F, Muche R. Systemic hypothermia in neonates with hypoxic-ischemic-encephalopathy: Efficacy outcomes of neo.nEURO.network RCT. *Pediatrics* 2010;**126**:e771–8.

17. Zhou WH, Cheng GQ, Shao XM, et al. Selective head cooling with mild systemic hypothermia after neonatal hypoxic-ischemic encephalopathy: a multicenter randomized controlled trial in China. *J Pediatr* 2010;**157**:367–72.

18. Davidson S, Jacobs S, Stewart M. 'Birth asphyxia': the NETS Victoria perspective. Canberra: 5th Annual Congress of the Perinatal Society of Australia and New Zealand; 2001.

19. Papile LA. Systemic hypothermia – a "cool" therapy for neonatal hypoxic-ischemic encephalopathy. *N Engl J Med* 2005;**353**:1619–20.

20. Robertson NJ, Kendall GS, Thayyil S. Techniques for therapeutic hypothermia during transport and in hospital for perinatal asphyxial encephalopathy. *Semin Fetal Neonatal Med* 2010;**15**:276–86.

21. Gray J, Geva A, Zheng Z, Zupancic JA. CoolSim: using industrial modeling techniques to examine the impact of selective head cooling in a model of perinatal regionalization. *Pediatrics* 2008;**121**:28–36.

22. Kattwinkel J, Cook LJ, Nowacek G, et al. Regionalized perinatal education. *Semin Neonatol* 2004;**9**:155–65.

23. Zanelli SA, Naylor M, Dobbins N, et al. Implementation of a 'Hypothermia for HIE' program: 2-year experience in a single NICU. *J Perinatol* 2007;**28**:171–5.

24. Fairchild K, Sokora D, Scott J, Zanelli S. Therapeutic hypothermia on neonatal transport: 4-year experience in a single NICU. *J Perinatol* 2010;**30**:324–9.

25. Anderson ME, Longhofer TA, Phillips W, McRay DE. Passive cooling to initiate hypothermia for transported encephalopathic newborns. *J Perinatol* 2007;**27**:592–3.

26. Hallberg B, Olson L, Bartocci M, Edqvist I, Blennow M. Passive induction of hypothermia during transport of asphyxiated infants: a risk of excessive cooling. *Acta Paediatr* 2009;**98**:942–6.

27. Thoresen M. Supportive care during neuroprotective hypothermia in the term newborn: adverse effects and their prevention. *Clin Perinatol* 2008;**35**:749–63.

28. Wyatt JS, Gluckman PD, Liu PY, et al. Determinants of outcomes after head cooling for neonatal encephalopathy. *Pediatrics* 2007;**119**:912–21.

29. Burnard ED, Cross KW. Rectal temperature in the newborn after birth asphyxia. *BMJ* 1958;**2**:1197–9.

30. Robertson NJ, Nakakeeto M, Hagmann C, et al. Therapeutic hypothermia for birth asphyxia in low-resource settings: a pilot randomised controlled trial. *Lancet* 2008;**372**:801–3.

31. Dahm LS, James LS. Newborn temperature and calculated heat loss in the delivery room. *Pediatrics* 1972;**49**:504–13.

32. Eicher DJ, Wagner CL, Katikaneni LP, et al. Moderate hypothermia in neonatal encephalopathy: efficacy outcomes. *Pediatr Neurol* 2005;**32**:11–7.

33. Horn AR, Woods DL, Thompson C, Eis I, Kroon M. Selective cerebral hypothermia for post-hypoxic neuroprotection in neonates using a solid ice cap. *S Afr Med J* 2006;**96**:976–81.

34. Horn A, Thompson C, Woods D, et al. Induced hypothermia for infants with hypoxic-ischemic encephalopathy using a servo-controlled fan: an exploratory pilot study. *Pediatrics* 2009;**123**:e1090–8.

35. National Perinatal Epidemiology Unit. UK TOBY cooling register, National Perinatal Epidemiology Unit, University of Oxford. [Accessed August 2010] Available from: http://www.npeu.ox.ac.uk/tobyregister.

36. Hoque N, Chakkarapani E, Liu X, Thoresen M. A comparison of cooling methods used in therapeutic hypothermia for perinatal asphyxia. *Pediatrics* 2010;**126**:e124–30.

37. Hobson A, Sussman C, Knight J, et al. Active cooling during transport of neonates with hypoxic-ischemic encephalopathy. *Air Med J* 2011;**30**:197–200.

38. Johnston ED, Becher JC, Mitchell AP, Stenson BJ. Provision of servo-controlled cooling during neonatal transport. *Arch Dis Child Fetal Neonatal Ed* 2012;**97**:F367–7.

39. O'Reilly KM, Tooley J, Winterbottom S. Therapeutic hypothermia during neonatal transport. *Acta Paediatr* 2011;**100**:1084–6; discussion e49.

40. Iwata S, Iwata O, Olson L, et al. Therapeutic hypothermia can be induced and maintained using either commercial water bottles or a "phase changing material" mattress in a newborn piglet model. *Arch Dis Child* 2009;**94**:387–91.

41. Thayyil S, Guhan AB, Marlow N, et al. Whole body cooling using phase changing material in neonatal encephalopathy: a pilot randomised controlled trial. EPAS 43506. 2010.

42. Azzopardi D, Brocklehurst P, Edwards D, et al. The TOBY Study. Whole body hypothermia for the treatment of perinatal asphyxial encephalopathy: a randomised controlled trial. *BMC Pediatr* 2008;**8**:17.

43. Azzopardi D, Strohm B, Edwards AD, et al. Treatment of asphyxiated newborns with moderate hypothermia in routine clinical practice: how cooling is managed in the UK outside a clinical trial. *Arch Dis Child Fetal Neonatal Ed* 2009;**94**:F260–4.

44. New South Wales Department of Health. Whole body cooling – neonates suspected moderate or severe hypoxic ischaemic encephalopathy (HIE). Policy Directive 2010_006. [January 22, 2010] Available from: http://www.health.nsw.gov.au/policies/pd/2010/pdf/PD2010_006.pdf.

45. Landry MA, Doyle LW, Lee K, Jacobs SE. Axillary temperature measurement during hypothermia treatment for neonatal hypoxic-ischaemic encephalopathy. *Arch Dis Child Fetal Neonatal Ed* 2012 [Epub ahead of print].

46. Barks JD. Technical aspects of starting a neonatal cooling program. *Clin Perinatol* 2008;**35**:765–75.

47. Gunn AJ, Gluckman PD, Gunn TR. Selective head cooling in newborn infants after perinatal asphyxia: a safety study. *Pediatrics* 1998;**102**:885–92.

48. Thoresen M. Cooling the newborn after asphyxia – physiological and experimental background and its clinical use. *Semin Neonatol* 2000;**5**:61–73.

49. Groenendaal F, Brouwer AJ. Clinical aspects of induced hypothermia in full term neonates with perinatal asphyxia. *Early Hum Dev* 2009;**85**:73–6.

50. Finer NN, Robertson CM, Richards RT, Pinnell LE, Peters KL. Hypoxic-ischemic encephalopathy in term neonates: Perinatal factors and outcome. *J Pediatr* 1981;**98**:112–7.

51. Sarnat HB, Sarnat MS. Neonatal encephalopathy following fetal distress. A clinical and electroencephalographic study. *Arch Neurol* 1976;**33**: 696–705.

## Chapter 10

# Whole body cooling for therapeutic hypothermia

Abbot R. Laptook

## Introduction

Hypothermia is currently recognized as the only therapy that has been demonstrated in rigorous randomized controlled trials to alter the outcome of late preterm and term infants with evidence of hypoxia–ischaemia accompanied by encephalopathy [1–6]. Hypothermia is a broad term when used in clinical care and can span profound reductions in temperature used for repair of congenital heart defects [7] to very mild reductions in temperature beyond the thermal neutral zone among infants with cold stress at birth [8]. Hypothermia as investigated for treatment of hypoxic–ischaemic encephalopathy (HIE) refers to a targeted temperature reduction regimen and is characterized by sequential phases of induction, maintenance and rewarming whereby each phase has specific temperature characteristics. There are currently two principal methods to achieve targeted temperature reduction: selective cooling with mild systemic hypothermia or whole body cooling. The following is an overview of whole body cooling which was used in four of the six large randomized trials of this therapy. This report will focus on two of the trials that used whole body cooling, the NICHD Body Cooling Trial [2] and the Total Body Hypothermia for Neonatal Encephalopathy Trial (TOBY) [3], since they share many similarities but also some differences. These two trials will be used as a template for discussion of specific aspects of this mode of therapeutic hypothermia and will provide an overview of whole body cooling to emphasize important background, rationale, implementation, monitoring and potentially unrecognized caveats regarding this therapy.

## Thermal characteristics of the brain during whole body cooling

Cooling the body is a straightforward method to cool the brain. Non-invasive measurements to record regional brain temperature are not readily available and necessitate the use of neonatal animals to determine thermal characteristics of the brain during whole body cooling. Newborn miniature swine have been used for this purpose since they are of a convenient size to facilitate insertion of temperature probes into the brain by means of burr holes and control of physiological variables to maintain a steady-state for temperature measurements [9]. Animals undergoing whole body cooling had the torso and extremities wrapped in a blanket (head was exposed to room temperature) which provided cooling or rewarming of the body by circulating water with different temperatures through the blanket. Temperatures were monitored from five sites including the deep rectum (5 cm depth), brain temperature (depths of 1 and 2 cm from the cortical surface), overlying the dura and from the scalp once resutured over the filled burr holes. Temperatures were recorded during a control period, during body cooling (continued until temperatures were in a steady state for 30 minutes) and body cooling with superimposed hypoxia (15 minutes of inhalation of 8% oxygen) and are plotted (Figure 10.1).

During the control period with the head exposed to ambient laboratory temperature (~ 23°C), there is a temperature gradient across the brain: 1.5 ± 1.2°C for the difference between the brain at a 2 cm depth and overlying the dura. Brain temperature (2 cm depth) closely approximates rectal temperature with a

*Neonatal Neural Rescue*, ed. A. David Edwards, Denis V. Azzopardi and Alistair J. Gunn. Published by Cambridge University Press. © Cambridge University Press 2013.

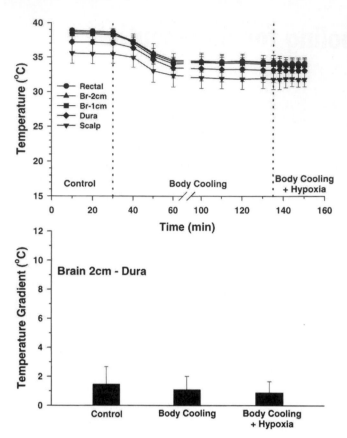

**Figure 10.1.** Thermal characteristics of body cooling. In the top panel temperatures of the rectum, brain (at a depth of 2 and 1 cm beneath the cortical surface), dura and scalp are plotted during control, body cooling and body cooling with superimposed hypoxia. Symbols for the different sites are indicated in the key. In the bottom panel temperature gradients between the brain at a 2 cm depth and dura is plotted during each of the three intervals. (With permission from Laptook, et al. *Pediatrics* 2001;**108**:1103–10.)

temperature difference of 0.26 ± 0.26°C. During body cooling, rectal temperature was reduced by 4°C and a similar magnitude of change in temperatures was measured at all brain sites. Consequently, the temperature gradient across the brain (brain 2 cm – dura) was slightly reduced to 1.1 ± 0.9°C. Thus, body cooling is characterized by homogeneous cooling of the cerebral cortex. During hypoxia superimposed on body cooling, the temperature gradient remained similar to control. An important characteristic of therapeutic hypothermia is maintenance of a constant brain temperature, because fluctuations of as little as 1–2°C in brain temperature can modify neurological outcome following hypoxia-ischaemia [10]. Given that therapeutic hypothermia may be used for infants with an unstable pulmonary status (e.g., meconium aspiration syndrome, pulmonary artery hypertension), it is reassuring that brain temperature is constant when hypoxia is superimposed on body cooling.

Based on the principles of thermal conduction, temperature gradients are expected across the brain of a newborn under control conditions. However, the magnitude of the gradient is a complex function that varies based on multiple variables such as tissue heat production, local blood flow, perfusing blood temperature, insulating temperature, ambient air temperature and non-central nervous system cranial blood flow. A study of newborn piglets indicated that the body weight of the animal influenced the temperature gradient across the brain [11]. Specifically, decreasing body weight was associated with lower peripheral brain temperatures measured at a 5 mm depth from the cortical surface. The latter observations may have implications for the extent of brain cooling achieved during therapeutic hypothermia and may in turn affect the extent of neuroprotection achieved.

# Temperature management of the at-risk neonate during and after resuscitation

## Resuscitation

All of the clinical trials to date have studied targeted temperature reductions within 6 hours of birth among infants who have been resuscitated, stabilized, evaluated for eligibility and completed the consent process [1–6]. The average age for randomization was 4–5 hours among these three trials with a relatively narrow time window among all enrolled infants. There are no data that have examined resuscitation combined with reductions in temperature in response to hypoxia–ischaemia among newborn infants. Although observations in animals indicate greater neuroprotection when therapeutic hypothermia is initiated either before or during [12] compared to following resuscitation [13] hypoxia–ischaemia, stabilization and diagnosis before initiating the treatment usually necessitates an interval of time for these processes. Furthermore, it is difficult at the time of a resuscitation to determine the root cause of the need for resuscitation (hypoxia–ischaemia versus other aetiology). Resuscitation should follow published guidelines for neonatal resuscitation and avoid extremes of temperature [14].

## After resuscitation

A contentious issue at present is the appropriate management of body temperature between resuscitation and possible initiation of targeted temperature reduction. This is especially important for clinicians outside of tertiary care centres who are responsible for stabilization and care of infants until transport to a centre that can provide therapeutic hypothermia. Given concerns regarding the duration of the therapeutic window, there has been enthusiasm for initiating cooling at referral hospitals and on transport principally with the use of body cooling. Two pragmatic trials have used cooling at referral hospitals and on transport as a means to extend the therapy to infants who are geographically beyond reaching a tertiary centre by 6 hours following birth [6,15]. These studies used body cooling which was achieved by removal of exogenous heat, application of cool gel packs and rewarming if there was an overshoot of the target temperature by means of exogenous heat and blankets. The TOBY trial also used cooling on transport for out-born infants, mostly by discontinuing warming [3]. Under conditions of conducting a clinical trial, trained study personnel followed preset protocols with monitoring of a core temperature site to guide the process of lowering the temperature. With completion of these trials dissemination of methods to initiate cooling on transport to a tertiary care facility for therapeutic

hypothermia has occurred. An example from the UK Cooling TOBY register [16] provides an algorithm to follow in conjunction with a transport consultant from a cooling centre (Figure 10.2).

However, in countries such as the United States, a systematic approach to cooling at referring hospitals and on transport is not well developed. It is unclear whether this reflects heterogeneity of the extent of regionalization of perinatal care, long distances over which infants are transported, or other factors. Recent observations from a 4-year experience of cooling at referral hospitals and on transport (removal of exogenous heat and if necessary application of cool gel packs) indicate that rectal temperatures on admission to a tertiary centre $< 32°C$ and $< 30°C$ occurred in 34% and 14% of infants, respectively [17]. The latter emphasizes the potential for harm when cooling is initiated under non-study conditions and may reflect several important issues: (1) initiation of targeted temperature management by health care providers with little experience in this therapy given that hypoxia–ischemia fulfilling treatment criteria is a relatively infrequent event, (2) the lack of systematic educational programmes provided by tertiary care centres to guide referring providers and (3) use of methods to reduce temperature that cannot be easily controlled even though temperature is being monitored. Ideally servo-control devices which are portable and can interface with other transport equipment should reduce the percentage of infants with excessively low temperatures on transport. An example of the performance of a prototype cooling/rewarming blanket compatible with transport equipment is shown in Figure 10.3 [18]. Manufacturers are starting to address such needs but the small market represented by newborn health care relative to adults may limit research development by industry. Some transport services in the United Kingdom now use specific cooling equipment to achieve whole body cooling during transport [19,20].

Important physiological changes in response to cooling are easily overlooked and may influence the extent of control of temperature with the above methodology used outside of tertiary centres. For example, the metabolic response to a fall in ambient temperature in newborn rat pups (chemical regulation, increases in oxygen consumption) differs during normoxia and hypoxia and thus impacts the rate of fall in temperature [21]. This is illustrated in Figure 10.4. Whether alterations in chemical regulation persist following hypoxia–ischaemia, or if such changes are

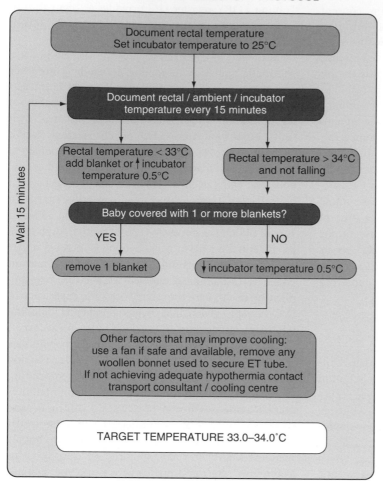

PASSIVE COOLING ON TRANSPORT PROTOCOL

Document rectal temperature
Set incubator temperature to 25°C

Document rectal / ambient / incubator
temperature every 15 minutes

Rectal temperature < 33°C
add blanket or ↑ incubator
temperature 0.5°C

Rectal temperature > 34°C
and not falling

Baby covered with 1 or more blankets?

YES

NO

remove 1 blanket

↓ incubator temperature 0.5°C

Wait 15 minutes

Other factors that may improve cooling:
use a fan if safe and available, remove any
woollen bonnet used to secure ET tube.
If not achieving adequate hypothermia contact
transport consultant / cooling centre

TARGET TEMPERATURE 33.0–34.0°C

**Figure 10.2.** Algorithm for cooling on transport. This is an example of a protocol for cooling on transport as part of the UK TOBY Cooling Register. The protocol is conducted by a transport team from centres that are experienced with providing therapeutic hypothermia and whose transport team has been trained with conducting such a protocol.

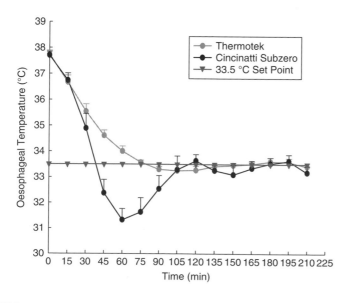

**Figure 10.3.** Prototype cooling blanket for transport. The profile of oesophageal temperatures from 4 neonatal swine is plotted over time. Each animal underwent a 3.5-hour interval of cooling to a set point temperature of 33.5°C with a commercially available cooling device (CSZ) and with a blanket under development. The latter has a more sophisticated servo algorithm which slows the rate of cooling as the oesophageal temperature approaches the set point. Please see plate section for colour version.

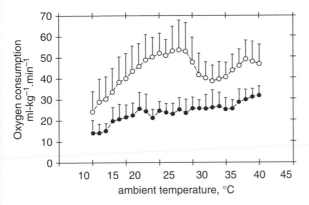

**Figure 10.4.** The effects of lowering ambient temperatures. The plot shows values of oxygen consumption of newborn rats over a range of ambient temperatures extending from 40°C to 15°C during normoxic conditions (open symbols) and hypoxic conditions (closed symbols). The typical metabolic response to a fall in ambient temperature during normoxia (increase in oxygen consumption) is abolished during hypoxia and oxygen consumption becomes linearly dependent on ambient temperature. (With permission from Mortola, et al. *Am J Physiol* 1992;**263**(Pt 2):R267–72.)

proportionate to the extent of hypoxia–ischaemia is unknown at present. Such knowledge gaps could contribute to the observation of greater falls in temperature among infants with severe compared to moderate hypoxic–ischaemic encephalopathy among infants who were cooled on transport [17]. Firm data to guide thermoregulatory practices for late preterm and term infants are lacking and have largely been extrapolated from preterm infants studied within nurseries without preceding hypoxia–ischaemia [22]. At present although core body temperature can be reduced by simple cooling modalities at referral hospitals and on transport, there is a growing recognition that implementation under non-study conditions can be accompanied by a substantial risk of unintended excessive cooling [23]. Initiating cooling on transport should ideally meet the following criteria: (1) presence of a medical provider able to determine encephalopathy, (2) personnel on transport trained in temperature control of encephalopathic infants, (3) use of a device that can control temperature and (4) use of alarms in conjunction with the device [24].

## Avoidance of elevated temperature

A less controversial issue but of critical importance in the management of infants following perinatal hypoxia–ischaemia is avoiding elevated temperature. Animal studies using 7-day-old rat pups demonstrate that elevations of core body temperature immediately following hypoxia–ischaemia increase the extent of brain injury compared with animals maintained at 36–37°C [25]. Similarly avoidance of elevated temperature reduced brain injury among 7 day rat pups with seizures occurring shortly after hypoxia–ischaemia [26]. Elevation of temperature even remote from hypoxia–ischaemia can be deleterious; temperature to 40°C at 24 hours following ischaemia in adult rats exacerbated the extent of neuronal injury compared to animals maintained at 37°C [27]. Complicating the interpretation of temperature effects on brain injury is that brain necrosis can result in elevated temperatures in newborns and adults. The latter may reflect expression of endogenous pyrogens such as interleukin-6 [28] or direct injury to thermoregulatory centres [29].

In the three clinical trials of targeted temperature management in newborns with HIE (CoolCap, NICHD, TOBY), there were infants in the non-cooled comparison arm with elevated temperatures. The percentage of infants with at least one core temperature value above 38°C was 31, 39 and 23% respectively for the CoolCap, NICHD and TOBY trials. In both the NICHD and CoolCap studies, secondary analyses indicated associations between elevated temperatures and an increase in the odds of death or disability at 18–22 months assessment [30,31]. Whether this association is causal is not clear. The association could be attributable to specific effects of an elevated temperature, the severity of the brain lesion, or both. In view of this association there is reasonable rationale for providing close monitoring of temperatures, avoiding ambient environments that may predispose to elevated temperatures and prompt, vigorous treatment if elevated temperatures occur. A similar approach has been adopted for adults with stroke [32].

## Targeted temperature management for HIE by means of body cooling

Any regimen to provide targeted temperature management following perinatal hypoxia–ischaemia, irrespective of the mode of cooling, can be characterized by three phases of induction, maintenance and rewarming. Induction is the interval of time in which temperature is reduced from presumably a normothermic range to the value of temperature that is desired or targeted to provide neuroprotection. Maintenance represents the interval of time over which the targeted temperature is continued. Rewarming is the duration over which a normothermic temperature is reestablished with resumption of typical thermal care practices in a NICU.

## Preparation for targeted temperature management

Both the NICHD and the TOBY trials used whole body cooling to provide targeted temperature management for infants with HIE. Both studies used commercially available systems: the Cincinnati Sub-Zero (CSZ) Blanketrol II Hypo-Hyperthermia system (Cincinnati, Ohio) in the NICHD trial and the Tecotherm TS 200 Total Body Cooling System (Tec Com GmbH, Halle, Germany) in the TOBY trial. Each system consists of a cooling unit, connecting tubes/hoses and a mattress. The CSZ system circulates water and the Tecotherm unit circulates an alcohol based cooling fluid through each system. Temperature probes monitoring core temperature sites interface with the devices. The CSZ product can have multiple blankets attached and preliminary studies (newborn piglets) demonstrated that circulating water through two blankets simultaneously (one pediatric size and one adult size) reduced the fluctuation in temperature above and below the set point compared to use of a single blanket [33]. The profiles of oesophageal and rectal temperature achieved in the NICHD and TOBY trials respectively are plotted in Figure 10.5. These systems are easy to use after appropriate education; oriented personnel can set up a cooling system within 15 minutes in preparation for patient use. In essence, fluid needs to be added to the cooling systems, hoses need to be attached with the blanket and the cooling system and a temperature probe needs to be inserted into a core body temperature site for monitoring. Both devices provide continuous displays of the temperature of the core body site being monitored and of the fluid circulating through the device.

## Time of initiation of targeted temperature management

The interval to initiation of hypothermia in newborn infants is based on experimental data. Gunn and colleagues performed a series of elegant studies in the late-gestation fetal sheep in which 30 minutes of brain ischaemia was followed by 72 hours of reduced brain temperatures initiated at three different time points following ischaemia [34–36]. Results of these studies indicated a therapeutic window of approximately 6 hours following an ischaemic event.

## Induction

In both the NICHD and TOBY trials all exogenous heat sources were turned off and the induction phase was characterized by a rapid fall in temperature (Figure 10.5). There are differences between the cooling systems used in these two trials. In the NICHD trial, blankets were pre-cooled to 5°C before placing an infant on the blanket; this was done to minimize the time to reach the target temperature (also known as the set point temperature) of 33.5°C for the oesophageal site. Most infants were cared for on radiant warmers, lying on paediatric size blankets which were positioned flat on the warmer surface without being draped over the infant. The cooling device for the NICHD trial was used in a servo-control mode (automatic control) such that the circulating water either heats or cools in response to the oesophageal temperature in an attempt to reach and maintain the desired target temperature. Due to the nature of the servo mechanism, the induction phase in the NICHD trial was characterized by a prominent overshoot of oesophageal temperature beyond the target temperature [37]. Specifically, the time to initially surpass 33.5°C occurred at 0.9 ± 0.5 hours (mean ± SD; range, .5–3.5 hours) after the initiation of cooling and the time to the maximum overshoot below the target temperature was 1.3 ± 1.0 hours. The maximum temperature overshoot was 1.4 ± 0.6°C (range, 0–4.1°C) below the target of 33.5°C.

In the TOBY trial, blankets were not pre-cooled and infants were positioned on the blanket within incubators with the power turned off. The cooling device and blanket used fluid that was temperature regulated by manual adjustment to keep the target rectal temperature between 33 and 34°C. The induction phase was also rapid but less so compared to the NICHD trial. To achieve cooling the bedside provider adjusted the temperature of the circulating fluid to 20°C; as the infant's temperature declined the temperature of the circulating fluid was incrementally raised to approximately 28°C and adjusted in 1–2°C steps to maintain rectal temperature close to 33.5°C. With this approach a manually controlled device provided good temperature control (Figure 10.5) but frequent adjustment of fluid temperature was required. Manual control requires more nursing time compared with monitoring a servo-controlled system. Since completion of the NICHD and TOBY trials, the profiles of targeted temperature reductions achieved with other hypo–hyperthermia systems have been

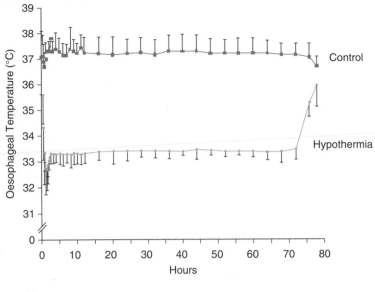

**Figure 10.5.** Oesophageal and rectal temp from two randomized trials of hypothermia. Part A shows the mean oesophageal temperature (±2 standard deviations) of infants in the control and hypothermia arm of the NICHD trial (with permission). Part B shows the rectal temperatures (±2 standard deviations) of infants in the control and hypothermia arm of the TOBY trial. (With permission, top: Shankaran, et al. NEJM 2005;**353**:1574–84; bottom: Azzopardi, et al. NEJM 2009;**361**:1349–58.). Please see plate section for colour version.

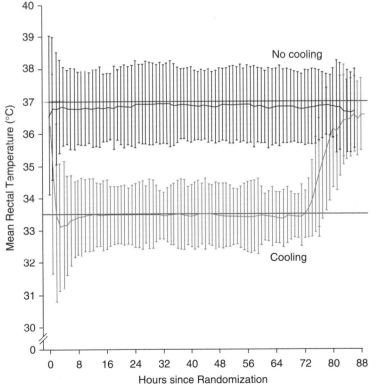

compared among small cohorts of infants. Newer devices with more sophisticated algorithms as part of the servo-control mechanism are being used in clinical practice and reports indicate little overshoot in temperature upon induction of therapy [38,39].

The rapid achievement of reduced temperatures during induction of both trials raises some important issues. Forcing body temperature below the physiological set point typically results in a vigorous thermoregulatory response characterized by heat conserving mechanisms (e.g., redistribution of cardiac output [40] and increased metabolic rate and heat production [41]). These responses may delay achieving the targeted temperature and potentially trigger physiological stress by associated metabolic alterations which accompany increased oxygen consumption (e.g. activation of thyroid and adrenal systems [42,43]). To a certain extent promoting a rapid drop in temperature minimizes the initiation and impact of counter-regulatory responses which may be more prominent if temperature were to fall gradually.

## Maintenance

The optimal target temperature and the duration of the maintenance of that temperature for this phase of the therapy remain unclear; values used in clinical trials have been inferred from animal studies but without systematic study in the perinatal period. Both the NICHD and TOBY trials demonstrated reasonably good control of core temperature during this phase of the therapy [2,3]. In the NICHD trial, mean oesophageal temperature was $33.4 \pm 0.4°C$ and in the TOBY trial mean rectal temperature was $33.5 \pm 0.5°C$. The slightly lower mean oesophageal temperature of the NICHD trial despite a target temperature of $33.5°C$ probably reflects patient care conducted predominantly on radiant warmers with exposure to the ambient NICU conditions. Consistent with this concept is the observation that 10 infants undergoing targeted temperature reductions in the NICHD trial had unexpected decreases in oesophageal temperature to $<32°C$ during the maintenance phase on at least one occasion (two infants had two episodes) [37].

The precision of temperature control may have a bearing on the extent of neuroprotection so it is desirable to use systems that maintain the target temperature with as little variation as possible. This has been evaluated among 34 infants in the UK TOBY Cooling Register which was established following completion of the TOBY trial to document the use of this therapy in the UK [38]. Half of the infants were treated with the manually controlled whole body cooling system (Tecotherm) and half were treated with a servo-control device (CritiCool, MTRE, Yavne, Israel). During maintenance the mean, 95% confidence interval and variance of rectal temperatures of infants undergoing manually controlled cooling was $33.6°C$ ($33.4°C$ to $33.8°C$, $0.1°C$) compared with $33.4°C$ ($33.3°C$ to $35.5°C$, $.04°C$) for infants undergoing servo-controlled cooling (means $P = 0.08$, equality of variance $P = 0.03$). In a study with a similar objective, the experience of infants undergoing targeted temperature management in a single centre was reviewed to compare modes of whole body cooling [39]. Infants undergoing whole body cooling with a servo-controlled device (n = 20) had less variability in their rectal temperatures compared with infants cared for with a manually controlled system; rectal temperature was maintained within $\pm 0.5°C$ of the target temperature 97% and 81% of the time for infants cared with a servo compared to a manually controlled system, respectively. Maintenance of temperature may also be affected by medications administered to infants undergoing targeted temperature reduction; muscle relaxants, sedatives and anti-convulsants have all been reported to be associated with reductions in temperature of infants undergoing hypothermia [44].

An important clinical issue is how the head should be cared for during whole body cooling. Data from adults indicate that heat loss from the head is a large portion of total heat loss in a cold environment [45]. Furthermore, there is little or no vasoconstriction in the head in response to cold exposure. Based on these observations, it has been speculated that wearing a hat may actually increase the temperature of the brain during hypothermia. Newborn swine have been used to examine this issue by examining the thermal characteristics of the brain during whole body hypothermia with and without a hat covering the head [46]. Animals wearing hats had higher cortical brain temperatures by a difference of $1.2 \pm 0.8°C$ compared with conditions of not wearing a hat during cooling; these observations were less prominent in deeper areas of the brain such as the basal ganglia. It would seem reasonable to refrain from the use of hats when undergoing whole body cooling. Related to this issue is whether the head should be in contact with the blanket during whole body cooling. This is pertinent to the temperature of the occiput for infants positioned supine on a cooling blanket or for all areas of the head when cared for with blankets that provide for body wraps including a hood for the head (e.g., Criticool, MTRE, Yavne, Israel). Whether a servo-controlled or manual controlled device is being used, there will be fluctuation in circulating fluid temperature in the blanket to maintain infants at the desired set point for core temperature. Fluctuations in cortical temperature can follow fluctuations in the temperature of the hood, in addition to limiting the extent of cortical cooling by acting as a barrier to heat dissipation [46]. Based on these considerations some clinicians believe that the head should not be in contact with the blanket when performing whole body cooling; definitive data to support this practice are lacking.

## Rewarming

The rate of rewarming is the component of a hypothermia regimen that has received the least investigation in the laboratory or clinical setting. The process of rewarming following the maintenance phase was similar between the NICHD and TOBY trials and aimed to raise core body temperature by no more than 0.5°C per hour. This rate of rewarming was picked somewhat arbitrarily. Using a servo-controlled device as in the NICHD trial, rewarming consisted of increasing the target temperature hourly until a set point temperature of 36.5°C was reached. In the TOBY trial the rectal temperature was allowed to increase by altering the temperature of the circulating fluid through the mattress to a maximum rectal temperature of 37 ± 0.2°C. Critical to the rewarming process is successful transition to the thermal practices of a specific NICU. Continued monitoring of a core body site (rectal, oesophageal) during which temperature control has reverted to standards of the NICU (e.g., radiant warmer, incubator or bassinet) would be a good practice to detect inadvertent elevated temperatures. It is unclear how long elevated temperatures may be hazardous to an injured brain and thus careful attention to thermal regulatory practices even remote from completion of targeted temperature management is prudent. NICU personnel are not frequently confronted with management of elevated temperatures, and, therefore, having an algorithm to guide interventions and monitoring will reduce the time infants may experience elevated temperatures.

## Trouble shooting

Whether one is using a servo-control or manually controlled device, there needs to be proper monitoring of the infants' temperatures and performance of the cooling system. Having a check list of potential problems and trouble shooting is helpful given that most NICUs do not provide this therapy very often and nurses may go through long intervals of time without use of cooling devices. A super-user model in which there are nursing or medical staff who may be used as a reference for any questions that arise may be needed in NICUs with less use of the therapy. Designating a core

body temperature that will trigger trouble shooting will help identify problems before there is potential impact on the infant. Problems can certainly occur at any time during targeted temperature management but are more likely to occur during the induction phase as opposed to during maintenance when there should be more of a steady state. Table 10.1 lists some common potential problems of a cooling device that providers need to be aware of especially when excessively low temperatures are encountered.

**Table 10.1.** Trouble shooting list for infants undergoing therapeutic hypothermia

| | Trouble shooting items | Potential action |
|---|---|---|
| 1 | Is the correct mode of cooling being used? | Verify whether the machine is set for manual or servo-(automatic) control mode. |
| 2 | Are the hoses inserted correctly? | Remove and re-insert connecting hoses to the cooling device and blanket. |
| 3 | Is there proper volume of fluid circulating in the system? | Add fluid to the system if applicable. |
| 4 | Are there obstructions to the flow of circulating fluid? | Examine the blanket and site where the hoses interface with the cooling device and blanket. |
| 5 | Is the temperature probe in the proper location? | Obtain a CXR to confirm probe placement if applicable (e.g, oesophageal probe). |
| 6 | Are specific parts of the cooling apparatus possibly defective? | Consider replacing the temperature probe, blanket and temperature probe adaptor one at a time to evaluate the response. |
| 7 | Is the cooling device itself defective? | Some devices provide warning signs indicating such. Consider having a back-up device. |

## Conclusion

Therapeutic hypothermia regimens which target reduction and maintenance of temperatures between 33°C and 34°C for late preterm and term infants with HIE have demonstrated a reduction in death or disability at 18–22 months of age [2,3,5,6]. Similar conclusions are derived from a meta-analysis that includes eight additional trials with a total of 1320 infants randomized to either hypothermia or normothermia [47]. Of note, 76% of the patients in the meta-analysis were enrolled in studies that used whole body cooling. Targeted temperature reductions for treatment of HIE may appear to be a simple and straightforward therapy leading some to conclude that any NICU can and should be able to offer this treatment. However, as noted in the Summary of the NICHD Workshop on Hypothermia and Perinatal Asphyxia [24], institutions offering hypothermia in non-research settings should implement studied and reported protocols and staff should be trained before initiating the therapy. Adoption of a whole body cooling protocol necessitates a decision of manual versus servo-control. As noted earlier, precision of temperature control appears to be superior with a servo-controlled device. Newer devices are being brought to the market that have more sophisticated servo-control devices than prior technology and provide remarkably constant core temperature. However, it is uncertain whether such differences in temperature alter neurodevelopmental outcome. More important is the impact of a servo-controlled device on the workload of bedside nursing staff. Servo-control frees the bedside provider from intermittent adjustments of the temperature of the circulating fluid and allows greater attention to the care of critically ill infants following perinatal hypoxia–ischaemia who often have dysfunction of multiple organs. Even with servo-control to regulate whole body cooling, close oversight of the cooling device is warranted to detect unanticipated problems that may limit the therapy.

The results of the clinical trials of targeted temperature management are extremely encouraging to date. Yet there are still important questions that remain to be resolved regarding this therapy. These include temperature regulation after resuscitation for infants at risk of HIE, cooling on transport, optimizing a targeted temperature regimen (duration and depth of temperature reduction) and the rate of rewarming.

## References

1. Gluckman PD, Wyatt JS, Azzopardi D, et al. Selective head cooling with mild systemic hypothermia after neonatal encephalopathy: multicentre randomised trial. *Lancet* 2005;**365**:663–70.

2. Shankaran S, Laptook AR, Ehrenkranz RA, et al. Whole-body hypothermia for neonates with hypoxic-ischemic encephalopathy. *N Engl J Med* 2005;**353**:1574–84.

3. Azzopardi DV, Strohm B, Edwards AD, et al. Moderate hypothermia to treat perinatal asphyxial encephalopathy. *N Engl J Med* 2009;**361**:1349–58.

4. Zhou WH, Cheng GQ, Shao XM, et al. Selective head cooling with mild systemic hypothermia after neonatal hypoxic-ischemic encephalopathy: a multicenter randomized controlled trial in China. *J Pediatr* 2010;**157**:367–72.

5. Simbruner G, Mittal RA, Rohlmann F, Muche R. Systemic hypothermia after neonatal encephalopathy: outcomes of neo.nEURO.network RCT. *Pediatrics* 2010;**126**:e771–8.

6. Jacobs SE, Morley CJ, Inder TE, et al. Whole-body hypothermia for term and near-term newborns with hypoxic-ischemic encephalopathy: a randomized controlled trial. *Arch Pediatr Adolesc Med* 2011;**165**:692–700.

7. Greeley WJ, Kern FH, Ungerleider RM, et al. The effect of hypothermic cardiopulmonary bypass and total circulatory arrest on cerebral metabolism in neonates, infants and children. *J Thorac Cardiovasc Surg* 1991;**101**:783–94.

8. Klaus MH, Fanaroff AA. The physical environment. In: Klaus MH, Fanaroff AA, editors. *Care of the high-risk neonate*. 5th edition. Philadelphia: Saunders; 2001. p. 130–46.

9. Laptook AR, Shalak L, Corbett RJ. Differences in brain temperature and cerebral blood flow during selective head versus whole-body cooling. *Pediatrics* 2001;**108**:1103–10.

10. Wass CT, Lanier WL, Hofer RE, Scheithauer BW, Andrews AG. Temperature changes of > or = 1 degree C alter functional neurologic outcome and histopathology in a canine model of complete cerebral ischemia. *Anesthesiology* 1995;**83**:325–35.

11. Iwata S, Iwata O, Thornton JS, et al. Superficial brain is cooler in small piglets: neonatal hypothermia implications. *Ann Neurol* 2006;**60**:578–85.

12. Laptook AR, Corbett RJ, Sterett R, et al. Modest hypothermia provides partial neuroprotection for ischemic neonatal brain. *Pediatr Res* 1994;**35**(Pt 1):436–442.

13. Laptook AR, Corbett RJ, Sterett R, et al. Modest hypothermia provides partial neuroprotection when used for immediate resuscitation after brain ischemia. *Pediatr Res* 1997;**42**:17–23.

14. Kattwinkel J, Perlman JM, Aziz K, et al. Part 15: neonatal resuscitation: 2010 American Heart Association Guidelines for Cardiopulmonary Resuscitation and Emergency Cardiovascular Care. *Circulation* 2010;**122**(Suppl 3):S909–19.

15. Eicher DJ, Wagner CL, Katikaneni LP, et al. Moderate hypothermia in neonatal encephalopathy: efficacy outcomes. *Pediatr Neurol* 2005;**32**:11–7.

16. University of Oxford National Perinatal Epidemiology Unit. The UK TOBY Cooling Register. www.npeu.ox. ac.UK/tobyregister Accessed 8/30/2010, 2010.

17. Fairchild K, Sokora D, Scott J, Zanelli S. Therapeutic hypothermia on neonatal transport: 4-year experience in a single NICU. *J Perinatol* 2010;**30**:324–329.

18. Wyckoff MH, Parikh N, Balachanadran N, Moya F, Laptook AR. *Improved temperature profile using a ThermoTek cooling system for induction of hypothermia compared to the Cincinnati Sub-Zero.* E-PAS2006;**59**:443.

19. Johnston ED, Becher JC, Mitchell AP, Stenson BJ. Provision of servo-controlled cooling during neonatal transport. *Arch Dis Child Fetal Neonatal Ed* 2012;**97**: F365–7.

20. O'Reilly KM, Tooley J, Winterbottom S. Therapeutic hypothermia during neonatal transport. *Acta Paediatr* 2011;**100**:1084–6.

21. Mortola JP, Dotta A. Effects of hypoxia and ambient temperature on gaseous metabolism of newborn rats. *Am J Physiol* 1992;**263**(Pt 2):R267–72.

22. Sinclair JC. Servo-control for maintaining abdominal skin temperature at 36C in low birth weight infants. *Cochrane Database Syst Rev* 2002(1):CD001074.

23. Hallberg B, Olson L, Bartocci M, Edqvist I, Blennow M. Passive induction of hypothermia during transport of asphyxiated infants: a risk of excessive cooling. *Acta Paediatr* 2009;**98**:942–6.

24. Higgins RD, Raju T, Edwards AD, et al. Hypothermia and other treatment options for neonatal encephalopathy: an executive summary of the Eunice Kennedy Shriver NICHD workshop. *J Pediatr* 2011;**159**:851–8 e851.

25. Fukuda H, Tomimatsu T, Kanagawa T, et al. Postischemic hyperthermia induced caspase-3 activation in the newborn rat brain after hypoxia-ischemia and exacerbated the brain damage. *Biol Neonate* 2003;**84**:164–71.

26. Yager JY, Armstrong EA, Jaharus C, Saucier DM, Wirrell EC. Preventing hyperthermia decreases brain damage following neonatal hypoxic-ischemic seizures. *Brain Res* 2004;**1011**:48–57.

27. Baena RC, Busto R, Dietrich WD, Globus MY, Ginsberg MD. Hyperthermia delayed by 24 hours aggravates neuronal damage in rat hippocampus following global ischemia. *Neurology* 1997;**48**:768–73.

28. Dinarello CA, Cannon JG, Mancilla J, Bishai I, Lees J, Coceani F. Interleukin-6 as an endogenous pyrogen: induction of prostaglandin E2 in brain but not in peripheral blood mononuclear cells. *Brain Res* 1991;**562**:199–206.

29. Thompson HJ, Hoover RC, Tkacs NC, Saatman KE, McIntosh TK. Development of posttraumatic hypothermia after traumatic brain injury in rats is associated with increased periventricular inflammation. *J Cereb Blood Flow Metab* 2005;**25**:163–76.

30. Laptook A, Tyson J, Shankaran S, et al. Elevated temperature after hypoxic-ischemic encephalopathy: risk factor for adverse outcomes. *Pediatrics* 2008;**122**:491–9.

31. Wyatt JS, Gluckman PD, Liu PY, et al. Determinants of outcomes after head cooling for neonatal encephalopathy. *Pediatrics* 2007;**119**:912–21.

32. Ginsberg MD, Busto R. Combating hyperthermia in acute stroke: a significant clinical concern. *Stroke* 1998;**29**:529–34.

33. Shankaran S, Laptook A, Wright LL, et al. Whole-body hypothermia for neonatal encephalopathy: animal observations as a basis for a randomized, controlled pilot study in term infants. *Pediatrics* 2002; **110** (Pt 1):377–85.

34. Gunn AJ, Gunn TR, de Haan HH, Williams CE, Gluckman PD. Dramatic neuronal rescue with prolonged selective head cooling after ischemia in fetal lambs. *J Clin Invest* 1997;**99**:248–56.

35. Gunn AJ, Gunn TR, Gunning MI, Williams CE, Gluckman PD. Neuroprotection with prolonged head cooling started before postischemic seizures in fetal sheep. *Pediatrics* 1998;**102**:1098–106.

36. Gunn AJ, Bennet L, Gunning MI, Gluckman PD, Gunn TR. Cerebral hypothermia is not neuroprotective when started after postischemic seizures in fetal sheep. *Pediatr Res* 1999;**46**:274–80.

37. Shankaran S, Laptook AR, McDonald SA, et al. Temperature profile and outcomes of neonates undergoing whole body hypothermia for neonatal hypoxic-ischemic encephalopathy. *Pediatr Crit Care Med* 2012;**13**:53–9.

38. Strohm B, Azzopardi D. Temperature control during therapeutic moderate whole-body hypothermia for neonatal encephalopathy. *Arch Dis Child Fetal Neonatal Ed* 2010;**95**:F373–5.

39. Hoque N, Chakkarapani E, Liu X, Thoresen M. A comparison of cooling methods used in therapeutic hypothermia for perinatal asphyxia. *Pediatrics* 2010;**126**:e124–30.

40. Mayfield SR, Stonestreet BS, Brubakk AM, Shaul PW, Oh W. Regional blood flow in newborn piglets during environmental cold stress. *Am J Physiol* 1986;**251**(Pt 1):G308–13.

41. Hey EN. The relation between environmental temperature and oxygen consumption in the new-born baby. *J Physiol* 1969;**200**:589–603.

42. Stern AI, Avron M. An adenosine 5'-diphosphate ribose:orthophosphate adenylyltransferase from Euglena gracilis. *Biochim Biophys Acta* 1966;**118**:577–91.

43. Stern L, Lees MH, Leduc J. Environmental temperature, oxygen consumption and catecholamine excretion in newborn infants. *Pediatrics* 1965;**36**:367–73.

44. Thoresen M. Supportive care during neuroprotective hypothermia in the term newborn: adverse effects and their prevention. *Clin Perinatol* 2008; **35**:749–763, vii.

45. Froese G, Burton AC. Heat losses from the human head. *J Appl Physiol* 1957;**10**:235–41.

46. Liu X, Chakkarapani E, Hoque N, Thoresen M. Environmental cooling of the newborn pig brain during whole-body cooling. *Acta Paediatr* 2011;**100**:29–35.

47. Edwards AD, Brocklehurst P, Gunn AJ, et al. Neurological outcomes at 18 months of age after moderate hypothermia for perinatal hypoxic ischaemic encephalopathy: synthesis and meta-analysis of trial data. *BMJ* 2010;**340**:c363.

# Selective head cooling

Paul P. Drury, Laura Bennet and Alistair J. Gunn

## Introduction

There is now overwhelming clinical evidence that mild to moderate post-asphyxial cerebral cooling can be associated with long-term neuroprotection, as reviewed in Chapter 4 and previous meta-analyses [1]. The key requirements for protection in clinical and preclinical studies are that hypothermia be initiated as soon as possible in the latent phase, within the first 6 hours, before secondary deterioration and that it be continued for a sufficient period in relation to the evolution of delayed encephalopathic processes, typically 48 hours or more (Chapter 7). Despite this remarkable progress, the optimal mode of cooling remains unresolved. Although the majority of clinical trials of therapeutic hypothermia have involved whole body cooling, much of the preclinical development of hypothermia was focused on head cooling with mild systemic hypothermia and the CoolCap (Natus Ltd, OR) remains the only system to have received FDA registration for treatment of hypoxic–ischaemic encephalopathy (HIE). The present chapter highlights the evidence for head cooling, outlines the technical procedures and critically reviews the evidence for its safety and effectiveness.

## Cooling the head "selectively"

To provide neuroprotection with the least possible risk of systemic adverse effects in sick, unstable neonates, ideally we would cool only the brain. Although this has been achieved experimentally using cardiac bypass procedures [2], it is clearly impractical in routine practice. Pragmatically, partially selective cerebral cooling can be obtained using a cooling cap applied to the scalp while the body is warmed by some method such as an overhead heater to limit the degree of systemic hypothermia [3–5]. In practice, mild systemic hypothermia is desirable during head cooling,

first to limit the steepness of the intracerebral gradient that would otherwise be needed (and thus avoiding the need for excessively cold cap temperatures) [6] and second to provide greater cooling of the brain stem. In the piglet, this approach has been demonstrated to achieve a substantial (median, 5.3°C) sustained decrease in deep intracerebral temperature at the level of the basal ganglia compared with the rectal temperature [7,8]. Similar results during brief head cooling have been reported by others in the fetal sheep [9], young adult cat [10], the newborn rat [11] and the piglet [12]. Although direct temperature measurements are not feasible in asphyxiated newborns, head cooling has been shown to increase the gradient between nasopharyngeal temperature, an index of the temperature at the base of the brain, and rectal temperature by nearly 1°C [3].

In many ways, this approach is an extension of normal physiology. Even in the healthy neonate, there is no single cerebral temperature, but a gradient from the warmer deep regions to the cooler surface [13]. The brain is a significant heat producer and is cooled by a combination of surface radiation and blood flow convection. Thus, the deep brain temperature is approximately 1° to 2°C higher than the surface of the head [14] and 0.7°C higher than core body temperature [13]. Consistent with these relationships, secondary hypoperfusion after asphyxia is associated with a further relative increase in deep brain temperature [13].

## Is head cooling safe?

Overall, the majority of potential safety issues appear to be generic to hypothermia, as discussed next. The only potential adverse effects that appear to be truly specific to head cooling are scalp oedema and local skin damage. Oedema was observed in 22% of cooled

*Neonatal Neural Rescue*, ed. A. David Edwards, Denis V. Azzopardi and Alistair J. Gunn. Published by Cambridge University Press. © Cambridge University Press 2013.

infants in the Fudan study [15] and 28% in the CoolCap study [16]. All cases rapidly resolved after rewarming, consistent with reduced venous return. Local pressure necrosis of the scalp occurred in a few very sick infants with the original CoolCap protocol, but no additional cases were seen after the frequency of removing the cap to check the scalp was increased to every 12 hours.

All remaining issues appear to be generic to systemic hypothermia. Hypothermia slows the atrial pacemaker and intracardiac conduction. Consequently, hypothermia to less than approximately 35.5°C is associated with mild, sustained physiological sinus bradycardia [5,16–18]. This relationship between heart rate and core temperature likely mainly reflects decreased metabolic demand with decreasing temperature. Although a fall in heart rate denotes a reduction in total cardiac output, experimentally a thermoregulatory increase in peripheral vascular tone balances the fall in heart rate and thus maintains blood pressure during cooling [19,20]. Systemic hypotension and requirement for blood pressure support were common in the CoolCap trial, and, overall, cooled infants were given more inotropes and volume expansion than non-cooled infants [21]. Detailed analysis of these data, however, showed that the requirement for inotropes was identical in cooled and control infants in the first 24 hours, but there was slower withdrawal of treatment from 24 to 72 hours such that cooled infants were receiving inotropes at a higher mean arterial blood pressure. This strongly suggests conservative approach to withdrawal of inotropes in cooled infants by (un-blinded) attending physicians, possibly partly in response to the reduced heart rate.

Some infants showed a markedly prolonged QT duration, above the 98th percentile corrected for age and heart rate, without arrhythmia, during cooling, that resolved with rewarming [22]. Although such isolated prolonged QT does not seem to be associated with an increased risk of ventricular arrhythmias, other therapies which lengthen the QT interval (such as macrolide antibiotics) should be avoided.

In contrast with the historical belief that hypothermia increases the risk of hypoglycaemia, hypothermia has been consistently associated with transient mild hyperglycaemia, both in adult [23] and infant trials [16], with no increase in the risk of hypoglycaemia. A similar transient rise in glucose concentrations has been observed in the piglet and near-term fetal sheep [24,25] and likely reflects hypothermia-induced catecholamine and cortisol release. Indeed, we and others have previously shown that hypothermia is associated with elevated ACTH, cortisol and glucose [26–28].

Hypothermia has profound anti-inflammatory effects, including neutropenia [29] and reduced neutrophil function [30], which in older adults seems to moderately increase the risk of pneumonia and bacteraemia [31,32]. There was no apparent increase in the rate of infection in the CoolCap trial, or other RCTs; however, it is important to appreciate that this may reflect routine screening and treatment for possible infection within the trials [16,18]. Thus, this potential risk must continue to be carefully monitored.

Historically, hypothermia has been associated with impaired coagulation in term infants [33]. Despite this, there was no increase in haemorrhagic complications in CoolCap or other large trials [16,18,34]. In part this may be due to confounding between other illnesses and risk of hypothermia in previous case series, but also in part because the primary effect of hypothermia is a linear increase in clotting times in proportion to the biochemical rate constant (i.e., 5% per degree) [35]; thus, the impact of mild therapeutic cooling of ~3°C will be associated with a modest prolongation of clotting times of 15%. In a smaller trial of whole body cooling, Eicher et al did find a reduced platelet count and an increase in plasma requirement in cooled infants [36]. Although it is not possible to rule out the possibility that this reflected slightly deeper cooling, to a rectal temperature of 33 °C vs. 33.5 °C [36], since this has not been replicated, most likely it was just a chance finding in a small study.

Given that prothrombin times are increased, however, modestly when measured at the patient's temperature [35], it is reasonable to ask whether there might be a risk for intracranial haemorrhage. Historically, intracranial haemorrhage has been shown in 24% of term infants with HIE [37]. With the exception of the TOBY trial which reported intracranial haemorrhage in 39% of the cooled infants and in 31% of the normothermia infants (not significantly different) [34], the majority of the other major trials found rates of less than 10%, with no differences between groups [15,16,18,36,38–40]. Moreover, in a larger case series of 86 infants with HIE and moderate to severely abnormal aEEG there was no difference in the incidence of intracranial haemorrhage between selective head and whole body cooling or no cooling assessed by magnetic resonance imaging [41]. Consistent with this reassuring finding, cerebral haemorrhage was not seen in piglets after cooling the cortex to less than 30°C [42,43]. An important caution is that head cooling has only been tested in term infants. It is unknown whether, in the setting of modern intensive care, selected preterm infants with evidence of acute metabolic acidosis on cord blood and clinical encephalopathy would be at risk of intracranial haemorrhage during head cooling [44]. It is encouraging that studies in preterm fetal sheep, at an equivalent stage of neural maturation, now suggest that head cooling, started 90 minutes after profound asphyxia, is associated with widespread neuroprotection [20]. However, at present hypothermia should not be used for preterm infants outside of controlled trials.

Finally, subcutanous fat necrosis has been associated with both asphyxia and hypothermia in neonates [45]. There have been case reports of this and related skin complications after profound hypothermia during cardiopulmonary bypass surgery or accidental hypothermia in neonates [46–51], but it remains unclear whether the association is with hypothermia or hypoperfusion injury. No cases occurred in CoolCap. This may reflect either no association with mild hypothermia, or a very infrequent complication.

# Eligibility for head cooling

As reviewed in Chapter 7, perhaps the most critical aspect of therapeutic hypothermia is to apply cooling as soon as possible, in the latent phase before the onset of secondary deterioration as shown by energy failure and seizures [9,20,24,52,53]. Table 11.1 outlines the criteria used for entry into the CoolCap trial. Although it is plausible that some benefit might be achieved despite small delays in starting treatment beyond 6 hours after birth [40], since in preclinical studies the window for effective intervention appears to be longer after milder injury [54], there is no strong evidence at present.

# Additional monitoring during cooling

As part of stepwise recruitment protocol, moderate or severe reduction in amplitude-integrated EEG amplitude was required to select infants for the initial CoolCap trial [16]. The amplitude-integrated EEG monitoring electrodes were then removed before the CoolCap was applied to prevent local pressure. However, subsequently other investigators have reported continued monitoring using single-channel

**Table 11.1.** Selection criteria for entry into the CoolCap trial

| Criterion A | Infants > 36.0 weeks' gestation* with ONE of the following: * for gestation age also use clinical assessment |
|---|---|
| ↓ | 1 Apgar score of <5 at 10 minutes after birth |
| | 2 Continued need for resuscitation, including endotracheal or mask ventilation, at ten minutes after birth |
| | 3 Acidosis defined as either umbilical cord pH or any arterial, venous or capillary pH within 60 minutes of birth less than pH 7.00 (<7.00) |
| | 4 Base deficit greater than or equal to (≥) 16 mmol/L in umbilical cord blood sample or any blood sample within 60 minutes of birth (arterial or venous blood) |
| Criterion B | Moderate to severe encephalopathy consisting of altered state of consciousness (lethargy, stupor or coma) and at least ONE or more of the following: |
| ↓ | 1 Hypotonia |
| | 2 Abnormal reflexes including oculomotor or pupillary abnormalities |
| | 3 Absent or weak suck |
| | 4 Clinical seizures, as recorded by trained personnel |
| Criterion C | At least 30 minutes duration of aEEG recording within the first 6 hours of life that shows abnormal background aEEG activity (al Naqeeb *et al*, 1999) or seizures (clinical or electrical) thus meeting ONE of the following: |
| ↓ | 1 Normal background with some electrical seizure activity |
| | 2 Moderately abnormal activity (upper margin of trace >10 μV and lower margin of trace <5 μV) |
| | 3 Suppressed activity (upper margin of trace <10 μV and lower margin of trace <5 μV) |
| | 4 Continuous seizure activity |

needle electrodes placed at P3-P4 during cooling without complications [55]. To date no studies have included other monitoring, such as near-infrared spectroscopy, during cooling. It is likely that additional monitoring equipment other than small aEEG electrodes would impede cooling and is not advisable.

## Cooling procedure

The key practical differences between head cooling and whole body cooling are the need first for manual control of cooling and second, to optimize the cooling environment to achieve a gradient between the head and the body. This means that head cooling needs more planning to deliver it effectively, although the amount of extra work or attention should not be excessive. Broadly, the general approach is to deliver maximal heat input to the baby's trunk and then adjust the temperature of the water being circulated through the cap to achieve the desired rectal temperature. Providing maximal heat to the body is important to achieve the maximal gradient between brain and body and to reduce the impact of changes in endogenous thermogenesis [56].

To allow maximal body warming, the infant should be placed directly under the radiant warmer with nothing impeding radiant warmth to the body; a reflective heat shield over the baby's head prevents inadvertent warming of the cap. Temperature probes are placed over the liver on the abdomen to control the radiant warmer and a regular rectal thermistor is placed 6 cm into the rectum and secured. In the CoolCap trial, a fully sheathed oesophageal probe was inserted into the nare to a depth of 5.5 cm and secured to measure nasopharyngeal temperature [16]; however, this probe has not been shown to provide immediately useful feedback at present.

The cap is then placed on the baby's head to allow cooled water to be circulated. The CoolCap provides a matrix where cooled water flows in from one end and out the other. The cap should be primed with distilled water and connected to the cooling machine using PVC or similar tubing prior to applying it. An appropriate sized cap is then fitted to the infant's head so that the face, forehead and ears are not covered. The cap is secured with a Velcro strap under the chin to hold the cap in place without being tight around the neck. A separate fabric cap is then placed over the plastic cooling cap and fastened with Velcro straps. This cap ensures

**Table 11.2.** Suggested starting cap and final radiant warmer temperatures

| Infant size | Suggested starting cap temperature | Suggested final radiant warmer servo temperature |
| --- | --- | --- |
| Small infants (<2.5 kg) | 12.0–15.0°C | ~37.0–37.5°C |
| Normal infants (≥2.5 kg, <4.0 kg) | 10.0–12.0°C | ~36.0–37.0°C |
| Large infants (≥4.0 kg) | 8.0–10.0°C | ~35.0–36.0°C |

the plastic cooling cap is held in place and provides an attachment point to secure the thermal cap. This cap partially covers the ears. The final cap is an insulating thermal cap which prevents both convective and radiant warming of the head. This cap attaches to the fabric cap by means of several Velcro attachments on the underside and outside respectively.

The ideal initial temperature of the cap will depend on several factors including infant's size, metabolic rate and medications, as suggested in Table 11.2. Although the optimal systemic temperature remains unclear, the published trials used a target rectal temperature range of 34–35°C. To allow rapid cooling at the start of treatment, the radiant warmer should initially be turned off and then re-started when rectal temperature reaches 35.5°C to avoid overshoot cooling. The recommended initial radiant heater servo setting is 37°C, which should be adjusted regularly to 0.5°C above the skin temperature measured by the radiant heater once the infant's temperature has stabilized, to maintain the heater at 100% output. In the CoolCap trial [16], typical final radiant warmer servo setting were ~37.0–37.5°C for small infants (<2.5 kg), 36.0–37.0°C for normal infants (>2.5, <4.0 kg) and 35.0–36.0°C for large infants (>4.0 kg). In no circumstances should the radiant warmer servo temperature be set higher than 37.5°C.

## Adjustments of cap temperature

Further adjustments of the cap temperature will almost always be required after hypothermia has been induced. During active cooling, temperature must be determined by the balance of endogenous heat production, external heat input from the overhead heater and heat removal.

In contrast with adults, infants preferentially use brown fat (non-shivering thermogenesis) instead of shivering to produce heat [57]. Post-asphyxial seizures are also an important source of both cerebral and peripheral thermogenesis [58]. Thus, factors that inhibit non-shivering thermogenesis or muscle activity, including hypoxia and commonly used anaesthetics and sedatives such as propofol, fentanyl and barbiturates [59,60] and have been associated with a fall in core body temperature in infants [60–64]. Furthermore, spontaneous changes in the metabolic rates of infants may occur more frequently during the evolution of hypoxic–ischaemic encephalopathy than previously recognized and also need to be met by appropriate adjustments in heat removal, i.e., by adjustment of the cap temperature.

Provided the infant is nursed with 100% radiant warmer input, typically the infant's rectal temperature will change slowly. Thus, changes in the cap temperature should be made in small steps, of 0.5 to 1°C at most. Furthermore, it is critical to allow sufficient time for compensation; typically it will take approximately 45 minutes for an infant to achieve steady state. Knowledge of the infant's size, condition, mediations and anticipated procedures or investigations all help predict the infant's response. For example, growth restricted infants and infants requiring inotrope support are likely to need a higher cap temperature due to reduced thermogenesis [56].

Rarely, a large infant or a very active infant will require more cooling than the cap can provide. If the cap will not reach 8°C in the first instance it may be useful to lower the room temperature by 1°C. If this does not adequately lower the temperature then practical steps should be taken, such as checking that the rectal temperature thermistor is correctly inserted, that the radiant warmer is in servo mode and the set-temperature is no higher than 37.5°C, that the cap is the appropriate size (use an extra-large cap if not already using one) and fits snugly, and that the water is circulating (the water alarm should be activated by any kinks). However, it is reasonable to note that active and large infants may require a skin set-point as low as 35.0°C.

## Management during medical procedures

The cap may need to be removed or the radiant heat maintaining the core body temperature may be obstructed by essential medical procedures such as X-rays or cardiac ultrasound. Similarly, longer procedures such as line placement which require draping the infant for longer than several minutes will tend to cause a cooling effect by reducing radiant heat input. One pragmatic approach is to position the infant's rectal temperature at the upper acceptable range around one hour before starting the procedure. If the procedure will be prolonged, the cap temperature may be increased or the cap removed completely and then restarted after the procedure.

## Rewarming

Following the 3 days of cooling, the rectal temperature should be raised to normal, in steps of no more than 0.5°C per hour. In the case of the CoolCare System, the cooling mode should be turned off and the monitor mode should be turned on before removing the CoolCap. The radiant warmer's set point is then adjusted to 35.0°C, or approximately 0.3°C above the rectal temperature and increased by approximately 0.5°C per hour, generally in increments of 0.2–0.3°C every 30 minutes.

## Transport

Many infants will need to be transferred to a regional centre with therapeutic hypothermia capability. In the cooling trials, the proportion of outborn infants was between 42% [18] and 82% [15]. Given the importance of starting cooling as soon as possible after birth, hypothermia during transfer needs to be considered. In peripheral hospitals where aEEG is not available, the decision to include therapeutic hypothermia in the management of the infant can be made based on criteria A and B alone (Table 11.1). Treatment can then be started peripherally and continued during transfer. As with standard intensive care, continuous monitoring of the infant's temperature with rectal thermistor is crucial to avoid overcooling. The optimal approach to cooling is unclear; however, passive cooling or active cooling with cool packs or even water-filled gloves can be used.

## Infant size and age

Given the contribution of non-shivering thermogenesis to heat production in the neonate, it is crucial to carefully monitor full-term small for gestational age (SGA) infants as they are likely to have less brown fat and they are easy to overcool [65]. A secondary analysis of the CoolCap trial showed that term low birth weight (< 25th percentile for term infants) infants with HIE had a better outcome that those ≥ 25th percentile of birth weight independent of cooling [66]. The mechanism is unknown, but speculatively, may have been related to lower non-shivering thermogenesis and thus relatively lower core temperatures. In contrast, therapeutic hypothermia showed greatest benefit in larger infants and was not associated with significant protection in the SGA infants [66]. Experimentally, cooling has been reported to be greater in smaller piglets for a given cap temperature [67]; however, others have shown neuroprotection in piglets with similar cortical cooling [43]. The reason for these contrasting results is not clear, but most likely was related to the level of head cooling that can be pragmatically achieved in the clinical setting. In the CoolCap trial smaller infants consistently required higher cap temperatures to stay in the target range for core body temperatures, thus they must have been exposed to less not greater cooling compared with larger infants. These findings further support the importance of achieving the maximum practical degree of head cooling for optimal results.

## Is selective head cooling "better or worse" than whole body cooling?

It is important to consider the direction of energy transfer, or heat sinks, between the two cooling modalities. Under normal conditions, the temperature of the cortex is around 0.5°C cooler than the deep grey matter structures [67], with natural cooling from scalp radiation. In newborn piglets Iwata et al found that selective head cooling was associated with a marked temperature gradient between cortex and deep brain structures which was reproducible at cap temperatures of 20, 15 and 10°C [67]. In contrast, whole body cooling has been associated with slightly higher brain than body temperatures [6,67], but relatively uniform temperatures throughout the brain. These data suggest that selective head cooling increases the natural temperature gradients, rather than reducing all regions to a similar temperature. Encouragingly, data in the piglet suggest that the optimal cooling temperature following hypoxia–ischaemia was lower for the cortex than for the deep grey matter [68]. Finally, a small case series suggested better cortical protection assessed by MRI in infants with selective head cooling compared to whole body cooling [41]. Thus, it remains plausible that head cooling might provide more optimal protection of the cortex, but similar or less protection of the basal ganglia.

Pragmatically, of the six major clinical trials reported to date only two used selective head cooling [15,16]. Their outcome at 18 months of age was broadly equivalent to the whole body cooling trials as reviewed in Chapter 20. To demonstrate a difference of 5% in a "head to head" study of whole body cooling and head cooling would require randomization of several thousand infants. Furthermore, given that the preclinical data suggest that any benefit would be for cortical protection, it is likely that long-term follow-up, well beyond infancy, would be needed to show a clinical difference.

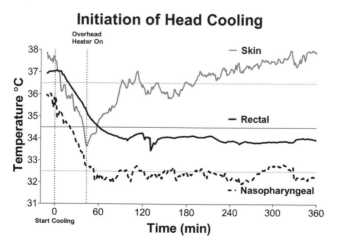

**Figure 11.1.** Example of the temperature gradients produced by selective head cooling. The cap is applied and the overhead heater is turned off at time 0. Note the broadly parallel falls in skin, rectal and nasopharyngeal temperatures. At the second vertical line, the overhead heater is turned on when the rectal temperature reaches 35°C. The skin temperature then rises and the rectal temperature reaches a stable plateau within the target range of 34 to 35°C. Note that the gradient between rectal and nasopharyngeal temperatures widens once the heater is turned on, by approximately 1°C, consistent with a greater fall in the temperature of the base of the brain than the core body temperature.

# Conclusion

On the clinical evidence available today, head cooling with mild systemic hypothermia and whole body cooling are supported by the pragmatic clinical trial evidence and are reasonable, easily implemented choices to apply therapeutic hypothermia in the neonatal intensive care unit. Furthermore, preclinical studies of both strategies are needed to establish ways to achieve further improvement in outcome. Because HIE is a relatively uncommon condition, it is clearly desirable whenever possible to centralise this treatment to larger intensive care units, to increase expertise in the use of hypothermia. Perhaps more importantly, it is clear that very large consortia of neonatal units will be needed to allow further improvements to current treatment protocols, such as the length or degree of hypothermia, to be incrementally tested.

# Acknowledgements

The authors' work reported in this chapter was supported by the Health Research Council of New Zealand, Lottery Health Board of New Zealand, the Auckland Medical Research Foundation and the March of Dimes Birth Defects Foundation. P. Drury is supported by the New Zealand Neurological Foundation W&B Miller Doctoral Scholarship.

# References

1. Edwards AD, Brocklehurst P, Gunn AJ, et al. Neurological outcomes at 18 months of age after moderate hypothermia for perinatal hypoxic ischaemic encephalopathy: synthesis and meta-analysis of trial data. *BMJ* 2010;**340**:c363.

2. Wass CT, Waggoner JR, Cable DG, et al. Selective convective brain cooling during normothermic cardiopulmonary bypass in dogs. *J Thorac Cardiovasc Surg* 1998;**115**:1350–7.

3. Gunn AJ, Gluckman PD, Gunn TR. Selective head cooling in newborn infants after perinatal asphyxia: a safety study. *Pediatrics* 1998;**102**:885–92.

4. Simbruner G, Haberl C, Harrison V, Linley L, Willeitner AE. Induced brain hypothermia in asphyxiated human newborn infants: a retrospective chart analysis of physiological and adverse effects. *Intensive Care Med* 1999;**25**:1111–7.

5. Battin MR, Penrice J, Gunn TR, Gunn AJ. Treatment of term infants with head cooling and mild systemic hypothermia (35.0 degrees C and 34.5 degrees C) after perinatal asphyxia. *Pediatrics* 2003;**111**:244–51.

6. Laptook AR, Shalak L, Corbett RJ. Differences in brain temperature and cerebral blood flow during selective head versus whole-body cooling. *Pediatrics* 2001;**108**:1103–10.

7. Thoresen M, Simmonds M, Satas S, Tooley J, Silver I. Effective selective head cooling during posthypoxic hypothermia in newborn piglets. *Pediatr Res* 2001;**49**:594–9.

8. Tooley J, Satas S, Eagle R, Silver IA, Thoresen M. Significant selective head cooling can be maintained long-term after global hypoxia ischemia in newborn piglets. *Pediatrics* 2002;**109**:643–9.

9. George S, Scotter J, Dean JM, et al. Induced cerebral hypothermia reduces post-hypoxic loss of phenotypic striatal neurons in preterm fetal sheep. *Exp Neurol* 2007;**203**:137–47.

10. Sefrin P, Horn M. Selective cerebral hypothermia following cardiac arrest in the cat. *Anaesthesist* 1991;**40**:397–403.

11. Towfighi J, Housman C, Heitjan DF, Vannucci RC, Yager JY. The effect of focal cerebral cooling on perinatal hypoxic-ischemic brain damage. *Acta Neuropathol (Berl)* 1994;**87**:598–604.

12. Gelman B, Schleien CL, Lohe A, Kuluz JW. Selective brain cooling in infant piglets after cardiac arrest and resuscitation. *Crit Care Med* 1996;**24**:1009–17.

13. Simbruner G, Nanz S, Fleischhacker E, Derganc M. Brain temperature discriminates between neonates with damaged, hypoperfused and normal brains. *Am J Perinatol* 1994;**11**:137–43.

14. Gunn AJ, Gunn TR. Effect of radiant heat on head temperature gradient in term infants. *Arch Dis Child Fetal Neonatal Ed* 1996;**74**:F200–3.

15. Zhou WH, Cheng GQ, Shao XM, et al. Selective head cooling with mild systemic hypothermia after neonatal hypoxic-ischemic encephalopathy: a multicenter randomized controlled trial in China. *J Pediatr* 2010;**157**:367–72, 72.e1–3.

16. Gluckman PD, Wyatt JS, Azzopardi D, et al. Selective head cooling with mild systemic hypothermia to improve neurodevelopmental outcome following neonatal encephalopathy. *Lancet* 2005;**365**:663–70.

17. Shankaran S, Laptook A, Wright LL, et al. Whole-body hypothermia for neonatal encephalopathy: animal observations as a basis for a randomized, controlled pilot study in term infants. *Pediatrics* 2002;**110**:377–85.

18. Shankaran S, Laptook AR, Ehrenkranz RA, et al. Whole-body hypothermia for neonates with

hypoxic-ischemic encephalopathy. *N Engl J Med* 2005;**353**:1574–84.

19. Walter B, Bauer R, Kuhnen G, Fritz H, Zwiener U. Coupling of cerebral blood flow and oxygen metabolism in infant pigs during selective brain hypothermia. *J Cereb Blood Flow Metab* 2000;**20**:1215–24.

20. Bennet L, Roelfsema V, George S, et al. The effect of cerebral hypothermia on white and grey matter injury induced by severe hypoxia in preterm fetal sheep. *J Physiol* 2007;**578**:491–506.

21. Battin MR, Thoresen M, Robinson E, et al. Does head cooling with mild systemic hypothermia affect requirement for blood pressure support? *Pediatrics* 2009;**123**:1031–6.

22. Gunn TR, Wilson NJ, Aftimos S, Gunn AJ. Brain hypothermia and QT interval. *Pediatrics* 1999;**103**:1079.

23. Bernard SA, Gray TW, Buist MD, et al. Treatment of comatose survivors of out-of-hospital cardiac arrest with induced hypothermia. *N Engl J Med* 2002;**346**:557–63.

24. Gunn AJ, Gunn TR, de Haan HH, Williams CE, Gluckman PD. Dramatic neuronal rescue with prolonged selective head cooling after ischemia in fetal lambs. *J Clin Invest* 1997;**99**:248–56.

25. Satas S, Loberg EM, Porter H, et al. Effect of global hypoxia-ischaemia followed by 24 h of mild hypothermia on organ pathology and biochemistry in a newborn pig survival model. *Biol Neonate* 2003;**83**:146–56.

26. Davidson JO, Fraser M, Naylor AS, et al. The effect of cerebral hypothermia on cortisol and ACTH responses after umbilical cord occlusion in preterm fetal sheep. *Pediatr Res* 2008;**63**:51–5.

27. Gunn TR, Butler J, Gluckman P. Metabolic and hormonal responses to cooling the fetal sheep in utero. *J Dev Physiol* 1986;**8**:55–66.

28. Thoresen M, Satas S, Loberg EM, et al. Twenty-four hours of mild hypothermia in unsedated newborn pigs starting after a severe global hypoxic-ischemic insult is not neuroprotective. *Pediatr Res* 2001;**50**:405–11.

29. Biggar WD, Bohn D, Kent G. Neutrophil circulation and release from bone marrow during hypothermia. *Infect Immun* 1983;**40**:708–12.

30. Biggar WD, Bohn DJ, Kent G, Barker C, Hamilton G. Neutrophil migration in vitro and in vivo during hypothermia. *Infect Immun* 1984;**46**:857–9.

31. Schubert A. Side effects of mild hypothermia. *J Neurosurg Anesthesiol* 1995;**7**:139–47.

32. Todd MM, Hindman BJ, Clarke WR, Torner JC. Mild intraoperative hypothermia during surgery for intracranial aneurysm. *N Engl J Med* 2005;**352**:135–45.

33. Chadd MA, Gray OP. Hypothermia and coagulation defects in the newborn. *Arch Dis Child* 1972;**47**:819–21.

34. Azzopardi DV, Strohm B, Edwards AD, et al. Moderate hypothermia to treat perinatal asphyxial encephalopathy. *N Engl J Med* 2009;**361**:1349–58.

35. Valeri CR, Feingold H, Cassidy G, et al. Hypothermia-induced reversible platelet dysfunction. *Ann Surg* 1987;**205**:175–81.

36. Eicher DJ, Wagner CL, Katikaneni LP, et al. Moderate hypothermia in neonatal encephalopathy: Safety outcomes. *Pediatr Neurol* 2005;**32**:18–24.

37. Fitzhardinge PM, Flodmark O, Fitz CR, Ashby S. The prognostic value of computed tomography as an adjunct to assessment of the term infant with postasphyxial encephalopathy. *J Pediatr* 1981;**99**:777–81.

38. Simbruner G, Mittal RA, Rohlmann F, Muche R. Systemic hypothermia after neonatal encephalopathy: outcomes of neo.nEURO.network RCT. *Pediatrics* 2010;**126**:e771–8.

39. Jacobs SE, Morley CJ, Inder TE, et al. Whole-body hypothermia for term and near-term newborns with hypoxic-ischemic encephalopathy: a randomized controlled trial. *Arch Pediatr Adolesc Med* 2011.

40. Li T, Xu F, Cheng X, et al. Systemic hypothermia induced within 10 hours after birth improved neurological outcome in newborns with hypoxic-ischemic encephalopathy. *Hosp Pract (Minneap)* 2009;**37**:147–52.

41. Rutherford MA, Azzopardi D, Whitelaw A, et al. Mild hypothermia and the distribution of cerebral lesions in neonates with hypoxic-ischemic encephalopathy. *Pediatrics* 2005;**116**:1001–6.

42. Tooley JR, Eagle RC, Satas S, Thoresen M. Significant head cooling can be achieved while maintaining normothermia in the newborn piglet. *Arch Dis Child Fetal Neonatal Ed* 2005;**90**:F262–6.

43. Tooley JR, Satas S, Porter H, Silver IA, Thoresen M. Head cooling with mild systemic hypothermia in anesthetized piglets is neuroprotective. *Ann Neurol* 2003;**53**:65–72.

44. Salhab WA, Perlman JM. Severe fetal acidemia and subsequent neonatal encephalopathy in the larger premature infant. *Pediatr Neurol* 2005;**32**:25–9.

45. Burden AD, Krafchik BR. Subcutaneous fat necrosis of the newborn: a review of 11 cases. *Pediatr Dermatol* 1999;**16**:384–7.

46. Chuang SD, Chiu HC, Chang CC. Subcutaneous fat necrosis of the newborn complicating hypothermic cardiac surgery. *Br J Dermatol* 1995;**132**:805–10.

47. Collins HA, Stahlman M, Scott HW, Jr. The occurrence of subcutaneous fat necrosis in an infant following induced hypothermia used as an adjuvant in cardiac surgery. *Ann Surg* 1953;**138**:880–5.

48. Duhn R, Schoen EJ, Siu M. Subcutaneous fat necrosis with extensive calcification after hypothermia in two newborn infants. *Pediatrics* 1968;**41**:661–4.

49. Glover MT, Catterall MD, Atherton DJ. Subcutaneous fat necrosis in two infants after hypothermic cardiac surgery. *Pediatr Dermatol* 1991;**8**:210–2.

50. Silverman AK, Michels EH, Rasmussen JE. Subcutaneous fat necrosis in an infant, occurring after hypothermic cardiac surgery. Case report and analysis of etiologic factors. *J Am Acad Dermatol* 1986;**15**:331–6.

51. Wiadrowski TP, Marshman G. Subcutaneous fat necrosis of the newborn following hypothermia and complicated by pain and hypercalcaemia. *Australas J Dermatol* 2001;**42**:207–10.

52. Gunn AJ, Gunn TR, Gunning MI, Williams CE, Gluckman PD. Neuroprotection with prolonged head cooling started before postischemic seizures in fetal sheep. *Pediatrics* 1998;**102**:1098 106.

53. Gunn AJ, Bennet L, Gunning MI, Gluckman PD, Gunn TR. Cerebral hypothermia is not neuroprotective when started after postischemic seizures in fetal sheep. *Pediatr Res* 1999;**46**:274–80.

54. Iwata O, Iwata S, Thornton JS, et al. "Therapeutic time window" duration decreases with increasing severity of cerebral hypoxia-ischaemia under normothermia and delayed hypothermia in newborn piglets. *Brain Res* 2007;**1154**:173–80.

55. Thoresen M, Hellstrom-Westas L, Liu X, de Vries LS. Effect of hypothermia on amplitude-integrated electroencephalogram in infants with asphyxia. *Pediatrics* 2010;**126**:e131–9.

56. Gunn AJ, Battin M. Hypothermic centralization: new use for old knowledge? *Pediatrics* 2000;**106**:133–4.

57. Gunn TR, Gluckman PD. Perinatal thermogenesis. *Early Hum Dev* 1995;**42**:169–83.

58. Meldrum BS, Horton RW. Physiology of status epilepticus in primates. *Arch Neurol* 1973;**28**:1–9.

59. Plattner O, Semsroth M, Sessler DI, et al. Lack of nonshivering thermogenesis in infants anesthetized with fentanyl and propofol. *Anesthesiology* 1997;**86**:772–7.

60. Wixson SK, White WJ, Hughes HC Jr, Lang CM, Marshall WK. The effects of pentobarbital, fentanyl-droperidol, ketamine-xylazine and ketamine-diazepam on core and surface body temperature regulation in adult male rats. *Lab Anim Sci* 1987;**37**:743–9.

61. Echizenya M, Mishima K, Satoh K, et al. Heat loss, sleepiness and impaired performance after diazepam administration in humans. *Neuropsychopharmacology* 2003;**28**:1198–206.

62. Clark SM, Lipton JM. Effects of diazepam on body temperature of the aged squirrel monkey. *Brain Res Bull* 1981;**7**:5–9.

63. Zachariah SB, Zachariah A, Ananda R, Stewart JT. Hypothermia and thermoregulatory derangements induced by valproic acid. *Neurology* 2000;**55**:150–1.

64. Nagarajan L, Johnston K, Williams S. Hypothermia and thermoregulatory derangements induced by valproic acid. *Neurology* 2001;**56**:139.

65. Gluckman PD, Sizonenko SV, Bassett NS. The transition from fetus to neonate – an endocrine perspective. *Acta Paediatr Suppl* 1999;**88**:7–11.

66. Wyatt JS, Gluckman PD, Liu PY, et al. Determinants of outcomes after head cooling for neonatal encephalopathy. *Pediatrics* 2007;**119**:912–21.

67. Iwata S, Iwata O, Thornton JS, et al. Superficial brain is cooler in small piglets: neonatal hypothermia implications. *Ann Neurol* 2006;**60**:578–85.

68. Iwata O, Thornton JS, Sellwood MW, et al. Depth of delayed cooling alters neuroprotection pattern after hypoxia-ischemia. *Ann Neurol* 2005;**58**:75–87.

# Hypothermic neural rescue for neonatal encephalopathy in mid- and low-resource settings

Nicola J. Robertson and Sudhin Thayyil

## Introduction

The most significant burden of neonatal encephalopathy (NE) occurs in low- and mid-resource settings [1]. The WHO World Health Report 2005 estimated that an annual 1 million survivors of "birth asphyxia" may develop cerebral palsy, learning difficulties or other disabilities [2]. Globally, perinatal asphyxia is responsible for 42 million disability life adjusted years – this is double that due to diabetes and three quarters of that due to HIV/AIDS [1]. Almost one quarter of the world's 4 million annual neonatal deaths are caused by perinatal asphyxia (Figures 12.1, 12.2) [3]: 99% of these deaths occur in low- and mid-resource settings especially those countries with higher neonatal mortality rates (Figures 12.1, 12.2). The potential benefits of therapeutic hypothermia (were it to be safe and effective in every setting) are potentially greater in low- and mid-resource settings where birth asphyxia is at least 10-fold higher than in the developed world. However, all the positive evidence about the safety and efficacy of cooling relates to high-income countries. Furthermore, there is a theoretical risk that problems such as immune suppression by hypothermia may be deleterious in a different setting; one pilot study in a low-resource setting [4] reported more deaths in the cooled group and the expensive high tech cooling devices used in the developed world are not appropriate for global use in low- and mid-resource settings.

In this chapter, we discuss risk factors, incidence and outcome of NE in mid- and low-resource settings and compare where possible with figures from high-income countries. There are clearly significant differences between settings in terms of risk factors, incidence and outcome. These differences emphasize the importance of considering both risk prevention and treatment to reduce NE in low- and mid-resourced settings. In addition, we

must remember that accidental hypothermia is a very significant problem in low- and mid-resource settings and leads to significant neonatal morbidity and mortality [5] and the differentiation between accidental and therapeutic hypothermia is a very important concept on a global scale. Therapeutic hypothermia involves a package of neonatal care that includes support, monitoring and maintenance of metabolic and physiological homeostasis with adequate sedation and supportive care. As therapeutic hypothermia is adopted as standard of care in high-income countries, considerable organizational procedures are being put in place, with training, guidelines, audit, education and well-trained staff. It is clear that some low- and mid-resource setting facilities cannot achieve even basic perinatal care and so many other improvements in perinatal care must be achieved first.

## Definition and epidemiology of NE in low- and mid-resource settings

### Definitions

*Neonatal encephalopathy* (NE) is the clinical manifestation of disordered neonatal brain function in the term infant in the early neonatal period, manifested by respiratory difficulties, depression of tone and reflexes, subnormal level of consciousness and often seizures [6]. Studies of developed world populations describe the aetiology of NE as being varied with many genetic, metabolic and infective conditions presenting with similar clinical signs [7–9]. The disorder is termed *hypoxic–ischaemic encephalopathy* (HIE) if there is evidence that intrapartum asphyxia is the cause of the encephalopathy resulting in neurologic depression or seizures [10]. An important recurrent concept, even in studies in developed world

---

*Neonatal Neural Rescue*, ed. A. David Edwards, Denis V. Azzopardi and Alistair J. Gunn. Published by Cambridge University Press. © Cambridge University Press 2013.

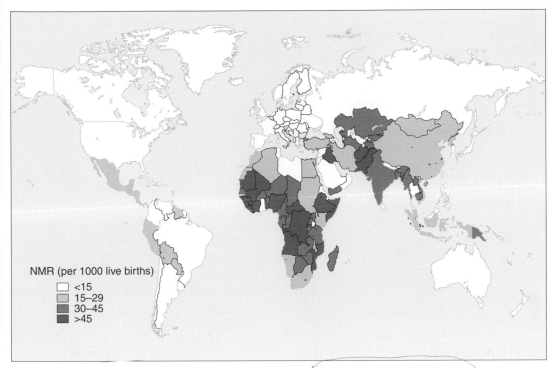

**Figure 12.1a.** Variation in neonatal mortality rate between countries (Zupan and Aahman WHO report 2005). Reproduced with permission from reference [3]. Please see plate section for colour version.

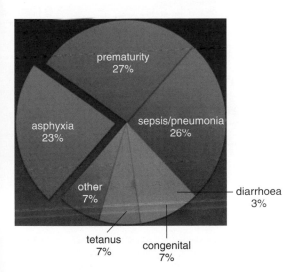

**Figure 12.1b.** Direct causes of neonatal deaths worldwide. Almost one quarter of deaths are attributed to perinatal asphyxia. Adapted from reference [3]. Please see plate section for colour version.

populations, is that the human injury of HIE is not clear cut; the aetiology, extent of hypoxia or ischaemia, maturational stage of the brain, regional cerebral blood flow and general health of the infant before the injury can all

impact on the extent of brain injury as well as the outcome following injury. Perinatal conditions that lead to hypoxia ischaemia, some of which are more likely in low- and mid-resource settings, are summarised in Table 12.1.

Accurate estimation of cases of NE or HIE is extremely difficult in low- and mid-resource settings; there is no single gold standard for accurate diagnosis of the condition due to low sensitivity and specificity of the markers used such as Apgar score, acidosis and fetal distress. Since 1996 there have been three consensus statements addressing the diagnosis of intrapartum asphyxia (Table 12.2) [10–12]. These consensus statements emphasize the use of multiple markers for the diagnosis; some signs are considered essential and others supportive. The two most recent statements use findings from cerebral imaging as supportive evidence of intrapartum asphyxia [10,12]. This is unlikely to be available in most low- and mid-resource settings.

# Risk factors

The case control study of NE in Western Australia showed that many cases of NE have origins before the

129

**Table 12.1.** Potential risk factors leading to intrapartum or postpartum hypoxia

|  | Factors leading to intrapartum hypoxia | Effect | Specific issues related to low- and mid-resource settings |
|---|---|---|---|
| Obstetric | Pre-eclampsia and eclampsia | Reduced placental flow | More common without fetal monitoring and optimal obstetric care |
|  | Separation of placenta from maternal circulation | Placental abruption |  |
|  | Compression of umbilical cord, impeding blood flow | Cord compression |  |
|  | Prolonged labour | Contractions associated with hypoxia |  |
|  | Breech presentation or shoulder dystocia | Fetal entrapment during labour |  |
| Postpartum | Failure of the infant to initiate respiration occurs in 5–10% of births worldwide | Postnatal hypoxia-ischaemia | Lack of adequate resuscitation is common in low- and mid-resource settings – and is the focus of active research and intervention |

Note: 60% of NE infants in a low-resource hospital setting (Kathmandu, Nepal) compared with 3% of controls had evidence of intrapartum compromise or were born after an intrapartum difficulty likely to result in intrapartum compromise [14].

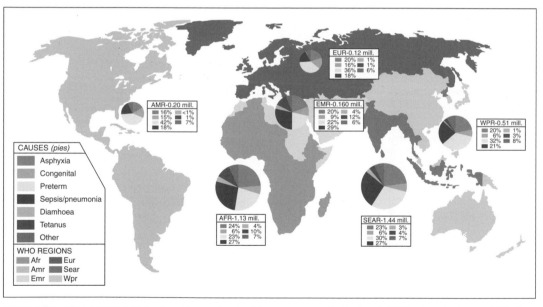

**Figure 12.2.** The estimated distribution of causes for 4 million neonatal deaths for the six WHO regions in the year 2000. The size of the circle represents the number of deaths in each region. Afr, Africa; Amr, Americas; EMR, Eastern Mediterranean; Eur, Europe; Sear, Southeast Asia; Wpr, Western Pacific. Reproduced with permission from Lawn *et al* [*Int J Epidemiol* 2006;**35**:706–18]. Please see plate section for colour version.

onset of labour. Intrapartum risk factors include maternal pyrexia, persistent occipito-posterior position and acute intrapartum events; however, in over 70% of cases of NE there was no evidence of intrapartum hypoxia [8,9]. This is very different to the situation in many low-income countries where mothers are stunted, do not access antenatal care, have high stillbirth rates and receive poor obstetric care. Under these conditions, intrapartum factors probably remain more important in the causation of NE [13]. For example, in the case controlled

**Table 12.2.** Three consensus statements on diagnosing intrapartum asphyxia

| American Academy of Pediatrics/ American College of Obstetrics and Gynecology (1996) [11] | International Cerebral Palsy Task Force (1999) [12] | American College of Obstetrics and Gynecology (2003) [10] |
|---|---|---|
| Essential<br>• Profound metabolic acidosis (pH < 7.0)<br>• Apgar score < 3 after 5 minutes<br>• Neonatal encephalopathy<br>• Multi-organ system dysfunction<br><br>Criteria suggestive of intrapartum timing | Metabolic acidosis in early neonatal blood sample (pH < 7.0) and base deficit ≥12 mmol/l<br>• Moderate or severe encephalopathy<br>• Cerebral palsy of spastic quadriplegia or dyskinetic type<br>• Sentinel event<br>• Abrupt change in fetal heart rate<br>• Apgar score < 6 beyond 5 min<br>• Multisystem involvement<br>• Imaging evidence | Metabolic acidosis (pH < 7.0) and base deficit ≥12 mmol/l<br>• Moderate or severe encephalopathy<br>• Cerebral palsy of spastic quadriplegia or dyskinetic type<br>• Exclusion of other pathologies of cerebral palsy<br>• Sentinel event<br>• Abrupt change in fetal heart rate<br>• Apgar score ≤3 beyond 5 min<br>• Multisystem failure within 72 hours of birth<br>• Imaging evidence |

study in Kathmandu, there was evidence of intrapartum hypoxia–ischaemia in 60% of encephalopathic infants. Independent risk factors for NE included short maternal stature, high maternal age, lack of antenatal care and multiple birth [14]; intrapartum risk factors included non-cephalic presentation, prolonged rupture of membranes, cord prolapse and uterine rupture.

The risk factor profile for NE differs considerably in low- and mid-income countries compared with high-income countries. Infection and inflammation is a particular area of concern and relevance to perinatal brain injury as it is known to lower the threshold and amplify hypoxic-ischaemic injury [15]. One-third of the 4 million neonatal deaths (<28 days) and 500,000 maternal deaths that occur annually worldwide are associated with infections [2,3] and in the areas with 28-day neonatal mortality rate (NMR) >45 per 1000 births, up to 50% of these deaths are due to infection [3]. Maternal intrapartum fever of > 37.5°C has been shown to increase the risk of perinatal brain injury independent of infection [9] and increase the risk of early-onset neonatal seizures at term [16]. There is substantial experimental evidence also that pre-existing intrauterine inflammation can exacerbate hypoxic–ischaemic injury [15,17]. A maternal intrapartum fever of > 38°C persisting > 1 hour is usually considered a clinical indicator of chorioamnionitis;

epidemiological studies suggest that chorioamnionitis is an independent risk factor for cerebral palsy among term and near-term infants [18]. Indeed, term infants exposed to maternal infection are predisposed to delivery room depression and NE [19].

It is possible that the "dual hit" of combined infection/inflammation and hypoxia–ischaemia [15,20] results in more severe brain injury and increase in the risk of cerebral palsy [21]. The dual hit may be one of the factors responsible for the worse neurological outcome even with mild or moderate NE reported from low- and mid-income countries [14]; studies are currently under way to investigate this.

## Incidence

Precise estimates of NE and HIE incidence are uncertain as there is a lack of data from low- and mid-income countries and a complete lack of data from community based settings where most of the burden of perinatal hypoxia–ischaemia falls. In 2006, an admission audit to the special care baby unit at Mulago Hospital, Kampala, Uganda, revealed a moderate to severe NE incidence of 17.9/1000 term live births (personal communication, M. Nakakeeto). In the Indian subcontinent, the Indian National Neonatal-Perinatal Database (NNPD) suggests an overall NE incidence of 14 per 1000 live births [22].

**Table 12.3.** Variation in risk for NE and NE case fatality for 193 countries organized according to five categories of neonatal mortality, as a marker of health system performance [1]

| | Category 1 Very low mortality NMR ≤5 | Category 2 Low mortality NMR 6–15 | Category 3 Moderate mortality | Category 4 High mortality NMR 31–45 | Category 5 Very high mortality NMR≥45 |
|---|---|---|---|---|---|
| Incidence of NE median (range) | 1.9 (0.7–6.0) | 6.7 (4.7–8.7) | 9.8 (3.6–10.2) | 13.4 (5.5–22.2) | 26.5 (26.5) |
| NE case fatality Median (range) | 21% (17–37) | 12% (12%) | 19% (10–28%) | 31% (20–33%) | No data |

*Note:* Country groupings for NMR are adapted from the Lancet neonatal survival series [3] – see Figure 1. Data adapted from Lawn *et al*, *Int J Gynecol Obstet* 2009;107:S5–S19.

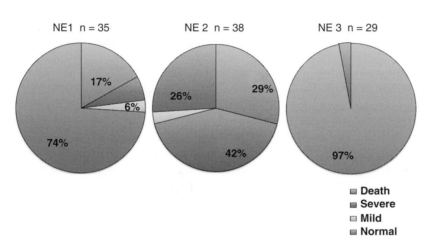

**Figure 12.3a.** Outcome of a cohort of 131 infants with NE (Stage 1–3) at 1 year of age in a maternity hospital in Kathmandu, Nepal. Reproduced from reference [14]. Please see plate section for colour version.

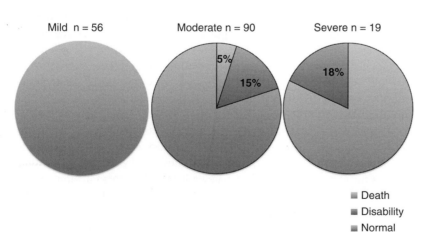

**Figure 12.3b.** Eight year outcome on death and disability in a cohort of infants with mild, moderate and severe encephalopathy at birth [24]. Comparing the outcomes (although tested at different ages) for a given Sarnat stage, significantly worse outcomes are seen in the low-resource setting in Kathmandu versus the Robertson and Finer study in the USA. For example, all infants with mild NE in the Robertson and Finer study had a normal outcome at 8 years whereas in the Ellis study 17% of infants died and 6% had a severe outcome at 1 year of age. 42% versus 15% of the moderate encephalopathy infants had disability or severe outcome (Ellis versus Robertson and Finer). 97% of those with severe NE in the Ellis study died. Please see plate section for colour version.

**Table 12.4.** Outcome of a cohort of 131 NE infants in Kathmandu, Nepal

| HIE Stage | Normal | Severe neuro-disability in survivors | Death | Composite outcome of death and severe neuro-disability |
|---|---|---|---|---|
| Stage I (n= 35) | 26 (74%) | 2/29 (6%) | 6 (17%) | 8 (23%) |
| Stage II (n=38) | 10 (26%) | 16/27 (42%) | 11 (29%) | 27 (71%) [95% CI 54% to 84%] |
| Stage III (n=29) | 1 (3%) | 0 | 28 (97%) | 28 (97%) |
| TOTAL (n=102) | | | | |

*Note:* All grades of NE severity carried an increased risk of neonatal death. Surviving infants with moderate NE had a high risk of major impairment and 97% of infants with severe NE died [23]. See Figure 12.3a and b.

As there is such a wide range in NMR across countries throughout the world, a recent systematic review for the Global Burden of Disease Project estimated the incidence of NE by NMR category. In very low mortality settings (NMR < 5) (see Figure 12.1, Table 12.3), the median incidence of NE is 1.9 per 1000 live births (range 0.7–6.0) compared with 26.5 per 1000 live births in the highest mortality settings (based on a single study) – a 14 fold disparity. Countries with NMR 6–15, 16–30 and 31–45 have an estimated median (range) incidence of NE of 6.7 (4.7–8.7), 9.8 (3.6–10.2) and 13.4 (5.5–22.2) [1]. South Asia and Africa, with large numbers of births and deaths, account for 73% of all intrapartum-related neonatal deaths worldwide.

## Outcome

The Global Burden of Disease Project estimated that the median neonatal case fatality for NE in very low mortality settings is 21% (range, 17%–37%) vs. 31% (range, 20%–33%) in the high mortality settings (NMR 31–45), although there is a complete lack of data from very high mortality settings (>45%) and no data from community settings, where the majority of intrapartum-related events are concentrated [1]. Across all NMR categories, approximately 25–29% of NE survivors may have a long-term moderate or severe impairment [1]. In the Kathmandu study, NE of all grades of severity carried an increased risk of neonatal death compared to developed-world settings (Figure 12.3a,b, Table 12.4) [23,24]. Almost 90% of the NE-associated deaths occurred during the neonatal period; surviving infants with moderate NE had a high risk of major impairment and no infant with severe NE survived. Ellis estimated a total prevalence of 1.1 per 1000 live births for major neurodevelopmental impairment at 1 year after NE

associated with possible birth asphyxia in term infants [23] in this low-income setting.

## Prevention of intrapartum-related deaths and morbidity

*Preventative* strategies are needed to reduce the burden of perinatal asphyxia in low- and mid-resource settings. However, as perinatal asphyxia is not completely preventable or always predictable, *treatment* strategies to minimize or reduce brain injury are also needed (see section on therapeutic hypothermia).

Delays in problem-recognition and care seeking, inadequate antenatal and intrapartum care and poor access to health facilities are common situations in low- and mid-resource settings and increase the prevalence and severity of intrapartum hypoxic events [25]. Prevention and treatment require an integrated approach that focuses on obstetrical and neonatal interventions and extends throughout life with strategies such as optimizing growth and nutrition of young girls and women. As well as the pathophysiological risk factors summarized above, economic, cultural, social and geographical factors (such as living at high altitude) influence the risk factors for asphyxia. Conditions that increase the risk of intrauterine hypoxia, such as pre-eclampsia or eclampsia, obstructed labour and low birth weight, are more prevalent in low-resource settings (Table 12.1). Interventions that prevent intrapartum complications (e.g. prevention and management of pre-eclampsia), detect and manage intrapartum problems (e.g. monitoring progress of labour with access to emergency obstetric care) and identify and resuscitate the non-breathing newborn (e.g. basic resuscitation) will reduce intrapartum-related mortality and morbidity.

## Improving obstetric care

Improving the quality of emergency obstetric care is an essential part of improving birth outcomes in low- and mid-resource settings. Training courses in emergency obstetrical care in the United Kingdom reduced the incidence of NE (relative risk [RR]: 0.51%, 95% confidence interval [CI]: 0.35–0.74) and low 5-minute Apgar scores (RR: 0.50%, 95% CI: 0.26–0.9) [26]– the impact is likely to be higher in low-middle resource settings with lower baseline standards of care. The major reductions in fetal and neonatal mortality in developed countries occurred before 1980 before routine use of ultrasound, Doppler and the high Caesarean delivery rates. Reducing cases of intrapartum stillbirth and neonatal deaths, therefore, requires well functioning obstetrical and neonatal care in which the mother and fetus are monitored for signs associated with fetal compromise, prenatally and in labour, and provided access to emergency obstetric and neonatal care [27].

## Resuscitation

Each year around 5–10% (~10 million) of newborn infants worldwide do not breathe immediately at birth and need basic resuscitation: tactile stimulation or airway clearing. Three to six percent (~6 million) of newborn infants require assisted ventilation at birth. The major burden of resuscitation is in low- and mid-resource settings where the health system capacity to provide neonatal resuscitation is inadequate. Neonatal resuscitation guidelines are reviewed by the International Liaison Committee on Resuscitation [28] and by Newton and English in the context of the low- and mid-resource setting [29]. Basic neonatal resuscitation is feasible and effective in resource-limited settings; stimulation and mask ventilation are the most important steps of resuscitation to reduce intrapartum-related deaths. Advanced procedures are rarely needed.

The Helping Babies Breathe (HBB) programme of the American Academy of Pediatrics is an example of a resuscitation-training programme aimed for global implementation in the resource-limited setting. A systematic review and meta-analysis determined that neonatal resuscitation training in mid- and low-resource country settings may avert approximately 30% of intrapartum-related neonatal deaths [30]. More effective and efficient training and implementation approaches are needed to sustain this.

A recent multicentre trial, the First Breath Study, found that basic neonatal resuscitation, with bag and mask, reduced stillbirths and perinatal mortality. The reduction in stillbirth was likely to be due to the improved recognition and intervention for severely depressed infants who would have otherwise been considered "stillborn"; this led to a 19% lower perinatal mortality rate. In addition, reductions in the proportions of births with a 5-minute Apgar score < 4 and with an abnormal neurologic examination at 7 days were observed [31].

Intrapartum-related neonatal deaths can be substantially reduced by improving the quality of services for all childbirths that occur in health facilities. For example, providing neonatal resuscitation for 90% of deliveries currently taking place in health facilities would save more than 93,000 newborn lives each year. There is much work to do, as a recent health service assessment in sub-Saharan Africa found only 15% of hospitals were equipped to provide basic neonatal resuscitation [30]. Training providers in neonatal resuscitation in health facilities may prevent 30% of deaths of full-term babies with intrapartum-related events [30]. Therefore, universal application of basic resuscitation may save hundreds of thousands of newborn lives currently lost each year and contribute to progress toward Millennium Development Goal 4. Neonatal resuscitation is a very cost-effective intervention with a cost of $208 per life saved – one of the most cost-effective perinatal care strategies.

## Post-resuscitation care

Post-resuscitation care may improve survival and long-term outcomes for newborns who have experienced intrapartum hypoxia and show signs of NE. Referral to a hospital neonatal unit for 12–24 hours of monitoring and essential and supportive newborn care is the first step in post-resuscitation care. Referral-level hospitals should be prepared to support breathing, maintain adequate oxygenation, provide an appropriate thermal environment (i.e., avoid hyperthermia) and ensure glucose and fluid balance [30].

## Challenges for therapeutic hypothermia in low- and mid-resource settings

As discussed in other sections of this book, several large clinical trials of therapeutic hypothermia in the

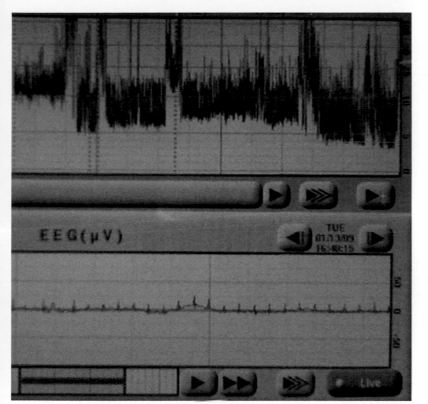

**Figure 8.1.** aEEG tracing obtained from occipito-parietal elctrodes from a comatose unresponsive infant. Note the initial part of the tracing would fall in the "normal range". The narrow band suggest some interference. The corresponding raw EEG tracing shows an EKG signal.

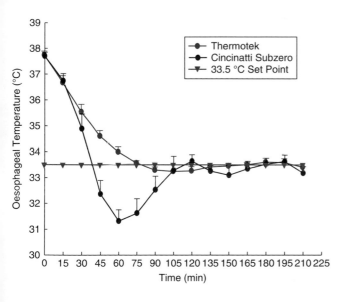

**Figure 10.3.** Prototype cooling blanket for transport. The profile of oesophageal temperatures from 4 neonatal swine is plotted over time. Each animal underwent a 3.5-hour interval of cooling to a set point temperature of 33.5°C with a commercially available cooling device (CSZ) and with a blanket under development. The latter has a more sophisticated servo algorithm which slows the rate of cooling as the oesophageal temperature approaches the set point.

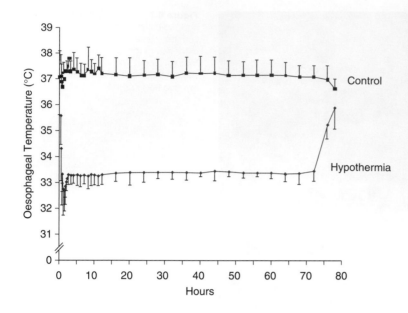

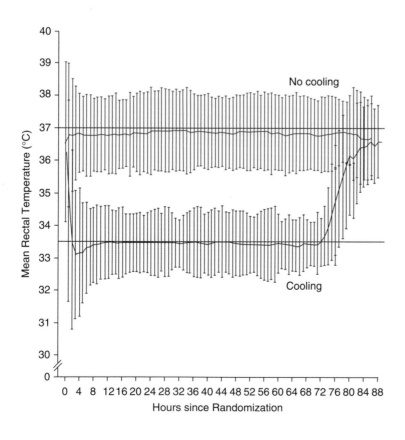

**Figure 10.5.** Oesophageal and rectal temp from two randomized trials of hypothermia. Part A shows the mean oesophageal temperature (±2 standard deviations) of infants in the control and hypothermia arm of the NICHD trial (with permission). Part B shows the rectal temperatures (±2 standard deviations) of infants in the control and hypothermia arm of the TOBY trial. (With permission).

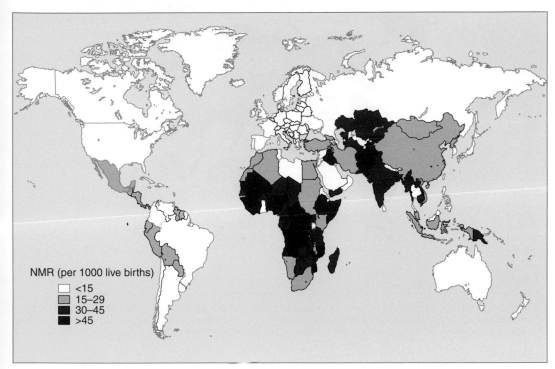

**Figure 12.1a.** Variation in neonatal mortality rate between countries (Zupan and Aahman WHO report 2005). Reproduced with permission from reference [3].

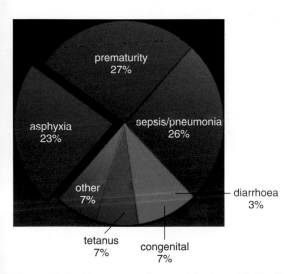

**Figure 12.1b.** Direct causes of neonatal deaths worldwide. Almost one quarter of deaths are attributed to perinatal asphyxia. Adapted from reference [3].

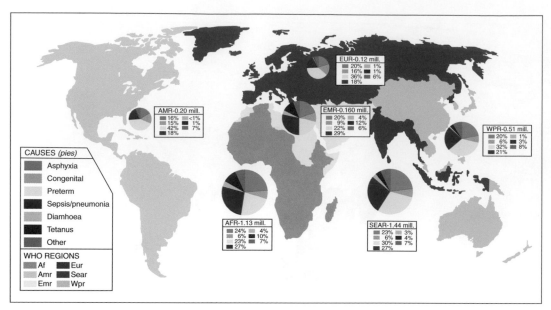

**Figure 12.2.** The estimated distribution of causes for 4 million neonatal deaths for the six WHO regions in the year 2000. The size of the circle represents the number of deaths in each region. Afr, Africa; Amr, Americas; EMR, Eastern Mediterranean; Eur, Europe; Sear, Southeast Asia; Wpr, Western Pacific. Reproduced with permission from Lawn et al [*Int J Epidemiol* 2006;**35**:706–18].

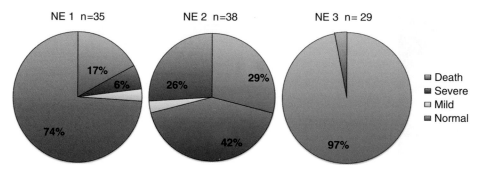

**Figure 12.3a.** Outcome of a cohort of 131 infants with NE (Stage 1–3) at 1 year of age in a maternity hospital in Kathmandu, Nepal. Reproduced from reference [14].

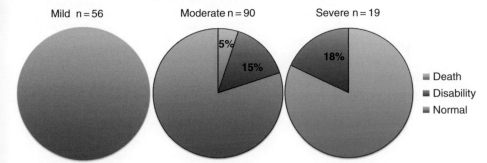

**Figure 12.3b.** Eight year outcome on death and disability in a cohort of infants with mild, moderate and severe encephalopathy at birth [24]. Comparing the outcomes (although tested at different ages) for a given Sarnat stage, significantly worse outcomes are seen in the low-resource setting in Kathmandu versus the Robertson and Finer study in the USA. For example, all infants with mild NE in the Robertson and Finer study had a normal outcome at 8 years whereas in the Ellis study 17% of infants died and 6% had a severe outcome at 1 year of age. 42% versus 15% of the moderate encephalopathy infants had disability or severe outcome (Ellis versus Robertson and Finer). 97% of those with severe NE in the Ellis study died.

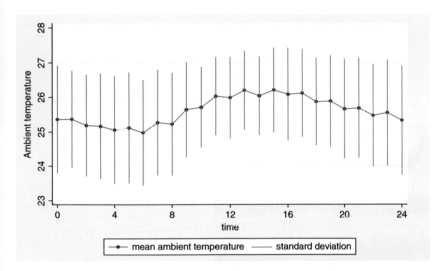

**Figure 12.4b.** Mean ambient temperature recorded in the special care baby unit in Mulago Hospital. The ambient temperature fluctuated very little between day and night.

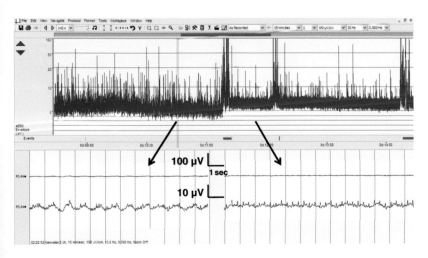

**Figure 13.2.** This mainly inactive/flat aEEG/EEG was recorded during the first hours of life in a severely asphyxiated infant. The initial aEEG looks like a very low voltage burst suppression pattern, although the lower border is lifted to 4–5 μVolt. Then there is an abrupt change in aEEG pattern when the baby was turned and the trace is lifted further to above 5 μVolt. The corresponding EEG samples are shown below. The upper EEG tracings are presented in a commonly used scale (100 μV/cm) and look almost entirely flat. When the scale is changed to 10 μV/cm, it is clear that the left trace is influenced by a suspected respiratory artefact (0.7–1 Hz) and the right trace is affected by a 3 Hz (corresponding to a heart rate of 180) artefact from the electrocardiogram. Such artefacts can consequently falsely lift the lower border of a flat/inactive aEEG/EEG tracing.

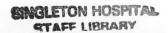

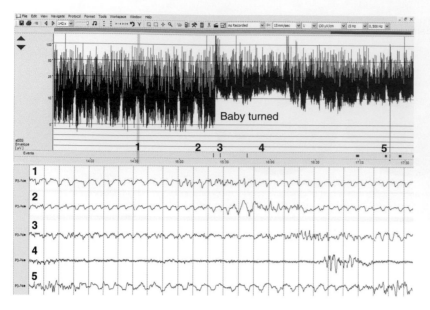

**Figure 13.3.** This term baby with moderate hypoxic–ischaemic encephalopathy and meconium aspiration was treated with high-frequency oscillation ventilation (HFOV) with frequency 10 Hz. The aEEG background in the 4-hour recording is discontinuous and shows repetitive seizures (at least 35–40 but they are difficult to count). The amplitude of the aEEG trace is "swaying" due to the HFOV artefact and this becomes even more pronounced when the baby is turned (resulting in pressure on the electrodes). The HFOV artefact on the burst suppression background is clearly seen in trace 4. Seizures may be more difficult to identify when the aEEG is influenced by artefacts from HFOV, but in this case they had a fairly similar appearance in the raw EEG (except for the 10 Hz HFOV artefact).

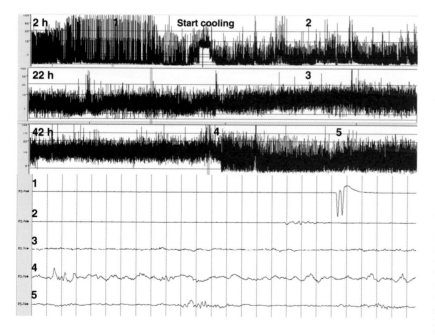

**Figure 13.4.** This term infant had a complicated delivery and was treated with moderate hypothermia starting at 5 hours of age. The aEEG samples each show 6 hours of recording, starting at 2, 22 and 42 hours, respectively. The 25 second-duration samples of EEG below correspond to the numbers in the aEEG traces. 1) Initially the infant was comatose and had no discernible electrocortical activity; the very regular burst suppression-like aEEG corresponds to a flat EEG interrupted by movements from gasping. 2) At 7 hours, the aEEG/EEG has intermittent very low voltage activity. 3) Around 25–26 hours, the aEEG amplitude increases, which corresponds to low voltage continuous activity; the baby seems to be more awake clinically. 4) The electrocortical activity is continuous with normal voltage at 44–45 hours, but two very brief suspected electroclinical seizures occurred and the infant was given midazolam, resulting in immediate depression and burst suppression pattern. 5) Two hours after the midazolam, a burst suppression pattern is still present.

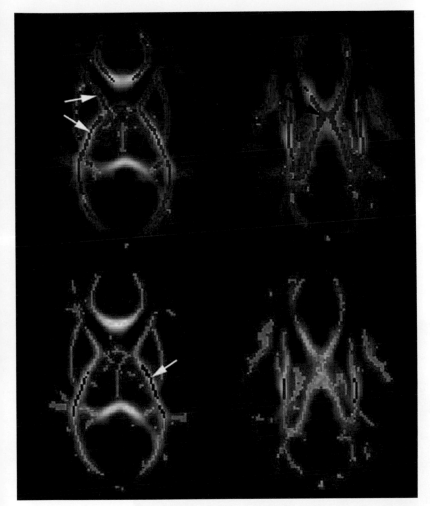

**Figure 14.10.** Tract-based spatial statistics (TBSS). Mean fractional anisotropy (FA) atlas. HIE non-cooled infants are compared with normal controls (top row). The blue regions represent areas of statistically reduced FA in the HIE group. There are multiple areas of white matter abnormality including the internal capsule (white arrows) and the corpus callosum (black arrow). HIE infants who were cooled are compared to normal controls (bottom row). There are still regions of reduced FA (blue) in the cooled HIE infants but these are less widespread and only involve the posterior limb of the internal capsule (left image) and the corona radiata (right image).

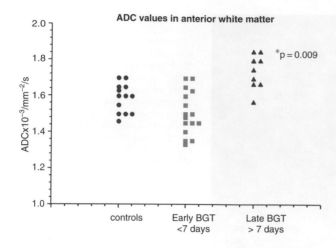

**ADC values in anterior white matter**

*p = 0.009

controls    Early BGT    Late BGT
            <7 days      > 7 days

**Figure 14.11d.** ADC values in the white matter of neonates with HIE and basal ganglia and thalamic lesions. ADC values in the white matter increase with time. ADC values would be expected to decrease with time in normal neonates as white matter water content decreases with maturation.

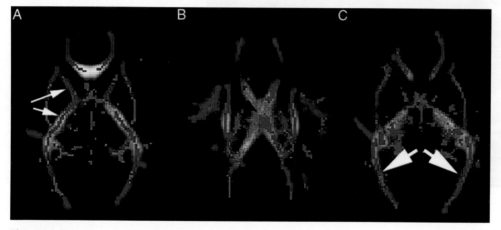

**Figure 20.3.** Axial images of mean FA of white matter tracts of infants with HIE. The group mean FA skeleton is shown in pink. Areas where the non-cooled group with HIE has a statistically lower FA than the cooled group are shown in blue: (a) internal capsules and external capsules (small white arrows), (b) body of the corpus callosum (black arrow), (c) optic radiations (large white arrows). Reproduced with permission from reference [49].

developed world have shown that cooling (1) decreases death and disability among infants with less severe aEEG abnormalities [32], (2) decreases death and moderate/severe disability and (3) increases the number of survivors without disability [33–35]. Therapeutic hypothermia under intensive care settings appears safe; although thrombocytopenia and arrhythmias are more frequent with therapeutic hypothermia, these can be corrected with appropriate clinical care [36,37]. Furthermore, there are suggestions that the favourable outcome of cooled infants at 18 months may be associated with favourable outcome at age 7–8; however, these studies are not yet published. Therapeutic hypothermia is now widely offered to infants with NE in high-income countries [38]. In the UK, in May 2010, the National Institute for Health and Clinical Excellence (NICE) recommended that *Therapeutic Hypothermia with Intracorporeal Temperature Monitoring for Hypoxic Perinatal Brain Injury* should be offered to "carefully selected infants", "in units experienced in the care of severely asphyxiated infants" who "enter the details of infants undergoing cooling into the UK TOBY cooling register" http://www.nice.org.uk/nicemedia/live/11315/48809/48809.pdf).

## Potential risks of extrapolating developed world trials to low- and mid-resource settings

There are several compelling reasons why the safety and efficacy data on therapeutic hypothermia from high-income countries should not be extrapolated to neonatal units in low- and mid-income countries. (1) Brain injury may already be established due to multiple antenatal insults (contributed to by maternal malnutrition and other co-morbidities), delayed hospital admissions often in obstructed labour, long delays in carrying out emergency Caesarean sections and lack of effective networks for neonatal transport. It is possible that the therapeutic window for hypothermia may, therefore, have passed [39]. (2) The incidence and profile of perinatal infections in this population are different. Cooling in the presence of infection might be deleterious as hypothermia may impair innate immune function, including neutrophil migration and function [40] (although it is reassuring that the neonatal cooling trials from high-income countries did not show a higher incidence of culture-proven sepsis in cooled infants) [33,34]. Hypothermia during sepsis in adult patients

has been associated with increased mortality, higher circulating levels of TNF-α and IL-618, prolongation of NF-KB activation and altered cytokine gene expression [41]. Hypothermia for head injury in adults increases the risk of pneumonia [42]. These factors may explain the higher morbidity and mortality associated with hypothermia in some clinical settings [41,43] and emphasize the need for careful monitoring of infection and mortality in cooled infants. In addition, convincing experimental [15,20] and epidemiological evidence suggests that the "dual hit" of combined infection and ischaemia results in more severe brain injury and increase in the risk of cerebral palsy [21]. It is not known if therapeutic hypothermia would be neuroprotective in such situations. (3) Hypothermia may not benefit encephalopathic infants with co-existing growth restriction from micronutrient deficiencies. (4) Cooling may be unsafe in the presence of meconium aspiration and pulmonary hypertension as facilities for advanced multi-organ support may not be available in resource-limited neonatal units. (5) Cooling equipment used in high-income countries is expensive, requires maintenance support and has recurring costs. Many "low tech" cooling methods like ice or frozen gel packs are labour intensive, and may result in marked temperature fluctuations and shivering [44], with a potential loss of neuroprotective efficacy.

## Pilot studies of therapeutic hypothermia

### Mulago Hospital, Kampala, Uganda

In 2007, we undertook a pilot feasibility study of whole body cooling at Mulago Hospital, Kampala, Uganda. We aimed to determine the feasibility of whole body cooling to 33–34°C for 72 hours by use of simple methods and inform a larger randomized controlled trial in this setting [4]. We also assessed the pattern, severity and evolution of brain tissue injury as seen on serial cranial ultrasound imaging and the feasibility of neurodevelopmental follow-up at 18–22 months of age [45]. In addition, we collected cranial ultrasound data on a cohort of over 100 well newborn Ugandan infants to provide baseline data for comparison with encephalopathic infants [46].

Inclusion criteria for the pilot study were gestational age at birth 37 weeks or more, requirement for resuscitation, and/or Apgar score less than 6 at 5 minutes plus an abnormal neurological assessment (a Thompson encephalopathy score >5 [47]) from 30 minutes to

3 hours after birth. Exclusions included apnoea or cyanosis, absent cardiac output for more than 10 minutes after birth and birth weight less than 2kg.

Infants in the therapeutic hypothermia group underwent whole body cooling with a mattress made of three commercially available water bottles (cost approximately US$10) laid sideways in the cot and filled with cool water from the tap in the neonatal unit (Figure 4); cooling with this simple method had been previously validated in an experimental model of

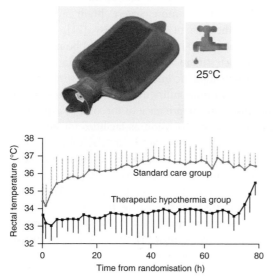

**Figure 12.4a.** Water bottles were filled with tepid tap water from the hospital and placed under the infant with a cotton sheet between the water bottle and the infant's back. This method of cooling achieved maintenance of the rectal temperature at 33.5°C for 72 hours. Reproduced with permission from reference [4].

perinatal asphyxia [48]. Infants wore only a nappy (diaper) and were otherwise naked or wrapped in cotton sheets or blankets. The tap water and ambient temperature of the neonatal unit had been measured previously; both were constant at 25–26°C with minimum diurnal or seasonal variation (Figure 12.4).

This study demonstrated several key points related to cooling in a low-resource setting. First, water bottles successfully maintained the core (rectal) temperature within target range (33–34°C); nursing input was needed and "targeted temperature management" was achieved by adding or removing blankets. Second, infants in both groups were hypothermic at randomization and it took > 15 hours for the rectal temperature to reach normothermia in the standard care group by standard methods (swaddling and gloves filled with warm water). This "endogenous hypothermia" could be an intrinsic neuroprotective response and was observed previously in asphyxiated infants some 50 years ago [49]. Non-shivering thermogenesis may be impaired in infants following birth asphyxia; under normal conditions the release of hormones that influence brown adipose tissue thermogenesis is under the control of the anterior hypothalamus [50]. Therefore, it is likely that disruption of this central control is responsible for the failure of asphyxiated neonates to generate endogenous heat through non-shivering thermogenesis [51]. Third, more deaths were seen in the cooled group: seven deaths in the therapeutic hypothermia group and one in the standard care group (RR 5.0) (95% confidence intervals 0.7–37). This is the only clinical trial of cooling to demonstrate mortality excess. The median age of death was

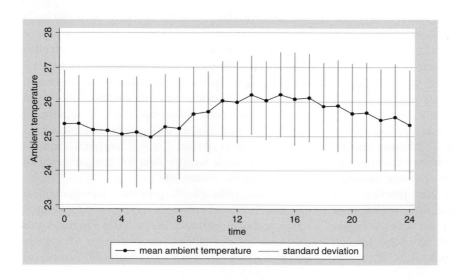

**Figure 12.4b.** Mean ambient temperature recorded in the special care baby unit in Mulago Hospital. The ambient temperature fluctuated very little between day and night. Please see plate section for colour version.

75 hours (range, 34–144 hours). Sepsis could have contributed to the excess of deaths in the cooled group although this cannot be proven because no blood cultures or blood indices suggestive of infection were available. However, it is important to seriously consider the impact cooling with co-existing sepsis might have on the morbidity and mortality of septic and encephalopathic infants – adult studies have shown higher circulating levels of TNF-α and IL-618, prolongation of NF-KB activation and altered cytokine gene expression [41] and increased risk of pneumonia [42]. It is also important to remember that "accidental neonatal hypothermia" with uncontrolled physiological homeostasis is a significant problem in low-resource settings and is associated with increased morbidity and mortality [5]. The excess in deaths could also be explained by the fact that more infants with Sarnat stage III were randomized to the therapeutic hypothermia group by chance than in the standard care group; evidence from Nepal has shown that, in settings where long-term ventilation and stabilization are not available, the mortality rate for infants with Sarnat stage III NE is 100% [23].

Future studies need to focus on identifying risk factors for NE (particularly the role of perinatal infection in the aetiology and outcome of NE) and effective dissemination of strategies for prevention and improvements in perinatal care. This study, although small, is important in emphasizing that the safety and efficacy of therapeutic hypothermia in mid- and low-resource countries has not been proven.

## India studies

In India and other mid-resource countries, most neonatal units do have good standards of basic intrapartum and neonatal care. In 2009, Guhan and colleagues performed a feasibility study of whole body cooling in a public sector hospital (~25,000 births per year) in South India (Calicut Medical College, Kozhikode, Kerala) (http://clinicaltrials.gov; NCT01138176) in two phases. The first phase was a prospective observational study (n = 22) to examine the clinical profile and brain tissue injury in outborn and inborn infants with NE admitted to the neonatal unit by serial cranial ultrasound (cUS) imaging (day 1, 3, 7), amplitude-integrated electroencephalogram (aEEG), EEG (day 3 to 4) and magnetic resonance imaging (MRI) (days 7 to 14). None of the infants had evidence of established brain injury at birth on cUS. Brain injury patterns on MRI were suggestive of an acute perinatal event, although a high incidence of white matter injury was seen on MRI, which may be related to co-existing perinatal infections [52,53].

The second phase was a pilot randomized controlled trial (n = 33) to examine the cooling efficacy of a low-tech "natural servo-controlled" cooling mattress made from phase changing material (PCM), which had been validated in our laboratory [48]. PCMs are passive heating and cooling substances, usually made of a salt hydrate, fatty acid and ester or paraffin, such as octadecane. They can be manufactured to have different "melting points". At room temperature, PCMs remain solid as long as the ambient temperature is below their melting point. When they come into contact with a warmer object, they absorb heat and in so doing change state to liquid. Conversely, liquid PCMs can solidify, giving off the heat, thus acting as a heat buffer to stabilize the temperature of whatever is in contact with them. PCMs act as natural servo-controlled devices and there is very little risk of over cooling. The nursing input is substantially lower than manual devices and ice packs. PCMs can be re-used and, therefore, appear to be an ideal cooling device in low-resource settings.

In the pilot study, PCM mattress (melting point 32°C) effectively induced and maintained cooling with a similar temperature stability to the Tecotherm device used in the TOBY trial [33,53]; minimal additional nursing interventions (e.g., use of blankets if rectal temperature [TR] < 33°C or additional PCM blocks if TR > 34°C) were required to maintain target temperature.

Several other small cooling studies have been performed in India over the past 5 years. At Sheri Kashmir Institute of Medical Sciences, Srinagar, Kashmir, India, 20 neonates with severe perinatal asphyxia were randomized to cooling with ice and 15 neonates served as controls. In babies with hypothermia, skin and rectal temperatures were maintained at 33.5°C for 72 hours followed by slow re-warming. The endpoint was death or abnormal neurological examination at the time of discharge. Although there were no significant differences between the patients who died in the two groups (15% vs. 33%, P > 0.05), hypothermic neonates were less likely to have abnormal neurological examination at discharge [54].

A pilot cooling study in a series of 20 infants (55% outborn) has recently been conducted in Christian Medical College, Vellore, using reusable ice gel packs obtained from the immunization clinic at no added expense [55]. These gel packs were wrapped in clean cloth to prevent cold injury to the skin. The mean time taken to achieve target rectal temperature was 52 ± 25 minutes; mean rectal temperature during cooling was 32.9 ± 0.11°C. The target temperature could be maintained for 72 hours. Adverse events observed during cooling were thrombocytopenia (25%), sinus bradycardia (25%), deranged bleeding parameters (20%), fat necrosis (15%), hyperglycaemia (15%), hypoglycaemia (10%), hypoxaemia (5%), life-threatening coagulopathy (5%) and death (5%). Shivering was noted in many of the babies, especially in the initial phase of cooling. The process was, however, relatively labour intensive.

Bharadwaj and Bhat recently reported a randomized controlled trial of while body cooling using frozen gel packs or standard care, in 134 infants with moderate or severe neonatal encephalopathy. Neonatal mortality was similar in the cooled and standard care infants −3 (4.8%) versus 6 (9.7%) (P = 0.49). In this study, cooled infants had a higher development quotient at 6 months on Amiel Tison assessment [56].

## South Africa studies

Several researchers have reported use of cooling with ice and frozen gel packs in South Africa in newborns [57,58]. In one study, infants frequently became agitated and exhibited shivering [57] and this method required intensive nursing input to prevent overcooling. Horn et al used a servo-controlled fan device to cool 10 infants with NE [44]. Infants were nursed on a servo-controlled radiant warmer, set to a target of 33.4 to 33.7°C. A servo-controlled fan connected to a rectal temperature probe was directed cephalo-caudally over the infants. There are several disadvantages of this method, including excessive shivering, patient discomfort and again high level of nursing monitoring. It is unclear if cooling would have occurred anyway by keeping babies naked in a cold room. Even though this method is described as suitable for use in low-resource settings, it does require a substantial amount of equipment including servo-controlled radiant warmers, air conditioning, and computer units, in addition to the fans.

These mid- and low-resource setting pilot cooling studies have shown that low-tech devices are mostly effective in the administration of therapeutic hypothermia, although some are relatively labour intensive and require close monitoring to maintain the target

**Table 12.5.** A summary of the cooling studies performed in mid- and low-resource settings

| Author | Country | Design | Sample size | Equipment | Temperature stability |
|---|---|---|---|---|---|
| Bhat [54] | India | RCT | 35 | Ice | Whole body cooling; rectal temperature 33.5°C |
| Bharadwaj and Vishnu Bhat [56] | India | RCT | 124 | Ice | Whole body cooling; rectal temperature 33.5°C (SD 0.6) |
| Thayyil [53] | India | RCT | 33 | Phase changing material | Whole body cooling; rectal temperature 33.5°C (SD 0.3) |
| Thomas [55] | India | Observational | 20 | Frozen vaccine carrier bags | Whole body cooling; rectal temperature 33°C (SD 0.5) |
| Robertson [4] | Uganda | RCT | 36 | Water bottles filled with tap water | Whole body cooling; rectal temperature 33.6°C (SD 0.69) |
| Horn [57] | South Africa | Observational | 5 | Cold gel packs to head | Selective head cooling; rectal temperature 33.9°C (SD 0.3 C) |
| Horn [44] | South Africa | Observational | 10 | Fans | Whole body cooling; rectal temperature 33.6°C (SD 0.2°C) |
| Lin [59] | China | RCT | 58 | Local head cooling equipment | Selective head cooling; rectal temperature 35°C (SD 0.6) |
| Zhou [60] | China | RCT | 194 | Local head cooling equipment | Selective head cooling; rectal temperature 34.5–35°C |

rectal temperature. None of these studies, however, have been adequately powered to study efficacy and safety of cooling in low- and mid-resource settings. A summary of cooling studies from low- and mid-income countries is in Table 12.5.

## Chinese studies

A single-centre randomized study was performed between 2001 and 2003 in the Children's Hospital of Wenzhou Medical College, China [58]. Entry criteria were: (1) gestational age >37 weeks; (2) Apgar scores < 6 at 5 minutes with first postnatal arterial blood gas pH < 7.10. Selective head cooling was achieved by applying a cooling cap device with circulating cold water at 10°C. Patients were kept under a radiant warmer with the targeted temperature set at 34–35°C for a total of 72 hours. A shield was used to block the cooling cap from the radiant heat during head cooling. An indwelling rectal temperature probe was used to monitor the temperature constantly and control infant temperature. A total of 58 patients (30 hypothermia, 28 control) completed the study. Hypothermia appeared to be tolerated in this study and attenuation of brain injury on imaging studies and neurological scores was reported [59].

A larger randomized controlled trial involving 12 centres in China was published in 2010; 194 infants were available for analysis (100 and 94 infants in the selective head cooling and control group, respectively). For the selective head cooling and control groups, respectively, the reported combined outcome of death and severe disability was 31% and 49% (odds ratio [OR]: 0.47; 95% confidence interval [CI]: 0.26–0.84; $P = 0.01$), the mortality rate was 20% and 29% (OR: 0.62; 95% CI: 0.32–1.20; $P = 0.16$) and the severe disability rate was 14% (11/80) and 28% (19/67) (OR: 0.40; 95% CI: 0.17–0.92; $P = 0.01$) [60].

## Future directions

Evidence from the cooling trials in high-income countries can only be safely applied to settings where population risk factors, infrastructure and facilities are comparable to trial centres informing the meta-analysis. We urge clinicians to remember the principle of *primum non nocere* and suggest that, until more safety and efficacy data are available on therapeutic hypothermia from low- and mid-resource settings, clinicians do not offer therapeutic hypothermia.

In low-resource settings with high NMR it is important to continue to focus on reducing intrapartum-related neonatal deaths and neonatal morbidity by improving the quality of services for all childbirths that occur in health facilities, identifying and addressing the missed opportunities to provide effective interventions to those who seek hospital-based care. For example, providing neonatal resuscitation for 90% of deliveries currently taking place in health facilities would save more than 93,000 newborn lives each year and reduce considerably neonatal morbidity and NE. Longer-term strategies must address the inequalities and inconsistencies in obstetric and perinatal care.

In some mid-resource settings with sufficient infrastructure and quality of obstetric and neonatal care, it may be possible to conduct large, adequately powered trials to determine the safety and efficacy of cooling. It is possible that unless a trial is performed that is relevant to mid-resource settings, there will be a creeping, uncertain introduction of hypothermia, with constant worries regarding residual safety concerns. It is possible that, given the sheer magnitude of the problem of perinatal asphyxia and NE worldwide, the establishment of an effective and safe therapy would have a high impact on medical practice throughout the world, save lives and reduce the burden on our societies.

# References

1. Lawn JE, Kinney M, Lee AC, et al. Reducing intrapartum related deaths and disability: can the health system deliver? *Int J Gynaecol Obstet* 2009;**107**(Suppl 1):S123–40, S140–2.

2. World Health Organization. *World Health Report: make every mother and child count*. Geneva, Switzerland: WHO; 2005.

3. Lawn JE, Cousens S, Zupan J; for the Lancet Neonatal Survival Steering Team. 4 million neonatal deaths: when? Where? Why? *Lancet* 2005;**365**:891–900.

4. Robertson NJ, Nakakeeto M, Hagmann C, et al. Therapeutic hypothermia for birth asphyxia in low-resource settings: a pilot randomised controlled trial. *Lancet* 2008;**372**:801–3.

5. Kumar V, Shearer J, Kumar A, Darmstadt G. Neonatal hypothermia in low resource settings: a review. *J Perinatol* 2009;**29**:401–12.

6. Nelson KB, Leviton A. How much of neonatal encephalopathy is due to birth asphyxia? *Am J Dis Child* 1991;**145**:1325–31.

7. Hankins G. The long journey: defining the true pathogenesis and pathophysiology of neonatal encephalopathy and cerebral palsy. *Obstet Gynaecol Surv* 2003;**58**:435–7.

8. Badawi N, Kurinczuk JJ, Keogh JM, et al. Antepartum risk factors for newborn encephalopathy: the Western Australian case-control study. *BMJ* 1998;**317**:1549–53.

9. Badawi N, Kurinczuk JJ, Keogh JM, et al. Intrapartum risk factors for newborn encephalopathy: the Western Australian case-control study. *BMJ* 1998;**317**:1554–8.

10. Force TACoOaGT. *Neonatal encephalopathy and cerebral palsy: defining the pathogenesis andpathophysiology*. Washington, DC: The American College of Obstetricians and Gynecologists, the American Academy of Pediatrics, 2003. p. 1–85.

11. Committee on Fetus and Newborn, American Academy of Pediatrics and Committee on Obstetric Practice, American College of Obstetricians and Gynecologists. Use and abuse of the Apgar score. *Pediatrics* 1996;**98**:141–2.

12. MacLennan A. A template for defining a causal relation between acute intrapartum events and cerebral palsy: international consensus statement. *BMJ* 1999;**319**:1054–9.

13. Ellis M, Costello A. Antepartum risk factors for newborn encephalopathy. Intrapartum risk factors are important in developing world. *BMJ* 1999;**318**:1414.

14. Ellis M, Manandhar N, Manandhar D, Costello A. Risk factors for neonatal encephalopathy in Kathmandu, Nepal, a developing country: unmatched case-control study. *BMJ* 2000;**320**:1229–36.

15. Eklind S, Mallard C, Leverin AL, et al. Bacterial endotoxin sensitizes the immature brain to hypoxic–ischaemic injury. *Eur J Neurosci* 2001;**13**:1101–6.

16. Lieberman E, Eichenwald E, Mathur G, Richardson D, Heffner L, Cohen A. Intrapartum fever and unexplained seizures in term infants. *Pediatrics* 2000;**106**:983–8.

17. Lehnardt S, Massillon L, Follett P, et al. Activation of innate immunity in the CNS triggers neurodegeneration through a Toll-like receptor 4-dependent pathway. *Proc Natl Acad Sci U S A* 2003;**100**:8514–9.

18. Wu YW, Escobar GJ, Grether JK, Croen LA, Greene JD, Newman TB. Chorioamnionitis and cerebral palsy in term and near-term infants. *JAMA* 2003;**290**:2677–84.

19. Nelson KB WR. Infection, inflammation and the risk of cerebral palsy. *Curr Opin Neurol* 2000;**13**:133–9.

20. Girard S, Kadhim H, Roy M, et al. Role of perinatal inflammation in cerebral palsy. *Pediatr Neurol* 2009;**40**:168–74.

21. Longo M, Hankins G. Defining cerebral palsy: pathogenesis, pathophysiology and new intervention. *Minerva Ginecol* 2009;**61**:421–9.

22. Network N. New India: WHO Collaborating Centre Newborn Training & Research, All India Institute of Medical Sciences, 2002–3. Available from: http://www.newbornwhocc.org/pdf/nnpd_report_2002-03.PDF.

23. Ellis M, Manandhar N, Shrestha PS, Shrestha L, Manandhar DS, Costello AM. Outcome at 1 year of neonatal encephalopathy in Kathmandu, Nepal. *Dev Med Child Neurol* 1999;**41**:689–95.

24. Robertson CM, Finer NN, Grace MG. School performance of survivors of neonatal encephalopathy associated with birth asphyxia at term. *J Pediatr* 1989;**114**:753–60.

25. Wall SN, Carlo W, Goldenberg R, et al. Reducing intrapartum-related neonatal deaths in low- and middle-income countries – what works? *Semin Perinatol* 2010;**34**:395–407.

26. Draycott T, Sibanda T, Owen L, Akande V, et al. Does training in obstetric emergencies improve neonatal outcome? *BJOG* 2006;**113**:177–82.

27. Goldenberg RL, McClure EM. Reducing intrapartum stillbirths and intrapartum-related neonatal deaths. *Int J Gynaecol Obstet* 2009;**107**:S1–3.

28. International Liaison Committee on Resuscitation. The International Liaison Committee on Resuscitation (ILCOR) consensus on science with treatment recommendations for pediatric and neonatal patients: pediatric basic and advanced life support. *Pediatrics* 2006;**117**:e955–77.

29. Newton O, English M. Newborn resuscitation: defining best practice for low-income settings. *Trans R Soc Trop Med Hyg* 2006;**100**:899–908.

30. Wall SN, Niermeyer S, English M, et al. Neonatal resuscitation in low-resource settings: what, who and how to overcome challenges to scale up? *Int J Gynaecol Obstet* 2009;**107**:S47–62.

31. Carlo WA, Goudar SS, Jehan I, et al. Newborn-care training and perinatal mortality in developing countries. *N Engl J Med* 2010;**362**:614–23.

32. Gluckman PD, Wyatt JS, Azzopardi D, et al. Selective head cooling with mild systemic hypothermia after neonatal encephalopathy: multicentre randomised trial. *Lancet* 2005;**365**:663–70.

33. Azzopardi D, Strohm B, Edwards A, et al. Moderate hypothermia to treat perinatal asphyxial encephalopathy. *N Engl J Med* 2009;**361**:1349–58.

34. Shankaran S, Laptook AR, Ehrenkranz RA, et al. Whole-body hypothermia for neonates with hypoxic-ischemic encephalopathy. *N Engl J Med* 2005;**353**:1574–84.

35. Simbruner G, Mittal RA, Rohlmann F, et al. Systemic hypothermia after neonatal encephalopathy: outcomes

of neo.nEURO.network RCT. *Pediatrics* 2010;**126**:e771–8.

36. Shankaran S, Pappas A, Laptook AR, et al. Outcomes of safety and effectiveness in a multicenter randomized, controlled trial of whole-body hypothermia for neonatal hypoxic-ischemic encephalopathy. *Pediatrics* 2008;**122**:e791–8.

37. Shah P. Hypothermia: a systematic review and meta-analysis of clinical trials. *Semin Fetal Neonatal Med* 2010;**15**:238–46.

38. Kapetanakis A, Azzopardi D, Wyatt J, Robertson N. Therapeutic hypothermia for neonatal encephalopathy: a UK survey of opinion, practice and neuro-investigation at the end of 2007. *Acta Paediatr* 2009;**98**:631–5.

39. Gunn A, Gunn T, Gunning M, et al. Neuroprotection with prolonged head cooling started before postischemic seizures in fetal sheep. *Pediatrics* 1998;**102**:1098–106.

40. Biggar W, Barker C, Bohn D, Kent G. Partial recovery of neutrophil functions during prolonged hypothermia in pigs. *J Appl Physiol* 1986;**60**:1186–9.

41. Fairchild KD, Singh IS, Patel S, et al. Hypothermia prolongs activation of NF-kappaB and augments generation of inflammatory cytokines. *Am J Physiol Cell Physiol* 2004;**287**:C422–31.

42. Gadkary CS, Alderson P, Signorini DF. Therapeutic hypothermia for head injury. *Cochrane Database Sys Rev* 2002;**1**:CD001048.

43. Arons MM, Wheeler AP, Bernard GR, et al. Effects of ibuprofen on the physiology and survival of hypothermic sepsis. Ibuprofen in Sepsis Study Group. *Crit Care Med* 1999;**27**:699–707.

44. Horn A, Thompson C, Woods D, et al. Induced hypothermia for infants with hypoxic-ischemic encephalopathy using a servo-controlled fan: an exploratory pilot study. *Pediatrics* 2009;**123**:e1090–8.

45. Robertson N, Hagmann C, Acolet D, et al. Pilot randomized trial of therapeutic hypothermia with serial cranial ultrasound and 18–22 month follow-up for neonatal encephalopathy in a low resource hospital setting in Uganda: study protocol. *Trials* 2011;**12**:138.

46. Hagmann C, Robertson N, Acolet D, et al. Cranial ultrasound findings in well newborn Ugandan infants. *Arch Dis Child* 2010;**95**:F338–44.

47. Thompson CM, Puterman AS, Linley LL, et al. The value of a scoring system for hypoxic-ischaemic encephalopathy in predicting neurodevelopmental outcome. *Acta Pediatr* 1997;**86**:757–61.

48. Iwata S, Iwata O, Olson L, et al. Therapeutic hypothermia can be induced and maintained using either commercial water bottles or a "phase changing material" mattress in a newborn piglet model. *Arch Dis Child* 2009;**94**:387–91.

49. Burnard E, Cross K. Rectal temperature in the newborn after birth asphyxia. *BMJ* 1958;**ii**:1197–9.

50. Morimoto A, Murakami N, Ono T, et al. Stimulation of ventromedial hypothalamus induces cold defense responses in conscious rabbits. *Am J Physiol* 1986;**250**:R560–6.

51. Cross K, Hey E, Kennaird D, et al. Lack of temperature control in infants with abnormalities of central nervous system. *Arch Dis Child Fetal Neonatal Ed* 1971;**46**:437–43.

52. de Vries LS, Verboon-Maciolek MA, Cowan FM. The role of cranial ultrasound and magnetic resonance imaging in the diagnosis of infections of the central nervous system. *Early Hum Dev* 2006;**82**:819–825.

53. Thayyil S, Ayer M, Guhan B, et al. Whole body cooling using phase changing material in neonatal encephalopathy: a pilot randomised control trial. *EPAS*:**4350**.6. 2010.

54. Bhat M. Therapeutic hypothermia following perinatal asphyxia. *Arch Dis Child Fetal Neonatal Ed* 2006;**91**:F464.

55. Thomas N, George K, Sridhar S, Kumar M, Kuruvilla K, Jana A. Whole Body Cooling in Newborn Infants with Perinatal Asphyxial encephalopathy in a Low Resource Setting: A Feasibility Trial. *Indian Pediatr* 2010;**48**:445–51.

56. Bharadwaj SK and Bhat BV. Therapeutic hypothermia using Gel packs for term neonates with hypoxic ischaemic encephalopathy in resource-limited settings: a randomized controlled trial. *J Trop Pediatr* (in press).

57. Horn A, Woods D, Thompson C, et al. Selective cerebral hypothermia for post-hypoxic neuroprotection in neonates using a solid ice cap. *S Afr Med J* 2006;**96**:976–81.

58. Horn A, Harrison M, Linley L. Evaluating a simple method of neuroprotective hypothermia for newborn infants. *J Trop Pediatr* 2010;**56**:172–7.

59. Lin Z, Yu H, Lin J, et al. Mild hypothermia via selective head cooling as neuroprotective therapy in term neonates with perinatal asphyxia: an experience from a single neonatal intensive care unit. *J Perinatol* 2006;**26**:180–4.

60. Zhou WH, Cheng GQ, Shao XM, et al. Selective head cooling with mild systemic hypothermia after neonatal hypoxic–ischaemic encephalopathy: a multicenter randomized controlled trial in China. *J Pediatr* 2010;**157**:367–72.

# 13

# Cerebral function monitoring and EEG

Lena Hellström-Westas

## Introduction

It has been known for many years that neonatal electroencephalography (EEG) is sensitive for demonstrating cerebral dysfunction and that the presence of severe EEG abnormalities is associated with brain damage and predictive of an increased risk for adverse neurodevelopmental outcome. However, it was not until interventions after hypoxic–ischaemic insults became an option for newborn infants that the predictive features of very early electrocortical activity became clinically important issues.

The present chapter is aimed as a practical guide for the clinician and will focus on development of major EEG activities and seizures in connection with cerebral insults. For a more detailed overview of the neonatal EEG development and maturational features, we refer to textbooks and comprehensive reviews [1–3].

## Technical aspects

A conventional neonatal EEG (cEEG) is usually recorded from 9 to 15 electrodes that are applied over the scalp according to the international 10–20 system, which is a method that defines the electrode positions in relation to the underlying cerebral cortex. The 10–20 system uses the nasion and the inion as landmarks and electrode positions are defined by 10% and 20% multiples of the distance between these positions. The electrode locations are defined by a capital letter followed by a number: F (frontal), C (central), T (temporal), O (occipital) and Z (midline), with even numbers indicating the right hemisphere and odd numbers the left side (Figure 13.1). A "bipolar montage" measures voltage gradients between two electrodes and is the most common method for clinical EEG recording, as compared to a "referential montage", which measures voltage difference against one reference lead or an average

of all leads. The voltage gradient, i.e., the EEG amplitude, increases with increasing electrode distance. This must be considered if voltage criteria are applied for assessment of EEG or amplitude-integrated EEG (aEEG).

Electrocardiogram (ECG), respiration, eye movements (electrooculogram, EOG) and muscle activity are usually recorded simultaneously with the EEG, which facilitates identification of seizures, artefacts and sleep stages. Video-EEG is the golden standard, since it is possible to review also behavioural signs and correlate this with the EEG and other recorded parameters. The duration of a cEEG examination usually varies between 20 and 60 minutes; it is preferable if the recording is long enough to include sleep–wake states (when present).

Different types of electrodes can be used for EEG recordings, e.g., disk or cup electrodes, self-adhesive stick-on electrodes or subdermal needle electrodes. Thin needle electrodes are very easy and quick to

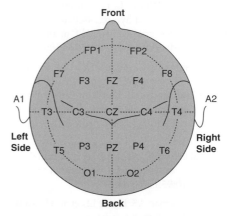

**Figure 13.1.** Electrode positions according to the international 10–20 system.

*Neonatal Neural Rescue*, ed. A. David Edwards, Denis V. Azzopardi and Alistair J. Gunn. Published by Cambridge University Press. © Cambridge University Press 2013.

apply after disinfection of the skin and they seem to cause very little discomfort. They have been used extensively for aEEG recordings in babies requiring intensive care treatment, e.g. for rapid initiation of good quality monitoring of infants with ongoing seizures, but surface electrodes are preferred in more stable infants. Self-adhesive stick-on electrodes can usually be very easily and gently applied in very preterm infants.

## Background activity

The term "background activity" refers to the dominating type of electrocortical activity during the EEG recording. "Continuous activity" is continuously ongoing with no major variations, although there may be some variability in amplitudes and frequencies. "Discontinuous activity" is characterized by periods of higher voltage ("bursts") alternating with periods of lower voltage activity ("interburst intervals", IBI). The normal background activity in the very preterm infant is mainly discontinuous, a pattern that has been called "tracé discontinu". With increasing maturation the background activity becomes more continuous; the duration of the interburst intervals decreases while the bursts increase in duration and decrease in amplitude. Electrocortical maturation proceeds in a parallel mode in preterm infants and in fetuses of comparable maturation. The terms conceptional age (CA), or postconceptional age (PCA), are often used in EEG terminology to describe an infant's maturation and is a summary of gestational age plus postnatal age in weeks.

The EEG of the normal term infant is synchronous (i.e. similar waveforms appear simultaneously over corresponding areas over the left and right hemispheres) and symmetrical (i.e. EEG amplitudes are the same in corresponding areas of the two hemispheres) and shows clear differences between sleep and wakefulness. The dominating EEG frequencies in term newborn babies are theta (4–8 Hz) and delta (0.5–4 Hz) activity, but alpha (8–13 Hz) and beta (13–30 Hz) activity are also present (the delineation of the frequency bands varies slightly between studies). The EEG background is continuous when the infant is awake or in active sleep (AS) and there is more discontinuous activity during quiet sleep (QS).

Discontinuous background patterns include the "tracé discontinu" in very immature infants, the normal "tracé alternant" (TA) pattern during quiet sleep in term infants and the abnormal burst suppression pattern, which is characterized by flat or very low voltage interburst intervals and lack of variability. Continuous very low voltage activity and flat or inactive (previously often called isoelectric) background patterns are characterized by extensive amplitude depression. They are often caused by severely abnormal conditions affecting the brain. The EEG amplitude can also be dampened by extra-cerebral factors, e.g. scalp oedema.

Filters are used when recording the EEG, to exclude extracerebral sources of activity such as movements, sweating, or electrical equipment. A low-pass filter excludes activity above a certain frequency, often 70 Hz, while the high-pass filter usually is set at 0.3–0.5 Hz and consequently lets activity above this threshold be recorded. Consequently, artefacts from high frequency oscillation ventilation (8–15 Hz), respiration (0.5–2 Hz), cardiac activity (2–3 Hz) and patting of the infant can affect the EEG recording. Very slow activity (<1 Hz), also called infraslow activity, can be recorded with special direct current amplifiers using high-pass filters set at very low frequencies, e.g., 0.05 Hz. It was suggested that this type of activity could be associated with modulation of cortical excitability [4]. Very few post-asphyctic infants have been recorded with this technology, but it was shown that very low-frequency activity (0–1 Hz) was more prominent in posterior regions and that presence of this activity possibly was related to a more favourable outcome [5]. Very fast, gamma activity (30–100 Hz), which has been linked to cognitive processes in adults, has not been demonstrated in newborn infants. Technology that records infraslow and ultrafast EEG activity has been called fullband EEG (fbEEG) [4].

## Sleep–wake cycling

Healthy term newborn babies have clearly delineated sleep–wake states that can be recorded by EEG even during the first hours of life [6]. The EEG in wakefulness and active sleep (AS, also called rapid eye movement sleep, REM) is very similar; it is continuous with mixed frequencies and amplitudes of around 25–50 µVolt, while the EEG during quiet sleep (QS, also called non-REM sleep) consists of either high-voltage slow activity (HVS), dominated by delta activity with amplitudes of 50–150 µVolt, or a discontinuous pattern called tracé alternant (TA) with 50–150 µVolt bursts of delta activity alternating with 25–50 µVolt theta activity [3]. Active sleep is further characterized by the presence of REMs, variable heart rhythm, irregular breathing, low muscle tone and occasional startles or muscle twitches, while quiet sleep is dominated by regular heart rate and respiration and low muscle activity. Indeterminate or transitional sleep occupies around 10–15% of total sleep time. Although sleep–wake states are not clearly delineated in very preterm infants < 30 conceptional weeks, variability in the electrocortical background, indicating immature sleep–wake cycling, can be seen in stable extremely preterm infants already at 24–25 gestational weeks.

## Cerebral function monitoring and the amplitude-integrated EEG (aEEG)

The main concept of cerebral function monitoring is the possibility of continuously recording and assessing brain function in intensive care patients at high risk for developing brain dysfunction. One of the first devices for continuous monitoring of brain function, the cerebral function monitor (CFM), was created in the 1960s for use in adults [7]. The CFM was based on a filtered, rectified and time-compressed single-channel EEG and was created for use in the intensive care unit. A main purpose of the CFM was to create a robust monitor with a stable trend recording of the EEG background with a minimum of artefacts. Furthermore, it should be easy to apply and interpret by the staff in the intensive care unit. In the early 1980s, it was subsequently shown that the CFM was excellent for monitoring brain function in newborn infants [8–10]. To distinguish the method of EEG processing from the name of a specific device, the method was later called amplitude-integrated EEG (aEEG) to denote that the display of the trend signal is based on the amplitude of the filtered and rectified EEG, although there is, from a technical aspect, no real "amplitude-integration" included in the signal processing. Today's monitors create the aEEG settings digitally and they also display and store the "raw" EEG, which makes it possible to review the signal later. This is a very important feature and clearly increases the accuracy of the new monitor as compared to the old CFM. Since the use of aEEG monitoring now also includes recording and assessment of the raw EEG, the term "limited channel EEG" has been suggested [11]. In this chapter, the abbreviation aEEG/EEG denotes that a limited channel EEG is recorded and should be assessed, together with the aEEG trend. The aEEG trend can be created in most digital standard EEG systems and some aEEG monitors can also be used for full EEG recordings. A comparison of various features in different monitors, including the asymmetric filter which is a key component in the aEEG, demonstrated that the aEEG trend is similar in the currently available monitors [12].

Monitors displaying the aEEG trend are increasingly used in intensive care units since they are simple to apply and easy to interpret and also because they add clinically relevant information about brain function in high-risk patients. However, the aEEG method also has limitations, which users must be aware of as is discussed below. It is strongly advised that the aEEG should be used as a complement to the cEEG or the video EEG and that neurophysiologists, or neurologists with expert knowledge in EEG, are involved in the monitoring. Our experience is that a consequence of using aEEG is an increasing the demand for cEEG recordings, since cerebral functional abnormalities are frequently detected during the monitoring with consequent need for more detailed information.

The aEEG background can be characterized both by patterns, based on EEG background activity (i.e. continuous, discontinuous, burst suppression, low voltage, inactive [13]) and by amplitudes. Overall, aEEG patterns correspond well with EEG background activity. However, it is sometimes difficult to distinguish whether the aEEG shows a discontinuous pattern or burst suppression. Usually burst suppression is characterized by a straight lower border with no variability, while the lower border amplitude is variable in discontinuous patterns. The amplitude classification was created by al Naqeeb et al as a method for rapid assessment of electrocortical background activity in high-risk infants that could be eligible for post-asphyctic intervention [14]. In this classification, electrocortical background activity in term infants is classified either as normal (minimum aEEG amplitude above 5 μVolt and upper amplitude above 10 μVolt), moderately depressed (minimum aEEG amplitude below 5 μVolt and upper amplitude above 10 μVolt), or suppressed (minimum aEEG amplitude below 5 μVolt and upper amplitude below 10 μVolt). An advantage with this method is that it is easy to learn for users with limited experience and that it has proved to be reliable in use in large multicentre trials (14). A limitation is that this classification does not include assessment of sleep–wake cycling [15]. Figure 13.2 also shows how the amplitude can be affected by artefacts and potentially misclassified if the EEG is not inspected carefully. Electrode positions need to be controlled, since increasing interelectrode distance is associated with higher voltage. Recent data also demonstrate that activity recorded from C3–C4

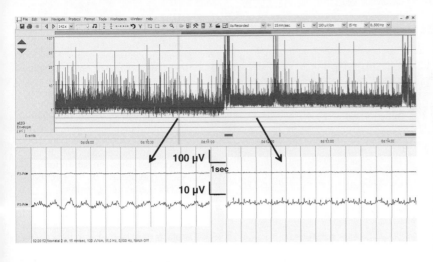

**Figure 13.2.** This mainly inactive/flat aEEG/EEG was recorded during the first hours of life in a severely asphyxiated infant. The initial aEEG looks like a very low voltage burst suppression pattern, although the lower border is lifted to 4–5 μVolt. Then there is an abrupt change in aEEG pattern when the baby was turned and the trace is lifted further to above 5 μVolt. The corresponding EEG samples are shown below. The upper EEG tracings are presented in a commonly used scale (100 μV/cm) and look almost entirely flat. When the scale is changed to 10 μV/cm, it is clear that the left trace is influenced by a suspected respiratory artefact (0.7–1 Hz) and the right trace is affected by a 3 Hz (corresponding to a heart rate of 180) artefact from the electrocardiogram. Such artefacts can consequently falsely lift the lower border of a flat/inactive aEEG/EEG tracing. Please see plate section for colour version.

seems to be of higher voltage than activity in P3–P4, although it is currently not known if this would influence the amplitude classification [12].

Several studies have now published "normal values" for the aEEG trend at different gestational ages [9,13,16]. Various measures have been assessed, including different types of patterns, as well as lower and upper aEEG amplitudes and variability due to sleep–wake cycling. The discontinuous EEG background during quiet sleep is easy to identify in the aEEG trend, with its broader bandwidth and lower minimum amplitude alternating with more continuous activity (more narrow bandwidth and higher minimum amplitude). The correspondence between clinically assessed sleep–wake states and aEEG pattern was previously evaluated in stable preterm infants at 32–34 weeks' conceptional age [17]. Several studies have shown that the strongest maturational feature is a progressive rise of the lower border amplitude, measured during the most continuous part of the tracing. Note that the aEEG appearance of wakefulness and active sleep are similar and that duration of indeterminate or transitional sleep is difficult to assess.

The aEEG background and amplitude can also be affected by extracerebral factors such as electrocardiogram, respiration and high frequency oscillation ventilation. Consequently, the "raw" EEG signal should always be assessed since it may reveal the reason for artefacts [15]. The "raw" EEG is also a necessary evaluation to confirm suspected seizures in the aEEG. However, brief seizures may be very difficult to

detect in the very time-compressed aEEG trend, see below. Figure 13.3 shows how high-frequency oscillation ventilation influences a seizure pattern in an infant with moderate hypoxic–ischaemic encephalopathy and subclinical seizures.

Traditionally, biparietal electrode positions (P3–P4) were used for aEEG monitoring in adults, since these electrodes are located above arterial border zones and consequently it was considered that these positions were the most sensitive to detect early cerebral dysfunction. However, the optimal electrode position in newborn infants has not been assessed, although studies investigating seizure distribution indicate that central positions are better than frontal (see below). Whether a single biparietal/bicentral channel, or two bilateral channels, should be used for clinical monitoring is also a matter for investigation. Two-channel recordings may be preferred in babies with lateralized brain injury and with two channels, it is also easier to assess possible artefacts.

## CFM/EEG in the diagnosis of neonatal encephalopathy and assignment of prognosis

### EEG response to hypoxic–ischaemic insults and prediction of outcome

If a hypoxic, ischaemic or hypoglycaemic insult becomes severe enough, the EEG becomes depressed

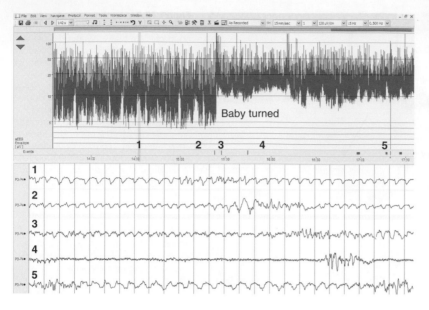

**Figure 13.3.** This term baby with moderate hypoxic–ischaemic encephalopathy and meconium aspiration was treated with high-frequency oscillation ventilation (HFOV) with frequency 10 Hz. The aEEG background in the 4-hour recording is discontinuous and shows repetitive seizures (at least 35–40 but they are difficult to count). The amplitude of the aEEG trace is "swaying" due to the HFOV artefact and this becomes even more pronounced when the baby is turned (resulting in pressure on the electrodes). The HFOV artefact on the burst suppression background is clearly seen in trace 4. Seizures may be more difficult to identify when the aEEG is influenced by artefacts from HFOV, but in this case they had a fairly similar appearance in the raw EEG (except for the 10 Hz HFOV artefact). Please see plate section for colour version.

as a sign of compromised neural function. The EEG response, which consists of slowing and amplitude depression, is not specific for a certain type of insult. The EEG depression may recover if oxygenation or glucose supplies are restored before irreversible neuronal injury has occurred. The degree of the EEG depression and the time to recovery reflects the severity of the insult and the extent of neuronal injury. In adult subjects, both EEG and aEEG have been used e.g. during carotid surgery to give early warning about cerebral ischaemia. Comparable data from newborn infants are scarce; to our knowledge a study by Roberton et al is the only study assessing EEG responses to hypoxia in newborn infants [18]. The infants were studied during weaning from mechanical ventilation; when hypoxia became marked, EEG slowing and amplitude depression was seen, which recovered when oxygenation improved. However, it is not possible to retrospectively estimate from the EEG the precise time when an acute insult occurred unless it was evident, either from continuous EEG-monitoring or as indicated by other variables, e.g. a sentinel event during delivery. However, the presence of chronic changes in the cEEG background (e.g. disorganized pattern, delayed maturation) indicates that the insult did not occur very recently, as shown by Watanabe et al [19].

# Prediction of outcome in asphyxiated infants

Several studies have demonstrated that aEEG/EEG and EEG background activity is a very sensitive predictor of later neurodevelopmental outcome in asphyxiated newborn infants as early as the first 3 to 12 hours of life [20–23]. Toet et al demonstrated that around 90% of infants will be correctly predicted by the aEEG/EEG background at 6 hours and around 80% of the infants at 3 hours [21]. The studies below mainly review data from non-cooled infants. However, with the introduction of interventions aiming at improving the outcomes, the predictive values of abnormal aEEG/EEG and EEG background features will be altered.

An early normal or slightly abnormal aEEG/EEG or cEEG background pattern is almost invariably associated with good outcome in asphyxiated infants [20–24]. Early appearance of sleep–wake cycling is also associated with better outcome in asphyxiated infants [20,21,24]. Osredkar et al demonstrated that sleep–wake cycling appearing before 36 postnatal hours in asphyxiated infants was associated with better outcome [25].

The ominous prognosis of inactive and burst suppression tracings has been shown in several publications. In 80 term infants (a majority suffered from fetal distress) who had cEEGs recorded during the first 24 hours of life, predictors of death or major sequelae were: inactive recordings after the first 10 postnatal hours and discontinuous recordings with longest IBI more than 40 seconds, shortest IBI longer than 2 seconds and longest burst duration 6 seconds or less [24]. Presence of SWC was associated with good outcome. Inactive or discontinuous traces were associated with cortical necrosis and injury to basal ganglia, cerebellum and brain stem on postmortem investigations. Menache et al demonstrated that a burst suppression pattern with predominant IBI more than 30 seconds was consistently associated with poor outcome, i.e. death or major sequelae [26]. Aso et al also investigated the correlation between EEG abnormalities and brain injury, diagnosed postmortem in 47 newborn infants [27]. Increasing EEG background abnormality correlated with the number of damaged brain structures; very little brain injury was found in infants with normal or moderately abnormal EEGs. In contrast, isoelectric tracings were associated with widespread brain injury, including the cerebral cortex, corpus striatum, thalamus, midbrain and pons in all patients. Burst-suppression was also associated with multifocal brain damage, but there were no common structures affected. The sensitivity of EEG asymmetry for focal brain injury was low (40%), but the specificity was relatively high (85%). Shah et al demonstrated a close correlation between the reduced aEEG amplitude and degree of brain damage in term encephalopathic infants [28]. A lower border aEEG amplitude below 6 µVolt was associated with brain injury on MRI with a very high sensitivity (92%). However, a lower border aEEG amplitude below 4 µVolt had a higher specificity as regards brain damage on MRI.

When the aEEG/EEG or EEG is recorded very shortly after hypoxic–ischaemic events in newborn infants, even the presence of extremely depressed electrocortical activity may be associated with good recovery. Toet et al demonstrated that severely depressed aEEGs by 3 hours of age could recover in some infants by 6 hours and be associated with good outcome [21]. Azzopardi et al also showed that outcome was good if a two-channel EEG was normalized by 12 hours of birth [22]. van Rooij et al demonstrated that the outcome was good in 50% of asphyxiated infants with burst suppression pattern at 6 hours, if the aEEG background changed to a continuous pattern at 24 hours [29]. Also Pressler et al demonstated that severely abnormal early EEGs may recover; three infants, out

of seven, with initially inactive EEGs that recovered within 8 to 12 hours had a normal outcome [30].

Murray et al demonstrated, in a cohort of asphyxiated infants with serial EEGs performed at 6, 12, 24 and 48 hours, that the predictive value of an abnormal EEG for adverse outcome was highest at 48 hours [23]. Early EEG features associated with abnormal outcome were background amplitude < 30 µVolt, interburst interval > 30 sec, seizures and absence of sleep–wake cycling.

Ter Horst et al evaluated aEEG recordings from asphyxiated infants during the first 72 hours [31]. The likelihood ratio for burst suppression or worse patterns for predicting adverse outcome was 2.7 (95% confidence interval [CI]: 1.4–5.0) during the first 6 hours and increased to 19 (95% CI: 2.8–128) between 24 and 36 hours, but was not significant after 48 hours. Normal voltage patterns (CNV and DNV) were predictive of normal neurologic outcomes up to 48 hours.

Several studies have consequently shown that, at around 6 postnatal hours, both the sensitivity and specificity for predicting outcome from the electrocortical background activity in asphyxiated infants is around 90%.

## Seizures

Seizures often appear within 24 hours after a severe hypoxic–ischaemic insult but due to individual susceptibility and when the exact timing of the insult not is known, it is not possible to use onset of seizures for timing of previous insults.

The diagnosis of neonatal seizures can be challenging and it was previously shown by video EEG that many clinically suspected seizures do not have corresponding EEG seizure activity [32,33]. Furthermore, a majority of neonatal seizures are actually subclinical, i.e., they can only be detected by aEEG/EEG [34]. "Electroclinical dissociation" is common, i.e., electroclinical seizures become subclinical after administration of antiepileptic medications [35]. Many of the earlier studies evaluating effects from antiepileptic medications did not take this into account.

A seizure is characterized by repetitive waveforms that increase and decrease in frequency and amplitude with a definite onset, peak and end. The duration varies from seconds to several minutes; in many studies a minimum duration of 10 seconds is used to define a seizure. Status epilepticus is usually defined as continuously ongoing or repeated seizures with duration of at least 30 minutes, or more than 50% of a conventional EEG recording. The possible ictal natures of brief (ictal/interictal) rhythmic discharges (BRD or BIRD) and periodic lateralized epileptiform discharges (PLED) have been discussed for many years. Their appearance is similar to epileptic seizure activity but BRD/BIRD are briefer and PLEDs lack the evolution of seizure activity and may continue mainly unchanged for many hours. Their presence is associated with brain injury, but their significance for infants with hypoxic–ischaemic encephalopathy is not known [36,37].

With long-term aEEG/EEG monitoring, it is also evident that seizure "architecture" is very variable and includes single and repetitive seizures as well as status epilepticus [13]. Subclinical seizures and status epilepticus may continue for many hours and sometimes days in encephalopathic infants. However, although a symptom of severe cerebral compromise and suggesting an increased risk for adverse outcome, the presence of seizures *per se* in asphyxiated infants does not seem to be predictive of worse outcome. Instead, several studies demonstrated that outcome is mainly related to the underlying brain injury as reflected by the overall background activity on which the seizures appear.

Several studies have shown that a majority of neonatal seizures will appear in temporal and central EEG leads [38–40]. However, the origin of neonatal seizure discharges shows a poor correlation with the underlying pathology [26,38]. It can be estimated that around 80% of seizures can be detected by limited-channel aEEG/EEG recordings using central–parietal leads [39,40]. Shellhaas *et al* compared seizure detection in 125 one-hour standard EEG recordings, containing 851 seizures, with a single-channel EEG (C3–C4) and a single-channel aEEG derived from C3–C4, respectively [39,41]. In total, 78% of the seizures in the standard EEG could be identified in the single-channel EEG. However, in the aEEG (without access to the EEG) five investigators detected only between 12 and 38% (mean 26%) of the seizures. The percentage of correctly detected seizures in the aEEG depended on the assessors' experience and on seizure duration, frequency and amplitude. Since many EEGs contained repeated seizures, 94% of EEGs with seizures could be identified by the single-channel EEG and between 22 and 57% (mean 40%) were detected by the aEEG (without EEG). These two studies also stress the need for adequate training and the importance of inspecting the "raw" EEG, when assessing aEEG/EEG recordings.

Fewer seizures will be detected if the electrodes are placed on the forehead. Wusthoff *et al* demonstrated that only 46% of seizures appeared in frontal leads (Fp3 between 12 and 38% Fp4), in contrast to 73% in C3 between 12 and 38% C4, in a study comprising 330 seizures from 125 neonatal cEEGs [42]. However, since repeated seizures may appear in one EEG, the same investigators also demonstrated that seizures located in Fp3 between 12 and 38% Fp4 actually were detected in 66% of the cEEG records, as compared to 90% of seizures in C3 between 12 and 38% C4 [42].

Bourez-Swart *et al* compared seizure detection from multichannel aEEGs derived from conventional EEGs [40]. They also found that a majority (68%) of seizures appeared in the centrotemporal regions, but despite this more seizures were detected in central leads than in temporal leads. They hypothesized that this could be due to larger amplitudes from propagated seizure activity in the central leads. With a single-channel aEEG (C3 between 12 and 38% C4), only 1 patient out of 12 was not identified as having seizures. The included infants had on average 20 seizures/hour detected in the EEG. The very high number of seizures can probably explain why the overall percentage of seizures detected by a single-channel aEEG (without EEG) was only 30%; very brief seizures are impossible to detect in the time-compressed aEEG trend.

When diagnosing seizures with aEEG/EEG, it is consequently necessary to assess the EEG trace and to have adequate training for the interpretation, since seizure-like artefacts (patting, hiccups, respiration) must also be excluded. Furthermore, unusual presentation of seizures in the aEEG trend must be recognized, e.g. continuously ongoing high-voltage seizure activity. Automated seizure detection alarms are currently being developed for many aEEG/EEG monitors and will probably be useful for daily clinical monitoring.

## aEEG/EEG for monitoring progress and treatment during hypothermia

### Early prediction of outcome

The predictive value of aEEG/EEG and cEEG will change in high-risk infants treated with hypothermia. Although an early normal continuous or slightly discontinuous aEEG/EEG pattern with sleep–wake cycling will still be associated with good outcome, delayed recovery of abnormal traces may also be associated with good outcome. However, only a few studies have yet addressed these issues [43–45]. Moderate hypothermia does not seem to alter the aEEG amplitude and consequently the altered predictive value is a consequence of the hypothermia intervention [46].

Hallberg *et al* recorded aEEG/EEG during cooling in 23 term infants; 20 of the infants were treated with phenobarbitone for clinical and/or electrographical seizures [44]. All five infants with a normal aEEG/EEG background pattern at 6 hours had a good outcome, but also 10 of the 15 infants with initial burst suppression aEEG pattern, or worse, at 6 hours had a normal outcome at one year. Four infants out of 10, with severely abnormal aEEG background at 24 hours, normalized between 36 and 48 hours and had a good outcome. Severe aEEG abnormalities were only predictive of adverse outcome after 36 hours. Figure 13.4 shows an aEEG trace with delayed recovery in a cooled baby that subsequently survived entirely healthy.

Thoresen *et al* compared the predictive value of aEEG/EEG in 31 non-cooled versus 43 cooled infants [45]. Comparable to previous studies, early normal or slightly abnormal aEEG patterns were associated with good outcome at 18 months; 24/28 infants with continuous or discontinuous aEEG patterns at 3 to 6 hours had a good outcome, and the four infants with adverse outcome were all non-cooled. The positive predictive value of an abnormal aEEG pattern between

3 and 6 hours was 84% in non-cooled infants and 59% in cooled infants. Infants with good outcome had normalized background pattern by 24 hours when treated with normothermia and by 48 hours when treated with hypothermia. The median time of onset of SWC associated with good outcome was 24 hours in non-cooled infants and 36 hours in cooled infants and never developing SWC always predicted poor outcome. Table 13.1 shows a summary of results from Hallberg *et al* and Thoresen *et al*.

Although experimental data indicate that moderate hypothermia is associated with a reduced number of seizures, seizures may still be quite prevalent in cooled newborn infants, although currently available data are scarce. In the only available study, including 20 infants treated with head cooling, 9 infants developed seizures (clinical and electrographical) before cooling and another 10 infants (in total 19/20) developed seizures, mainly subclinical, during cooling [47]. Seizure frequency increased between 24 and 36 hours and reached a peak on the second day of life. Experimental data indicate that seizures may also increase during rewarming after hypothermia treatment, as indicated by studies in fetal sheep [48]. Consequently, it is important to continue aEEG/EEG monitoring during and after rewarming. Findings in another experimental study of fetal sheep indicate that the amplitude of seizures may

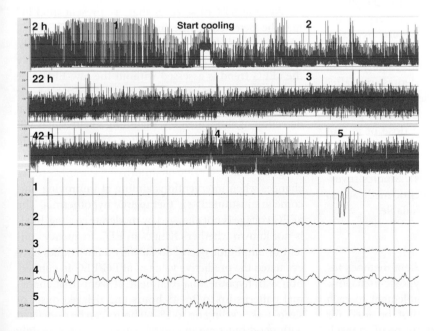

**Figure 13.4.** This term infant had a complicated delivery and was treated with moderate hypothermia starting at 5 hours of age. The aEEG samples each show 6 hours of recording, starting at 2, 22 and 42 hours, respectively. The 25 second-duration samples of EEG below correspond to the numbers in the aEEG traces. 1) Initially the infant was comatose and had no discernible electrocortical activity; the very regular burst suppression-like aEEG corresponds to a flat EEG interrupted by movements from gasping. 2) At 7 hours, the aEEG/EEG has intermittent very low voltage activity. 3) Around 25–26 hours, the aEEG amplitude increases, which corresponds to low voltage continuous activity; the baby seems to be more awake clinically. 4) The electrocortical activity is continuous with normal voltage at 44–45 hours, but two very brief suspected electroclinical seizures occurred and the infant was given midazolam, resulting in immediate depression and burst suppression pattern. 5) Two hours after the midazolam, a burst suppression pattern is still present. Please see plate section for colour version.

**Table 13.1.** Altered predictive values of aEEG background patterns after induction of hypothermia

|  | 6 Hours | 24 Hours | 48 Hours | 72 Hours |
|---|---|---|---|---|
| CNV/DNV present | HT 100% (19/19) NT 82% (9/11) | HT 97% (33/34) NT 79% (11/14) | HT 92% (44/48) NT 65% (11/17) | HT 85% (44/52) NT No additional infants |
| SWC present | HT 100% (2/2) NT 100% (1/1) | HT 100% (11/11) NT 86% (6/7) | HT 100% (17/17) NT 80% (8/10) | HT 79% (27/34) NT 55% (12/22) |

*Note:* The table shows the chance of surviving with good outcome at 12–18 months in relation to the time after birth when CNV/DNV or SWC develops and in relation to hypothermia (HT) or normothermia (NT) treatment, respectively. Combined HT data from Hallberg *et al* and Thoresen *et al*; NT data from Thoresen *et al* [44,45]. Figures are percentage of infants with good outcome, below and within brackets are the actual numbers of infants.

be dampened during cooling [49]. The clinical implication of this finding is not known; it may suggest that seizures could be more difficult to identify on EEG/aEEG if the amplitude is lower but this is not certain and remains to be tested.

# Effects on aEEG/EEG of medications

Sedative and antiepileptic medications depress cerebral activity. The degree and duration of depression depends on the type of medication, the given dose, the maturaty of the baby and probably also the illness severity. Bjerre *et al* showed that recovery of the aEEG background pattern after a severe hypoxic–ischaemic insult is possible, despite increasing blood concentrations of phenobarbital [8]. Shany *et al* assessed the duration of aEEG depression after administration of common antiepileptic medications, including lorazepam, diazepam, midazolam, phenobarbital and lidocaine [50]. A single dose of any of these medications resulted in a mean 2.5-hour depression of aEEG background activity, with a relatively large range (15 minutes to 15 hours). Studies investigating pharmacokinetics of antiepileptic medications in cooled infants are currently not available.

# Conclusion

The EEG and the aEEG/EEG are excellent methods for assessing brain function after hypoxic–ischaemic insults and should be used as a complement to each other. However, these methods cannot be used for retrospective estimation of the exact timing of an insult

unless aEEG/EEG or EEG monitoring was available during the insult. The presence of chronic changes in the EEG indicates that the insult is not entirely fresh. If the timing of an insult can be reasonably decided, e.g. as in acute perinatal asphyxia, then acute changes in the EEG and aEEG are superb early prognostic indicators. Background patterns associated with high risk for neurodevelopmental impairment or death include inactivity, low voltage and burst suppression, while a continuous normal voltage background and presence of sleep–wake cycling are predictive of normal outcome.

Around 80% of seizures that are present in cEEG may be detected in the limited-channel aEEG/EEG, when recorded from central or parietal leads. However, a majority of seizures are missed if only the aEEG trend is assessed without the raw-EEG, due to the heavily time-compressed trend. Whether one or two channels of aEEG/EEG should be used for optimal detection of abnormalities, including seizures, has not yet been fully evaluated. However, two channels will increase the ability to rule out artefacts.

The predictive value of abnormal EEG/aEEG traces changes when interventions aiming at improving outcome are instituted, e.g. therapeutic hypothermia. The aEEG voltage is not changed by moderate cooling, but it is not known whether changes in EEG frequency content or amplitude occur. So far only a few studies have evaluated the predictive value of aEEG/EEG in connection with hypothermia treatment. It seems that abnormal patterns up to 36–48 hours and delayed onset of sleep–wake cycling up to 48–60 hours can be associated with good outcome in cooled babies. Seizures, mainly subclinical, may still be common in cooled infants and consequently it is important to continue aEEG/EEG monitoring during hypothermia treatment including rewarming and initially during normothermia.

# References

1. Lombroso CT. Neonatal polygraphy in full-term and premature infants: a review of normal and abnormal findings. *J Clin Neurophysiol* 1985;**2**:105–55.

2. Mizrahi EM, Hrachovy RA, Kellaway P. *Atlas of neonatal encephalography*, 3rd edition. Philadelphia: Lippincott Williams & Wilkins; 2004. p. 1–250.

3. André M, Lamblin MD, d'Allest AM, et al. Electroencephalography in premature and full-term infants. Developmental features and glossary. *Neurophysiol Clin* 2010;**40**:59–124.

4. Vanhatalo S, Palva JM, Holmes MD, et al. Infraslow oscillations modulate excitability and interictal epileptic activity in the human cortex during sleep. *Proc Natl Acad Sci U S A* 2004;**101**:5053–7.

5. Thordstein M, Löfgren N, Flisberg A, et al. Infraslow EEG activity in burst periods from post asphyctic full term neonates. *Clin Neurophysiol* 2005;**116**:1501–6.

6. Korotchikova I, Connolly S, Ryan CA, et al. EEG in the healthy term newborn within 12 hours of birth. *Clin Neurophysiol* 2009;**120**:1046–53.

7. Maynard D, Prior PF, Scott DF. Device for continuous monitoring of cerebral activity in resuscitated patients. *Br Med J* 1969;**4**:545–6.

8. Bjerre I, Hellström-Westas L, Rosén I, Svenningsen N. Monitoring of cerebral function after severe asphyxia in infancy. *Arch Dis Child* 1983;**58**:997–1002.

9. Viniker DA, Maynard DE, Scott DF. Cerebral function monitor studies in neonates. *Clin Electroencephalogr* 1984;**15**:185–92.

10. Archbald F, Verma UL, Tejani NA, Handwerker SM. Cerebral function monitor in the neonate. II: Birth asphyxia. *Dev Med Child Neurol* 1984;**26**:162–8.

11. Shah DK, Mackay MT, Lavery S, et al. Accuracy of bedside electroencephalographic monitoring in comparison with simultaneous continuous conventional electroencephalography for seizure detection in term infants. *Pediatrics* 2008;**121**:1146–54.

12. Quigg M, Leiner D. Engineering aspects of the quantified amplitude-integrated electroencephalogram in neonatal cerebral monitoring. *J Clin Neurophysiol* 2009;**26**:145–9.

13. Hellström-Westas L, Rosén I, de Vries LS, Greisen G. Amplitude-integrated EEG: Classification and interpretation in preterm and term infants. *Neoreviews* 2006;**7**:e76–87.

14. al Naqeeb N, Edwards AD, Cowan FM, Azzopardi D. Assessment of neonatal encephalopathy by amplitude-integrated electroencephalography. *Pediatrics* 1999;**103**:1263–71.

15. Hagmann CF, Robertson NJ, Azzopardi D. Artifacts on electroencephalograms may influence the amplitude-integrated EEG classification: a qualitative analysis in neonatal encephalopathy. *Pediatrics* 2006;**118**:2552–4.

16. Thornberg E, Thiringer K. Normal pattern of the cerebral function monitor trace in term and preterm neonates. *Acta Paediatr Scand* 1990;**79**:20–5.

17. Greisen G, Hellström-Vestas L, Lou H, Rosén I, Svenningsen NW. Sleep-waking shifts and cerebral blood flow in stable preterm infants. *Pediatr Res* 1985;**19**:1156–9.

18. Roberton NR. Effect of acute hypoxia on blood pressure and electroencephalogram of newborn babies. *Arch Dis Child* 1969;**44**:719–25.

19. Watanabe K, Hayakawa F, Okumura A. Neonatal EEG: a powerful tool in the assessment of brain damage in preterm infants. *Brain Dev* 1999;**21**:361–72.

20. Hellström-Westas L, Rosen I, Svenningsen NW. Predictive value of early continuous amplitude integrated EEG recordings on outcome after severe birth asphyxia in full term infants. *Arch Dis Child Fetal Neonatal Ed* 1995;**72**:F34–8.

21. Toet MC, Hellstrom-Westas L, Groenendaal F, Eken P, de Vries LS. Amplitude integrated EEG 3 and 6 hours after birth in full term neonates with hypoxic-ischaemic encephalopathy. *Arch Dis Child Fetal Neonatal Ed* 1999;**81**:F19–23.

22. Azzopardi D, Guarino I, Brayshaw C, et al. Prediction of neurological outcome after birth asphyxia from early continuous two-channel electroencephalography. *Early Hum Dev* 1999;**55**:113–23.

23. Murray DM, Boylan GB, Ryan CA, Connolly S. Early EEG findings in hypoxic-ischemic encephalopathy predict outcomes at 2 years. *Pediatrics* 2009;**124**:e459–67.

24. Pezzani C, Radvanyi-Bouvet MF, Relier JP, Monod N. Neonatal electroencephalography during the first twenty-four hours of life in full-term newborn infants. *Neuropediatrics* 1986;**17**:11–8.

25. Osredkar D, Toet MC, van Rooij LG, et al. Sleep-wake cycling on amplitude-integrated electroencephalography in term newborns with hypoxic-ischemic encephalopathy. *Pediatrics* 2005;**115**:327–32.

26. Menache CC, Bourgeois BF, Volpe JJ. Prognostic value of neonatal discontinuous EEG. *Pediatr Neurol* 2002;**27**:93–101.

27. Aso K, Scher MS, Barmada MA. Neonatal electroencephalography and neuropathology. *J Clin Neurophysiol* 1989;**6**:103–23.

28. Shah DK, Lavery S, Doyle LW, et al. Use of 2-channel bedside electroencephalogram monitoring in term-born encephalopathic infants related to cerebral injury defined by magnetic resonance imaging. *Pediatrics* 2006;**118**:47–55.

29. van Rooij LG, Toet MC, Osredkar D, et al. Recovery of amplitude integrated electroencephalographic background patterns within 24 hours of perinatal asphyxia. *Arch Dis Child Fetal Neonatal Ed* 2005;**90**: F245–51.

30. Pressler RM, Boylan GB, Morton M, Binnie CD, Rennie JM. Early serial EEG in hypoxic ischaemic encephalopathy. *Clin Neurophysiol* 2001;**112**:31–7.

31. ter Horst HJ, Sommer C, Bergman KA, et al. Prognostic significance of amplitude-integrated EEG during the first 72 hours after birth in severely asphyxiated neonates. *Pediatr Res* 2004;**55**:1026–33.

32. Mizrahi EM, Kellaway P. Characterization and classification of neonatal seizures. *Neurology* 1987;**37**:1837–44.

33. Murray DM, Boylan GB, Ali I, et al. Defining the gap between electrographic seizure burden, clinical expression and staff recognition of neonatal seizures. *Arch Dis Child Fetal Neonatal Ed* 2008;**93**:F187–91.

34. Clancy RR, Legido A, Lewis D. Occult neonatal seizures. *Epilepsia* 1988;**29**:256–61.

35. Boylan GB, Rennie JM, Pressler RM, et al. Phenobarbitone, neonatal seizures and video-EEG. *Arch Dis Child Fetal Neonatal Ed* 2002;**86**:F165–70.

36. Shewmon DA. What is a neonatal seizure? Problems in definition and quantification for investigative and clinical purposes. *J Clin Neurophysiol* 1990;**7**:315–68.

37. Oliveira AJ, Nunes ML, Haertel LM, Reis FM, da Costa JC. Duration of rhythmic EEG patterns in neonates: new evidence for clinical and prognostic significance of brief rhythmic discharges. *Clin Neurophysiol* 2000;**111**:1646–53.

38. Patrizi S, Holmes GL, Orzalesi M, Allemand F. Neonatal seizures: characteristics of EEG ictal activity in preterm and fullterm infants. *Brain Dev* 2003;**25**:427–37.

39. Shellhaas RA, Clancy RR. Characterization of neonatal seizures by conventional EEG and single-channel EEG. *Clin Neurophysiol* 2007;**118**:2156–61.

40. Bourez-Swart MD, van Rooij L, Rizzo C, et al. Detection of subclinical electroencephalographic seizure patterns with multichannel amplitude-integrated EEG in full-term neonates. *Clin Neurophysiol* 2009;**120**:1916–22.

41. Shellhaas RA, Soaita AI, Clancy RR. Sensitivity of amplitude-integrated electroencephalography for neonatal seizure detection. *Pediatrics* 2007;**120**:770–7.

42. Wusthoff CJ, Shellhaas RA, Clancy RR. Limitations of single-channel EEG on the forehead for neonatal seizure detection. *J Perinatol* 2009;**29**:237–42.

43. Mariani E, Scelsa B, Pogliani L, Introvini P, Lista G. Prognostic value of electroencephalograms in asphyxiated newborns treated with hypothermia. *Pediatr Neurol* 2008;**39**:317–24.

44. Hallberg B, Grossmann K, Bartocci M, Blennow M. The prognostic value of early aEEG in asphyxiated infants undergoing systemic hypothermia treatment. *Acta Paediatr* 2010;**99**:531–6.

45. Thoresen M, Hellström-Westas L, Liu X, de Vries LS. Effect of hypothermia on amplitude-integrated electroencephalogram in infants with asphyxia. *Pediatrics* 2010;**126**:e131–9.

46. Horan M, Azzopardi D, Edwards AD, Firmin RK, Field D. Lack of influence of mild hypothermia on amplitude integrated-electroencephalography in neonates receiving extracorporeal membrane oxygenation. *Early Hum Dev* 2007;**83**:69–75.

47. Yap V, Engel M, Takenouchi T, Perlman JM. Seizures are common in term infants undergoing head cooling. *Pediatr Neurol* 2009;**41**:327–31.

48. Gerrits LC, Battin MR, Bennet L, Gonzalez H, Gunn AJ. Epileptiform activity during rewarming from moderate cerebral hypothermia in the near-term fetal sheep. *Pediatr Res* 2005;**57**:342–6.

49. Bennet L, Dean JM, Wassink G, Gunn AJ. Differential effects of hypothermia on early and late epileptiform events after severe hypoxia in preterm fetal sheep. *J Neurophysiol* 2007;**97**:572–8.

50. Shany E, Benzaquen O, Friger M, Richardson J, Golan A. Influence of antiepileptic drugs on amplitude-integrated electroencephalography. *Pediatr Neurol* 2008;**39**:387–91.

# Magnetic resonance imaging in hypoxic–ischaemic encephalopathy and the effects of hypothermia

Mary A. Rutherford and Serena Counsell

## Introduction

Magnetic resonance (MR) imaging is an ideal tool to assess the neonatal brain following a hypoxic–ischaemic event, providing complementary information to cranial ultrasound. It can identify alternative or additional diagnoses such as congenital malformations or antenatal injury and an optimal examination allows the timing, the site and severity of perinatally acquired injury to be determined. This in turn may be used to predict neurodevelopmental outcome for the majority of neonates. The provision of diagnostic and prognostic information is, however, often hampered by poor image quality, inappropriately timed examinations and inaccurate interpretation of the scans. Image quality may be impaired by motion artefact, poor signal to noise ratio or inappropriate sequence choice.

In the new era of interventions, such as hypothermia, designed to prevent or modify perinatally acquired brain injury it is necessary to determine whether imaging practice needs to be altered during or following therapy to ensure it fulfils its potential as a diagnostic and prognostic tool. Hypothermia has become standard of care in the neonate with hypoxic–ischaemic encephalopathy (HIE) and the demand for MR examination of the neonatal brain to predict prognosis is increasing rapidly. In parallel with its clinical role, MRI is able to assess the neurobiological effects of a new intervention, providing surrogate data for later outcomes and thereby avoiding the delays inherent in long-term follow-up studies [1–3].

This chapter will address the practical issues of acquiring and interpreting brain images in neonates with perinatal brain injury, review the current literature on the effects of hypothermia on imaging appearances and finally detail some of the advanced imaging techniques and their potential role in future intervention studies.

## Practical issues

The following paragraphs resemble the instructions inside a new appliance box, mundane but essential to exploit the abilities of magnetic resonance imaging (MRI) to a maximum.

## Sedation

Neonates are uncooperative and a successful examination relies on a still baby. To this end, neonates may be imaged during natural sleep, following a feed or more successfully under light sedation with, for instance, chloral hydrate. We use a dose of chloral hydrate between 25 and 50 mg/kg orally, by means of nasogastric tube or rectally [4]. We keep the infant nil by mouth for at least an hour before administration as this will aid absorption of the chloral hydrate. We give the chloral approximately 15 minutes before the start of the examination. Neonates will then usually sleep through a 30–45 minute examination. Severely encephalopathic neonates may require less sedation or may already be sedated by anticonvulsant medication. All neonates, sedated or not, should be monitored from onset of sedation to waking. MR-compatible pulse oximetry and electrocardiography (ECG) is required during the scan itself. A nurse or doctor, familiar with the hazards of an MR environment and trained in neonatal resuscitation, should be in attendance throughout the scan.

*Neonatal Neural Rescue*, ed. A. David Edwards, Denis V. Azzopardi and Alistair J. Gunn. Published by Cambridge University Press. © Cambridge University Press 2013.

## Safety

We always use ear protection as excessive noise may wake the sleeping infant and could potentially harm the developing auditory system. We use mouldable dental putty as individualized earplugs and neonatal earmuffs (Natus minimuffs, www.natus.com). Infants may move even when asleep: moulded air bags or foam placed snugly around the infant's head will keep this to a minimum. Swaddling the infants will keep them warm and also reduce movements. Full metal checks need to be carried out with particular attention, in this population, to the presence of intravenous scalp lines, long lines, electroencephalography (EEG) electrodes, metallic endotracheal tube holders, splints, intraventricular shunts and metal fasteners on baby clothes [5]. All staff involved in neonatal imaging need to be trained in MR safety.

## Hardware and software adaptations

Image quality is governed by the signal to noise ratio. This is maximized by using a closely fitting coil. In the absence of a dedicated neonatal head coil, an adult knee coil may be used. Phased array coils may provide improved benefit in terms of signal to noise, although lack of homogeneity may be an issue. Placement of the neonatal head in the centre of the coil will minimize heterogeneity. Infants with severe encephalopathy may be ventilator dependent in the first few days from delivery and it may, therefore, be necessary to perform an MR examination using MR compatible ventilator equipment. In the absence of this, a neonate can be safely hand bagged during a short MR examination. A larger adult type coil may then be necessary to accommodate the endotracheal tube.

## Sequences

The majority of neonatal studies have been performed at 1 or 1.5 Tesla but 3 Tesla scanners are increasingly available and starting to replace many 1.5 Tesla systems particularly for brain imaging. Most MR sequences designed for imaging the adult brain will need to be adapted to obtain good quality images of the immature brain with its higher water content. The exact imaging parameters depend on the specific system and magnet strength being used. Our parameters for neonatal brain imaging at 1.5 and 3 Tesla are shown in Table 14.1.

The following sequences provide an optimal neonatal examination:

- T1 (longitudinal relaxation time) weighted sequence acquired in the transverse plane. This is ideal for assessing the basal ganglia and thalami and provides the best views of the posterior limb of the internal capsule (Figure 14.1).
- T2 (transverse relaxation time) weighted sequence acquired in the transverse plane. This is better than T1 weighted imaging for identifying early ischaemic change and provides excellent grey/white matter contrast in the very immature brain (Figure 14.1).
- T1 weighted sequence acquired in the sagittal plane. This permits accurate assessment of the cerebellar vermis and the corpus callosum and improves the detection of subdural haemorrhage and sinus thrombosis. A volume acquisition is recommended as it provides thin slices and can be reformatted into any plane. It can also be used for absolute quantification of brain structures.

**Table 14.1.** Suggested MRI sequence parameters

| 1.5 T scanner | | | |
|---|---|---|---|
| **Sequence** | T2 TSE | 3DT1 TFE | DWI EPI |
| **Plane** | trans | sag | trans |
| TR (ms) | 4500 | 30 | 6000 |
| TE (ms) | 210 | 4.5 | 90 |
| Flip angle | 90 | 30 | 90 |
| Slice thick (mm) | 4 | 1.6 | 5 |
| NSA | 2 | 1 | 1 |
| Time (min) | 4:30 | 5:45 | 0:30 |
| **3 T scanner** | | | |
| **Sequence** | T2 TSE | 3DT1 FFE | DTI EPI |
| **Plane** | trans | sag | trans |
| TR (msec) | 8000 | 17 | 8000 |
| TE (msec) | 160 | 4.6 | 49 |
| Flip angle | 90 | 13 | 90 |
| Slice thick (mm) | 2 | 0.8 | 2 |
| NSA | 1 | 1 | 1 |
| SENSE | ×2 | | ×2 |
| Time (min) | 4:40 | 4:20 | 3:0+ |

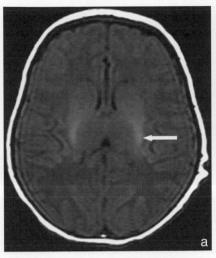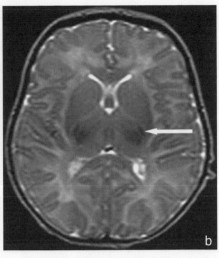

**Figure 14.1.** Normal term born neonate. T1 and T2 weighted images acquired in the axial plane. Level of the basal ganglia. There is high signal intensity in approximately half of the posterior limb of the internal capsule on the T1 weighted image (a). The corresponding low signal from myelin is slightly less on the T2 weighted image (b).

- Diffusion weighted imaging which is essential for early (< 5 days) identification of ischaemic tissue. Diffusion tensor imaging obtained in at least six non-collinear directions allows further quantification of tissue microstructure with measurements of both anisotropy and diffusivity (see below).
- A venogram to exclude the presence of sinus thrombosis and differentiate this from subdural haemorrhage.
- Angiography to look at both cerebral and neck vessels, pathology which may be implicated in focal stroke.
- MR proton spectroscopy to identify lactate and confirm tissue injury. In addition metabolite ratios, specifically Lactate/Naa, from basal ganglia and thalamic tissue may be used to predict abnormal outcome [6].

In an unsettled infant, motion resistant sequences should be used such as single shot acquisition sequences or propeller filling of k space [7].

## Clinical history

The pattern of injury sustained by a neonate may be influenced by their gestation and predicted by the clinical history and the clinical presentation [8–11]. In some cases, a specific insult may be recognised, such as hypoglycaemia or an acute

hypoxic–ischaemic event such as a uterine rupture, but in many cases the aetiology is not clear. Infants who develop neonatal seizures but who do not require aggressive resuscitation at delivery are more likely to have sustained white matter and cortical lesions such as a focal stroke or parasagittal infarction [8] Within this group, there are also more likely to be neonates with alternative or additional pathologies, e.g. cerebral malformations, metabolic disorders, or hypoglycaemia [12] (Figure 14.2). Infants with a global hypoxic–ischaemic insult, particularly if it is acute such as following a sentinel event, are likely to sustain basal ganglia and thalamic lesions [10] (Figures 14.3–14.5). However, in the absence of an acute event approximately 50% of neonates with HIE will also have significant white matter lesions [13] (Figure 14.6). The clinical presentation, therefore, serves as a guide to the lesions that will have been sustained. The majority of information to date on the relationship between clinical presentation and lesion pattern has been acquired in non-cooled infants. However, with cooling now becoming standard practice in neonates with HIE the effects of hypothermia can be assessed [1,14–19].

## Timing of scans

Perinatal brain lesions are at their most visually obvious on conventional T1 and T2 weighted imaging between 1 and 2 weeks from the time of injury.

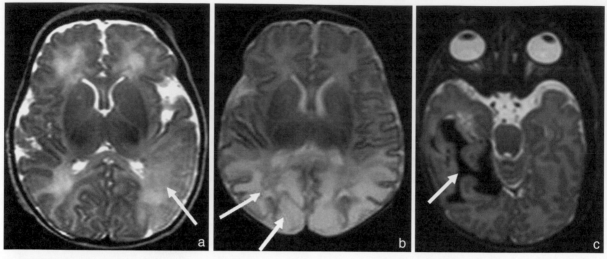

**Figure 14.2.** White matter and cortical injury. Neonates with less severe depression at delivery may show predominantly white matter and cortical injury. (a) Middle cerebral artery infarction seen as a loss of grey–white matter differentiation in the left parietal and temporal lobe (arrow). (b) Bilateral parasagittal infarction associated with hypoglycaemia seen as bilateral loss of grey–white matter differentiation in posterior parietal, occipital and temporal lobes. (c) Focal haemorrhagic lesion seen as abnormal low signal intensity involving mainly white matter in the right temporal lobe.

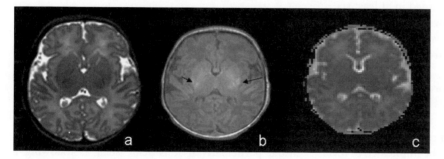

**Figure 14.3.** Mild basal ganglia and thalamic (BGT) lesions in a term born neonate with HIE imaged on day 7 with (a) T2 weighted (b) T1 weighted and (c) diffusion ADC map. Treated with hypothermia. There are small regions of increased signal intensity within the lateral lentiform nucleus on T1 weighted imaging (b, arrows). There are no corresponding abnormal signal intensities on the T2 weighted or diffusion weighted images. Myelination within the PLIC has a normal appearance.

Imaging within the first few days may show only subtle abnormalities in the presence of significant brain injury, which are difficult to interpret particularly for the inexperienced radiologist. Early image examinations should always include a diffusion-weighted sequence, which is reliable for detecting infarcted white matter (Figure 14.8) but less able to detect the full extent of injury to the basal ganglia and thalami (Figure 14.9). The DWI visual appearances of infarcted tissue are obvious very early and may last for 2 weeks, by which time abnormalities on conventional imaging will be at their most obvious [20]. Whilst there is theoretical concern that the presence of hypothermia may delay the evolution of lesions,

particularly on diffusion weighted imaging, there is as yet no evidence to demonstrate this. In addition, there are several reports of overt abnormalities on diffusion imaging during the early hypothermic period [16]. Imaging at this time can be performed without interrupting the hypothermia treatment and may be useful for management decisions in the severely injured neonate [18].

There is a predictable evolution of perinatal brain lesions (Figures 14.3–14.7) and serial conventional imaging may, therefore, allow the timing of injury to be assessed. Repeat imaging may also be useful to document atypical evolution of imaging abnormalities, particularly when an additional or different

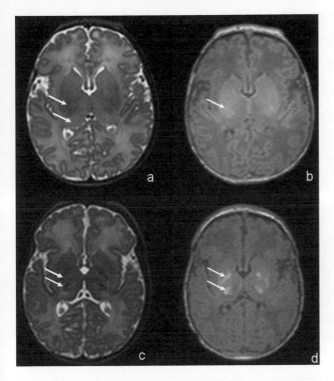

**Figure 14.4.** Moderate basal ganglia and thalamic (BGT) lesions in a term born neonate imaged on day 4 (a, b) and day 18 (c, d) with T2 weighted (a, c) and T1 weighted sequences (b, d). Abnormalities within the basal ganglia and thalami and PLIC are subtle on day 4. There is decreased myelin within the PLIC on T1 weighted imaging (b, arrow) and some increase in signal intensity in the thalami, but this appears normal on T2 weighted images (a, arrow). Adjacent to the PLIC there is abnormal increased signal intensity within the globus pallidus on T2 weighted imaging (a). By day 18 there are obvious abnormal increased signal intensities within the BGT (arrows). On T1 weighted imaging there is no myelin detected within the PLIC. On T2 weighted images there are abnormal high and low signal intensities within the thalami (lower arrow), myelin is lost within the PLIC and there is abnormal low signal intensity within the globus pallidus (upper arrow) (c).

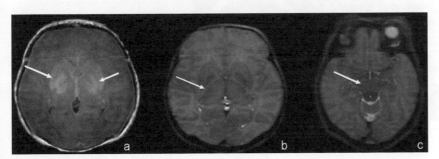

**Figure 14.5.** Severe basal ganglia and thalamic (BGT) lesions in a term born neonate imaged on day 3. There was a history of decreased fetal movements before delivery. There is marked swelling of the entire brain including the BGT. There is diffuse increased signal intensity within the BGT on T1 weighted images (arrow) (a). Myelin in the PLIC is reduced. On T2 weighted images there is no myelin visualized within the PLIC (arrow) and there is generalized increased signal intensity within the BGT with a loss of detail but abnormal decreased signal intensity within the globus pallidus. There is swelling and abnormal increased signal intensity with loss of detail within the mesencephalon of the brainstem (c) (arrow).

diagnosis such as a metabolic disorder is suspected. In some metabolic disorders, there are additional congenital malformations of the brain such as hypoplasia or agenesis of the corpus callosum in non-ketotic hyperglycinaemia. A normal scan or an isolated delay in myelination in an infant with persisting seizures should raise the possibility of a metabolic disorder or an epileptic encephalopathy.

Infants with severe encephalopathy should always have brain imaging, but this may be practically difficult and it may not be possible to perform before an infant dies. In such circumstances and particularly if no autopsy is performed post-mortem, MR imaging should be considered. It may allow confirmation of abnormalities consistent with a hypoxic–ischaemic insult or suggest an alternative diagnosis, information

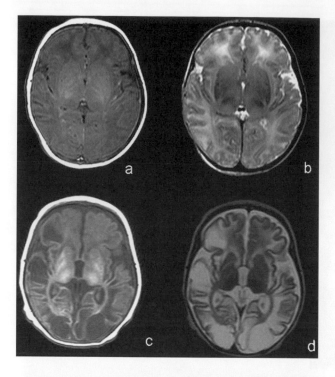

**Figure 14.6.** Severe basal ganglia and thalamic (BGT) and white matter lesions in a term born (38+5 weeks GA) neonate with HIE. Imaged on day 5 (a, b) and day 15 (c, d) with T1 weighted (a, c) and T2 weighted (b, d) sequences. There is some loss of grey white matter differentiation within the hemispheres on day 5. There is abnormal signal intensity within the PLIC and loss of detail in the BGT on T1. On T2 there is abnormal low signal intensity within the lentiform nuclei. There is some low signal intensity within the PLIC consistent with myelin but this does not appear normal for age. By day 15 there is overt cystic infarction throughout both hemispheres. In addition there is overtly abnormal increased signal intensity within the BGT on T1 weighted images 9 (c).

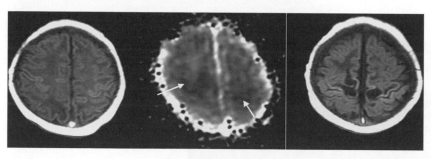

**Figure 14.7.** Cortical and subcortical injury. Term born neonate with HIE. Axial images at the level of the central sulcus. T1 weighted sequence and diffusion ADC map at 3 days of age. There is no overt abnormal signal intensity on T1 weighted imaging (a). On diffusion imaging there is obvious abnormal low signal intensity in and around the central sulci bilaterally (arrows). Follow-up images at three weeks show overt abnormal signal intensity (SI) within the cortex (high SI) and subcortical white matter (low SI). This infant also sustained severe injury to the basal ganglia and thalami (images not shown).

that is clearly important for counselling parents and for medicolegal proceedings.

## Interpreting scans

The correct interpretation of images requires a thorough knowledge of the normally developing brain (Figure 14.1) and of the range of perinatally acquired lesions and their evolution. Perinatal injury is often symmetrical and may be confused with normal appearances and *vice versa*, by those not experienced in neonatal brain imaging. It may be appropriate to send images to a centre that regularly

performs neonatal brain MR examinations for a confirmatory report or second opinion.

## Patterns of injury and prediction of outcome

In neonates with a global acute hypoxic–ischaemic insult, lesions are usually detected within the basal ganglia and thalami with abnormal signal intensity in the intervening posterior limb of the internal capsule (PLIC) (Figures 14.3–14.5). Abnormal signal intensity within the PLIC is an excellent predictor of abnormal outcome in term infants with HIE [3,21]. Basal ganglia and

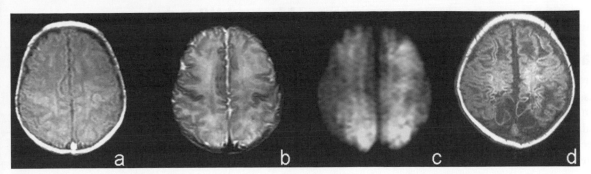

**Figure 14.8.** Diffusion weighted imaging in white matter infarction. Term born neonate with HIE imaged at 3 days (a, b, c) and 3 weeks (d) T1 weighted (a, d) and T2 weighted sequences (b) and raw diffusion image (c) at the level of the centrum semiovale. There is very subtle loss of grey white matter differentiation on T1 weighted images (a) which is more obvious, posteriorly on T2 weighted images (b). There is, however, overt diffuse abnormal high signal intensity, posterior more than anterior, on diffusion image consistent with widespread ischaemic change and impending infarction. This was confirmed on follow-up scan at 3 weeks (d).

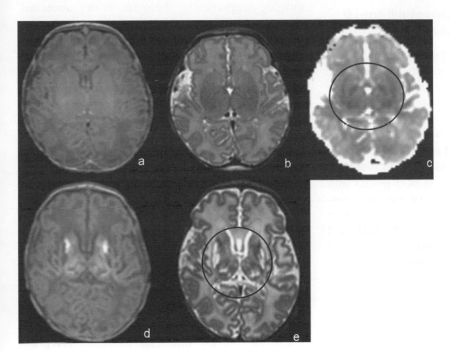

**Figure 14.9.** Diffusion weighted imaging in basal ganglia and thalamic (BGT) lesions. Term born neonate with HIE imaged on day 3 (a, b, c) and day 22 (d, e) T1 weighted (a) and T2 weighted (b) images show some loss of detail within the BGT and abnormal lack of signal from myelin in the PLIC. On diffusion ADC map there are small multifocal areas of abnormal low signal intensity (encircled), consistent with restricted diffusion in the BGT. At follow-up there is severe widespread cystic infarction of the entire BGT (encircled). These BGT changes were more severe than predicted from day 3 diffusion scan alone.

thalami (BGT) lesions give rise to motor impairment in the form of cerebral palsy. The severity of the BGT lesions dictates the severity and nature of the cerebral palsy [3,10,21] (Figures 14.3–14.5). Lesions in the BGT are often accompanied by injury to the cortex and sub-cortical white matter, most typically around the central sulcus. These changes are most obvious after the first week from injury (Figure 14.7). In approximately 50% of neonates with BGT lesions, there will be more extensive white matter abnormalities (Figures 14.5–14.8). The motor outcome for these children is still dictated by

the BGT lesions but white matter involvement may exacerbate any cognitive deficit. However, infants with severe BGT lesions have severe cognitive impairment regardless of the severity of additional early white matter involvement. Infants with severe BGT lesions all develop a secondary microcephaly with reduction in white matter that appears to be a secondary process [22].

In some infants who present with what is thought to be HIE, there is no BGT involvement but only white matter lesions (Figure 14.7). These may be haemor-rhagic. These lesions give rise to tissue atrophy and later cognitive impairment. The more severe the white matter lesions, the worse the cognitive outcome [13].

## Imaging following hypothermia

There are very few published studies using imaging to assess the effects of hypothermia following perinatal brain injury [1,14–19]. There are several important questions to ask about the effect of hypothermia or indeed any new intervention designed to modify or prevent brain injury, namely:

- Is the pattern of lesions altered in terms of both frequency and type of lesion?
- Is the evolution of the lesions altered?
- Is there evidence to support a decrease in brain injury?
- Can the pattern of lesions acquired still provide accurate information on later outcome?

Hypothermia is instituted at present within the first 6 hours from delivery with the intent that a therapeutic effect would be immediate in the prevention of acute lesions. The longer term effects of hypothermia on brain lesion evolution and brain development have not been systematically studied. Two small early studies looked at the effect of both head and whole body cooling on the pattern of injury detected with neonatal MRI. The first demonstrated a decrease in BGT lesions with both head and whole body cooling but was not a controlled trial [14]. The second demonstrated a decrease in cortical lesions with cooling over both the body and under the head as required [15]. Neither study reported an increase in haemorrhage or thrombosis or a pattern of lesions considered unusual for neonates with HIE. A more recent imaging study was performed within the multicentre randomized controlled TOBY trial [23]. This demonstrated that cooling was associated with a decrease in both white matter and BGT lesions. More convincingly, it was associated with an increase in normal brain appearances. The median postnatal age at scan within both groups was 8 days and the ability for the scan to predict outcome was not altered by treatment with cooling; accuracy of prediction (0.84 (0.74–0.94) in the cooled infants compared with 0.81 (0.71–0.91) in the non-cooled infants. The issue of changes in the evolution of scan findings is more difficult to address within the TOBY trial but no obvious delays in lesion evolution were noted. It has also been reported that, in neonates with lesions, diffusion images are already abnormal during cooling [16].

## Advanced MR techniques

### Diffusion weighted imaging

Diffusion weighted imaging (DWI) provides a measure of the random motion of water within a tissue. Quantification of this motion or diffusivity can be measured with an apparent diffusion coefficient (ADC). The ability of DWI to assess tissue injury in the immature brain was initially reported in neonates with perinatal stroke. In white matter infarction visual abnormalities on DWI are at their most obvious 1 to 4 days after delivery at a time when conventional imaging may not be that abnormal (Figures 14.7, 14.8) [14,24,25]. Abnormal signal intensity gradually reduces by the end of the first week as the conventional imaging appearances become more abnormal. Typically ADC values within white matter infarction fall to less than 50% of their normal value. However, within a lesion the values may be quite variable. Similar results with DWI can be shown whether white matter infarction is focal as in middle cerebral artery infarction or if it arises as part of a more global under perfusion, so-called parasagittal injury. The evolution of the diffusion abnormality in focal white matter infarction is consistent with and appears to be similar to that seen in adults, although it has been suggested that ADC values may pseudonormalize more quickly than in the adult patient [24]. However, as the aetiology of perinatal stroke is poorly understood and seizures may not become clinically obvious until 48 hours, it is difficult to time the exact onset of ischaemia. In infants with HIE and a more global hypoxic–ischaemic insult, the most frequent site of injury as previously discussed is to the central grey matter. There are fewer studies using DWI in infants with HIE and these have had conflicting results [14,25–29]. As for unilateral infarction DWI will have largely normalized by the end of the second week, both visually and in terms of ADC values. In infants with HIE, ADC values were significantly reduced in the first week following severe injury to either white matter or BGT ($P < 0.0001$) but values normalized at the end of the first week and then increased during week 2. However, the fractional anisotropy (FA) value may continue to fall providing a detection of injury beyond 2 weeks [30]. We have found that ADC values $< 1.1 \times 10^{-3}/\text{mm}^2$ were always associated with white matter (WM) infarction and values $< 0.8 \times 10^{-3}/\text{mm}^2$ with thalamic infarction [20].

Early visual analysis may be particularly misleading when there has been widespread injury to WM and BGT probably because there is no normal tissue for comparison. A visual clue may be found by observing the appearance of the usually normally appearing cerebellum [20,31]. In these infants, measuring the ADC values will correctly detect the presence of ischaemic tissue.

Of importance is the evidence that early visual appearances of DWI and the ADC values may be either normal or small and focal in the presence of isolated but clinically significant BGT lesions (Figure 14.8). Repeat diffusion studies over the first two weeks from injury show that within the BGT abnormal areas of restriction may vary from one structure to the next [26]. Characteristically, the sequence of BGT abnormality starts in the ventrolateral nuclei of the thalami, then affects the putamen and finally the globus pallidus where abnormal signal intensity may still be obvious 2 weeks after the injury. A single diffusion examination may, therefore, underestimate the total lesion load within the BGT.

## Diffusion tensor imaging

Diffusion tensor imaging (DTI) may improve the ability to detect abnormal tissue by providing us with another parameter: the anisotropy or directional diffusivity within a tissue. Anisotropy increases with age as myelination decreases radial diffusivity perpendicular to WM tracts. Anisotropy is variably deranged following acute focal infarction in adults. We have shown that during the first week from delivery FA values in the WM were significantly decreased in not only infants with severe abnormality but also those with moderate abnormality. Of interest, given the phenomenon of pseudonormalization with ADC values, is that FA values in severe WM lesions were also significantly reduced during the second and third weeks [30]. In addition, anisotropy was significantly decreased in the first week throughout the BGT and became progressively more abnormal within the region of the ventrolateral nuclei. FA was, therefore, significantly abnormal in both severe and moderate WM and BGT lesions with no pseudonormalization. This suggests that a combination of ADC and FA values derived from DTI combined with visual analysis of conventional imaging offers the best approach at present for identifying and timing all abnormal tissue.

Two post-acquisition approaches to quantification of DTI data are being increasingly used to study the immature brain [32]. Tract-based spatial statistics (TBSS) is an automated, observer-independent approach for assessing FA in the major WM tracts on a voxel-wise basis across groups of subjects [33], which has been previously applied to investigate microstructure in preterm infants at term equivalent age [34]. More recently, it has been applied to assess the effect of hypothermia in a small group of neonates with HIE and demonstrated a significant improvement in FA values in multiple WM tracts in neonates treated with hypothermia [2] (Figure 14.10).

Whilst the signature lesion in HIE is the BGT, there is often additional WM involvement acutely and in all neonates with severe BGT WM abnormalities develop over the first few weeks, presumably as a result of axonal degeneration [22]. The ability of TBSS of WM tracts to assess a treatment effect is likely, therefore, to extend beyond the neonatal period. Indeed, FA values in WM, assessed by TBSS in the neonatal period, are correlated with early neurodevelopmental performance [34]. Probabilistic tractography also exploits data on FA but provides an assessment of connectivity. It has been widely used to study the preterm brain [35–37], but there are few studies in the term infant with HIE [37]. Whilst TBSS provides a sensitive tool for assessing the difference between groups of neonates, tractography increases our understanding about the individual effects of injury on brain connectivity and, therefore, provides an insight into brain repair and plasticity as well as the association of structure with later function [36,37].

## MR spectroscopy

Within the routine MR examination, it is possible to obtain MR spectroscopy. On most commercial scanners, the intrinsic coil will allow the collection of proton spectroscopy data. Phosphorus spectroscopy, originally used to establish the concept of primary and secondary energy failure in neonates with HIE, requires a specific coil [38]. A recent meta-analysis has shown that metabolite ratios obtained from proton spectroscopy provide an excellent measure of outcome [5], demonstrating a valuable role for MRS in intervention trials.

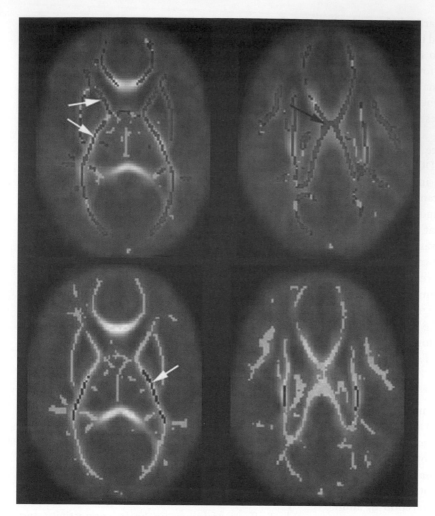

**Figure 14.10.** Tract-based spatial statistics (TBSS). Mean fractional anisotropy (FA) atlas. HIE non-cooled infants are compared with normal controls (top row). The blue regions represent areas of statistically reduced FA in the HIE group. There are multiple areas of white matter abnormality including the internal capsule (white arrows) and the corpus callosum (black arrow). HIE infants who were cooled are compared to normal controls (bottom row). There are still regions of reduced FA (blue) in the cooled HIE infants but these are less widespread and only involve the posterior limb of the internal capsule (left image) and the corona radiata (right image). Please see plate section for colour version.

## The future

Potential therapies at present concentrate on acute intervention, but there is evidence to suggest ongoing injury in the neonate with HIE that may be amenable to later treatments. In a study of infants who had sustained BGT lesions perinatally, we found that WM appearances, which were initially normal, with normal ADC, deteriorated during the second week (Figure 14.11). ADC values instead of decreasing within the WM as would normally happen with increasing postnatal age actually increased [22]. This phenomenon can be witnessed when looking at serially obtained conventional images when WM eventually atrophies (Figure 14.11). These late changes are consistent with delayed injury occurring as a consequence of an initial insult to the BGT. This suggests that there may still be scope for intervening during the first few days after a perinatal hypoxic ischaemic insult. These interventions may have to be targeted towards WM and possibly to different mechanisms of cell death, e.g. apoptosis and necrosis.

## Acknowledgements

We would like to thank all the staff of the Robert Steiner MR Unit, Hammersmith Hospital and the neonatal units of Hammersmith and Queen Charlotte's Hospital. We are also grateful to the Biomedical Research Centre, The Medical Research Council and Philips Medical Systems for their support.

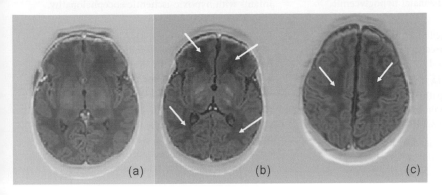

**Figure 14.11.** Delayed abnormalities in white matter following basal ganglia and thalamic injury. T1 weighted imaging in a neonate with HIE and basal ganglia and thalamic lesions (a) at 4 days. At 18 days, there has been marked decrease in signal intensity within the white matter (b, c) (arrows). (d) ADC values in the white matter of neonates with HIE and basal ganglia and thalamic lesions. ADC values in the white matter increase with time. ADC values would be expected to decrease with time in normal neonates as white matter water content decreases with maturation. Please see plate section for colour version of (d).

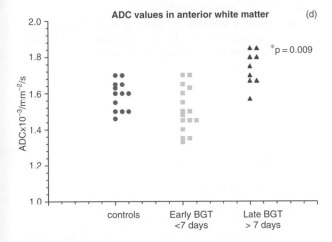

# References

1. Shankaran S, Barnes PD, Hintz SR, et al; for the Eunice Kennedy Shriver National Institute of Child Health and Human Development Neonatal Research Network. Brain injury following trial of hypothermia for neonatal hypoxic-ischaemic encephalopathy. *Arch Dis Child Fetal Neonatal Ed* 2012;**97**:F398–F404.

2. Porter EJ, Counsell SJ, Edwards AD, et al. Tract-based spatial statistics of magnetic resonance images to assess disease and treatment effects in perinatal asphyxial encephalopathy. *Pediatr Res* 2010;**68**:205–9.

3. Martinez Biarge M, Diez-Sebastian J, Rutherford M, et al. Outcomes after central grey matter injury in term perinatal hypoxic-ischaemic encephalopathy. *Neurology* 2011;**76**:2055–61.

4. Cowan FM. Sedation for magnetic resonance scanning of infants and young children. In: Whitwam JG, McCloy RF, editors. *Principles and practice of sedation.* London: Blackwell Healthcare; 1998. 15.3 p. 206–213.

5. Pennock J. Patient preparation, safety and hazards in imaging infants and children. In: Rutherford MA, editor. *MRI of the neonatal brain.* London: Saunders; 2002. www.mrineonatalbrain.com.

6. Thayyil S, Chandrasekaran M, Taylor A, et al. Cerebral magnetic resonance biomarkers in neonatal encephalopathy: a meta-analysis. *Pediatrics* 2010;**125**:e382–95.

7. Malamateniou C, Malik S, Counsell S. et al. Motion compensation techniques in MR neonatal and fetal imaging. *AJNR Am J Neuroradiol* 2012 May 10 [Epub ahead of print].

8. Mercuri E, Cowan F, Rutherford M, et al. Ischaemic and haemorrhagic brain lesions in newborns with seizures and normal Apgar scores. *Arch Dis Child Fetal Neonatal Ed* 1995;**73**:67–74.

9. Burns CM, Rutherford MA, Boardman JP, et al. Patterns of cerebral injury and neurodevelopmental

outcomes after symptomatic neonatal hypoglycemia. *Pediatrics* 2008;**122**:65–74.

10. Okereafor A, Allsop J, Counsell SJ, et al. Patterns of brain injury in neonates exposed to perinatal sentinel events. *Pediatrics* 2008;**12**:906–14.

11. Logitharajah P, Rutherford MA, Cowan FM. Hypoxic-ischemic encephalopathy in preterm infants: antecedent factors, brain imaging and outcome. *Pediatr Res* 2009;**66**:222–9.

12. Cowan F, Rutherford M, Groenendaal F, et al. Origin and timing of brain lesions in term infants with neonatal encephalopathy. *Lancet* 2003;**361**:713–4.

13. Martinez-Biarge M, Bregant T, Wusthoff C, et al. White matter and cortical injury in hypoxic-ischaemic encephalopathy: antecedent factors and two year outcome. *J Pediatr* 2012 [Epub ahead of print].

14. Rutherford MA, Counsell S, Allsop J, et al. Diffusion weighted MR imaging in term perinatal brain injury: a comparison with site of lesion and time from birth. *Pediatrics* 2004;**114**:1004–14.

15. Rutherford MA, Azzopardi D, Whitelaw A, et al. Mild hypothermia and the distribution of cerebral lesions in neonates with hypoxic-ischemic encephalopathy. *Pediatrics* 2005;**116**(4):1001–6.

16. Cheong JL, Coleman L, Hunt RW, et al; for the Infant Cooling Evaluation Collaboration. Prognostic utility of magnetic resonance imaging in neonatal hypoxic-ischemic encephalopathy: substudy of a randomized trial MRI in neonatal hypoxic-ischemic encephalopathy. *Arch Pediatr Adolesc Med* 2012;**166**:634–40.

17. Wintermark P, Hansen A, Soul J, et al. Early versus late MRI in asphyxiated newborns treated with hypothermia. *Arch Dis Child Fetal Neonatal Ed* 2011;**96**:F36–44.

18. Massaro AN, Kadom N, Chang T, et al. Quantitative analysis of magnetic resonance images and neurological outcome in encephalopathic neonates treated with whole-body hypothermia. *J Perinatol* 2010;**30**:596–603.

19. Wintermark P, Labrecque M, Warfield SK, et al. Can induced hypothermia be assured during brain MRI in neonates with hypoxic-ischemic encephalopathy? *Pediatr Radiol* 2010;**40**:1950–4.

20. Bednarek N, Mathur A, Inder T, et al. Impact of therapeutic hypothermia on MRI diffusion changes in neonatal encephalopathy. *Neurology* 2012;**78**:1420–7.

21. Rutherford MA, Pennock JM, Counsell SJ, et al. Abnormal magnetic resonance signal in the internal capsule predicts poor neurodevelopmental outcome in infants with hypoxic-ischemic encephalopathy. *Pediatrics* 1998;**102**:323–8.

22. Rutherford MA, Counsell SJ, Allsop J, et al. Delayed abnormalities in diffusion following perinatal hypoxia-ischaemia to the brain: a marker for secondary injury and a late therapeutic window? *Early Hum Dev* 2004;**77**:119–20.

23. Rutherford M, Ramenghi LA, Edwards AD, et al. Assessment of brain tissue injury after moderate hypothermia in neonates with hypoxic–ischaemic encephalopathy: a nested substudy of a randomised controlled trial. *Lancet Neurol* 2010;**9**:39–45.

24. Kuker W, Mohrle S, Mader I, et al. MRI for the management of neonatal cerebral infarctions: importance of timing. *Childs Nerv Syst* 2004;**20**:742–8.

25. Mader I, Schoning M, Klose U, et al. Neonatal cerebral infarction diagnosed by diffusion-weighted MRI: pseudonormalization occurs early. *Stroke* 2002;**33**:1142–5.

26. Barkovich AJ, Miller SP, Bartha A, et al. MR imaging, MR spectroscopy and diffusion tensor imaging of sequential studies in neonates with encephalopathy. *AJNR Am J Neuroradiol* 2006;**27**:533–47.

27. Forbes KP, Pipe JG, Bird R. Neonatal hypoxic-ischemic encephalopathy: detection with diffusion-weighted MR imaging. *AJNR Am J Neuroradiol* 2000;**21**:1490–6.

28. Wolf RL, Zimmerman RA, Clancy R, et al. Quantitative apparent diffusion coefficient measurements in term neonates for early detection of hypoxic-ischemic brain injury: initial experience. *Radiology* 2001;**218**:825–33.

29. McKinstry RC, Miller JH, Snyder AZ, et al. A prospective, longitudinal diffusion tensor imaging study of brain injury in newborns. *Neurology* 2002;**59**:824–33.

30. Ward P, Counsell S, Allsop J, et al. Reduced fractional anisotropy on diffusion tensor magnetic resonance imaging after hypoxic-ischemic encephalopathy. *Pediatrics* 2006;**117**:e619–30.

31. Vermeulen RJ, Fetter WP, Hendrikx L, et al. Diffusion-weighted MRI in severe neonatal hypoxic ischaemia: the white cerebrum. *Neuropediatrics* 2003;**34**:72–6.

32. Counsell SJ, Tranter SL, Rutherford MA. Magnetic resonance imaging of brain injury in the high-risk term infant. *Semin Perinatol* 2010;**34**:67–78.

33. Smith SM, Johansen-Berg H, Jenkinson M, et al. Acquisition and voxelwise analysis of multi-subject

diffusion data with tract-based spatial statistics. *Nat Protoc* 2007;2:499–503.

34. Tusor N, Wusthoff C, Smee N, et al. Prediction of neurodevelopmental outcome after hypoxic-ischemic encephalopathy treated with hypothermia by diffusion tensor imaging analyzed using tract-based spatial statistics. *Pediatr Res* 2012;**72**:63–9.

35. Anjari M, Srinivasan L, Allsop JM, et al. Diffusion tensor imaging with tract-based spatial statistics reveals local white matter abnormalities in preterm infants. *Neuroimage* 2007;**35**:1021–7.

36. Bassi L, Ricci D, Volzone A, et al. Probabilistic diffusion tractography of the optic radiations and visual function in preterm infants at term equivalent age. *Brain* 2008;131(Pt 2):573–82.

37. Counsell SJ, Dyet LE, Larkman DJ, et al. Thalamo-cortical connectivity in children born preterm mapped using probabilistic magnetic resonance tractography. *Neuroimage* 2007;**34**:896–904.

38. Azzopardi D, Wyatt JS, Cady EB, et al. Prognosis of newborn infants with hypoxic-ischemic brain injury assessed by phosphorus magnetic resonance spectroscopy. *Pediatr Res* 1989;**25**:445–51.

## Chapter 15

# Novel uses of hypothermia

Seetha Shankaran and Rosemary Higgins

## Introduction

This chapter will review novel uses of hypothermic neural rescue. To understand novel uses of hypothermia in neonates, it is helpful to examine novel uses of hypothermia in adult and paediatric patients as applications in one patient group often lead to use in other groups. In most applications of hypothermia neural rescue, there is evidence of benefit in preclinical models. This chapter will cover "novel uses" defined as new or promising applications of hypothermia that do not have safety and efficacy in the clinical setting established as yet.

## Novel uses of hypothermia in adults

### Hypothermia in focal cerebral ischaemia in adults

Adults who suffer acute focal ischaemia currently are managed in the Neuro Intensive Care Stroke Units with supportive management and therapy aimed at recanalization of occluded cerebral vessels with thrombolytic therapy administered within a short therapeutic window. In the preclinical model of acute transient cerebral ischaemia, hypothermia may be protective, if applied early. Reduction in infarct size is noted after middle cerebral artery occlusion with cooling to 30–33°C for 60–180 minutes [1]. In models of permanent focal ischaemia, neuroprotection with hypothermia has not been clearly demonstrated, especially if delayed in onset. The optimum depth of hypothermia in the rat model of focal cerebral ischaemia was 34°C versus 32°C or > 34°C for evaluation of infarct size and 34°C versus all other temperatures for functional outcome, thus indicating a possible U-shaped curve for effectiveness [2]. Rewarming following post-ischaemic treatment with hypothermia at 33°C has been examined in the rat model of focal ischaemia by comparing rapid (within 20 minutes) versus slow rewarming. Infarct size was smaller following slow rewarming compared to normothermia or fast rewarming [3].

There have been multiple trials with induced hypothermia in sedated (six trials) and awake patients (six trials) following stroke in adults with uncertain results. Small patient numbers (ranging from 4 to 50), differences in target temperature (32°C or 33°C), time to treatment (ranging from one to 9 hours in awake patients and < 5 to 28 hours in sedated patients) and duration of cooling (< 1 to 3 days) make comparisons difficult between studies [4]. Reductions in mortality rate or intracranial hypertension, or improvement in neurological outcome were not observed consistently across studies.

Few studies have investigated combination therapy of an agent to recanalize occluded vessels such as recombinant tissue plasminogen activator (rtPA) and hypothermia in adult stroke. Surface and endovascular cooling have been used with rtPA therapy in adults with ischaemic stroke; although the combination therapy was well tolerated, efficacy was not established due to small sample size of the studies [5]. An ongoing trial is evaluating thrombolysis in acute stroke patients treated with hypothermia using endovascular cooling and intravenous tPA along with anti-shivering protocols [7]. It should be noted, however, that the effect of thrombolytic therapy is temperature dependent [8] and the risk of haemorrhage is high. Another challenge is that adults often do not present soon after a stroke has occurred and the vast majority of stroke patients do not meet criteria for rtPA therapy or mechanical thrombectomy.

*Neonatal Neural Rescue*, ed. A. David Edwards, Denis V. Azzopardi and Alistair J. Gunn. Published by Cambridge University Press. © Cambridge University Press 2013.

# Hypothermia in severe traumatic brain injury

Hypothermia as a treatment for traumatic brain injury (TBI) has been evaluated in the preclinical arena. Cooling to 32–35°C has been found to diminish the degree of neural damage, decrease mortality and improve neurological outcome in animal models [9,10]. The large randomized controlled trial of 392 adult patients with TBI treated with hypothermia to 33.0°C or normothermia resulted in increased length of hospital stay with critical complications in the hypothermia group without any overall treatment effect measured by the Glasgow Outcome Scale. There were subgroup effects: those who were <45 years of age, hypothermic on admission to hospital and randomized to the hypothermia arm showed greater improvement at 6 months post-TBI compared with adults of same age who were hypothermic on admission and randomized to normothermia and allowed to passively re-warm [11]. Therefore, an ongoing randomized controlled trial designed to evaluate hypothermia for 48 hours initiated within 2.5 hours of injury among 240 patients with TBI age 16–45 years is ongoing with the primary outcome of Glasgow Outcome Scale at 6 months after injury. The target temperature will be 35.0°C for phase 1 patients (Glasgow Coma Scale 3–8 on initial evaluation) and 33.0°C for those patients with Glasgow Coma Scale ≤ 8 post-resuscitation (phase II). Hypothermia will be achieved by surface cooling, cooled ventilated air and instillation of ice water into the stomach. Rewarming will be slow (0.25°C per hour) and fever in the normothermia group managed per protocol with acetaminophen and surface cooling [12]. In the preclinical setting of TBI, hypothermia followed by slow rewarming appears to provide maximal protection when evaluated histologically and by imaging techniques, whereas hypothermia followed by rapid rewarming reverses any protective effects and exacerbates both pathological and functional consequences [13].

# Hypothermia after spinal cord injury

In the rat model subjected to contusion-induced spinal cord injury, hypothermia results in improved locomotor function and decreased histopathological damage [14]. Similar beneficial effects have been noted in the rabbit model of spinal cord injury [15]. In adults, a recent report of a series of 14 patients (age 16 to 62 years) with cervical spinal cord injury treated with intravascular cooling to 33°C has been published [16]. The time between injury and induction of hypothermia was 9.2 ± 2.2 hours, time to target temperature was 2.7 ± 0.42 hours and duration of cooling 47.6 ± 3.1 hours. Although feasibility of cooling following spinal cord injury has been noted in adults, no randomized controlled trial has been performed to date to evaluate safety and efficacy.

# Hypothermia in hepatic encephalopathy

Since hypothermia has been noted to decrease elevated intracranial pressure (ICP) following some TBI studies, a novel use of hypothermia to reduce/prevent elevated ICP related brain injury in patients with hepatic encephalopathy awaiting liver transplant has been reported [17]. Fourteen comatosed patients with increased ICP unresponsive to standard therapy responded with reduction of ICP by 50% following hypothermia to 32–33°C for 10–118 hours. Thirteen patients were able to undergo liver transplant and had neurological recovery. Hypothermia potentially limits the delivery of ammonia to the brain [18]. The US Acute Liver Failure Study Group observed that hypothermia appear to be promising as a "bridge" to liver transplantation in these select patients.

# Hypothermia for refractory status epilepticus

A subset of adults who have return of spontaneous circulation following cardiac arrest develop post-anoxic status epilepticus (SE) characterized by prolonged myoclonic or convulsive seizures or non-convulsive status in coma. Refractory SE has an increased risk of mortality. Hypothermia has been noted to have significant anti-seizure activity in the preclinical setting [19,20]. Two recent reports review case series (four patients in one report and six in another) of hypothermia for refractory SE. Corry *et al* report that four adults with SE refractory to anticonvulsants who were treated with endovascular cooling to 31–35°C, had seizure suppression on EEG. Adverse effects included shivering, coagulopathy without bleeding and venous thromboembolism [21]. Rossetti and colleagues attempted to evaluate predictors of awakening from post-anoxic SE after hypothermia [22]. They concluded that preservation of brain stem, somatosensory evoked potentials and EEG reactivity may be associated with favourable outcome among patients with post-anoxic SE treated with hypothermia.

# Novel uses of hypothermia in paediatrics

## Hypothermia after paediatric cardiac arrest

There are currently limited data on use of hypothermia for paediatric cardiac arrest. The American Heart Association guidelines (2005) for cardiopulmonary resuscitation and emerging cardiovascular care suggest hypothermia therapy be considered in children who remain comatose after resuscitation. A 2-year retrospective five-centre study revealed that 29 of 79 paediatric patients with cardiac arrest were treated with hypothermia ($33.7 \pm 1.3°C$ for $20.8 \pm 11.9$ hours). Mortality rate was similar between patients treated with hypothermia and those without this intervention (when adjustments were made for propensity score, duration of arrest and need for extracorporeal membrane oxygenation, ECMO). No differences in hypothermia-related adverse events were noted between groups [23]. After multi-centre cohort studies evaluating risk factors, clinical characteristics and outcomes of in-hospital paediatric cardiac arrest [24] and in-hospital versus out-of-hospital cardiac arrest [25], the Pediatric Emergency Care Applied Research Network and NICHD have initiated a multi-centre randomized controlled trial of whole body cooling to $32-34°C$ for 48 hours to evaluate improvement in neurobehavioural outcome (measured by Vineland Score) 1 year post-arrest [NCT00880087 and NCT00878644].

## Hypothermia after paediatric TBI

Based on experimental data that hypothermia improves survival and neurological outcome [9,26], an international, multicentre randomized controlled trial of hypothermia ($32.5°C$ for 24 hours) initiated within 8 hours of injury was compared to normothermia among 225 children with TBI. The primary outcome at 6 months following TBI (severe disability, persistent vegetative state or death) was noted among 31% of patients in the hypothermia group as compared to 22% of patients in the normothermia group, relative risk (RR) 1.41 (0.89–2.22). The authors concluded that research was necessary to evaluate whether earlier implementation of cooling or longer duration of cooling would improve outcome [27]. Therefore, a trial is currently ongoing (Pediatric Traumatic Brain Injury Consortium: Hypothermia) funded by National Institute of Neurological Disorders and Stroke (NINDS) and will enroll 340 subjects; the intervention is cooling to $32°-33°C$ for 48 hours followed by slow warming and the primary outcome is mortality 3 months post-injury [28].

## Hypothermia for junctional ectopic tachycardia in paediatrics

A novel use for hypothermia in paediatrics is post-cardiotomy junctional ectopic tachycardia (JET). This therapy was evaluated in a recent pilot study. Ten patients with JET were cooled using cooling blankets and 4°C normal saline infusion to a target temperature of 32–34°C. The median heart rate decreased from 187 to 158 and all patients had atrioventricular synchrony restored with conversion to normal rhythm or with successful atrial pacing [29]. Further studies with adequate sample size should evaluate this therapy.

## Hypothermia for refractory status epilepticus in children

Febrile refractory status epilepticus (RSE) in children is often caused by presumed encephalitis and is associated with a high morbidity. In addition, hyperthermia that often accompanies status may aggravate epileptic brain damage. As noted earlier, use of hypothermia in adult RSE has been explored. At the 2010 Pediatric Academic Societies meeting, a retrospective, single-centre case series of 32 children treated with hypothermia (32 to 34°C, n = 14) or normothermia (n = 18) and general anaesthesia/sedation was reported [30]. Treatment with hypothermia increased recovery (assessed by the Pediatric Cerebral Performance Category Scale) among all 14 children treated with hypothermia compared to 11 of 18 children in the normothermia group. Novel use of hypothermia in febrile RSE study needs further study.

# Novel uses of hypothermia in neonates

## Hypothermia during cardiorespiratory failure

Neonates with severe hypoxic respiratory failure who fail aggressive ventilatory support and inhaled prostaglandin therapy are placed on extracorporeal membrane oxygenation (ECMO). These infants are at risk for neurodevelopmental sequelae due to acute deterioration in clinical status before and during the ECMO.

Since hypothermia is now considered "usual care" as neuroprotection for neonatal HIE, hypothermia during ECMO has been evaluated in a pilot study of feasibility and safety [31,32]. Currently a randomized controlled trial is ongoing among neonates with severe cardio respiratory failure requiring ECMO ($\geq 35$ weeks gestation, $\leq$ three weeks of age, with $\geq 2000$ g birth weight, no evidence of bleeding disorder, no congenital or acquired central nervous system disorder, with a potentially reversible condition that did not require greater than 7 consecutive days of high pressure ventilation before ECMO). Infants with congenital diaphragmatic hernia, postoperative cardiac support and those who have received cooling before ECMO are excluded. Cooling was achieved through the water heater in the ECMO circuit maintained at $34.0°C$ for 48 hours, followed by rewarming at $0.5°C$ every hour. Primary outcome is neurodevelopmental outcome at 2 years. The sample size is 118 infants and the follow-up phase of the study is ongoing [33].

## Hypothermia as adjunct treatment in hyperammonaemia and encephalopathy

Urea cycle disorders as well as disorders of organic acid metabolism can cause severe hyperammonaemia and encephalopathy and neonates with these disorders are at risk for brain injury. Supportive therapy includes alternate pathway therapy and dialysis. Based on the reports of hypothermia use in adults with acute liver failure and hepatic encephalopathy, a multicentre randomized controlled trial of usual treatment and usual treatment with hypothermia for hyperammonaemia secondary to disorders of urea cycle or organic aciduria has been planned [34]. Hypothermia will be achieved with whole body cooling and will be maintained for 24 to 72 hours after dialysis. Outcomes include time to decrease ammonia levels < 200, time to normalization of EEG, brain injury on MRI after 7–10 days and developmental outcome at 6–9 and 18–21 months of age.

## Hypothermia for advanced necrotizing enterocolitis

Neonatal necrotizing enterocolitis (NEC) with multiorgan dysfunction is associated with a high mortality and morbidity rate. In the animal model of intestinal ischaemia and reperfusion, hypothermia to 32 to $33.0°C$ decreases intestinal injury and other organ dysfunction when applied during the period of ischaemic injury and results in improved survival when applied following reperfusion [35,36]. The feasibility and safety of hypothermia in preterm neonates with NEC and multiorgan dysfunction was evaluated in a pilot study of 15 neonates, with 5 neonates per group cooled to 35.0, 34.5 and $33.5°C$, respectively, for 48 hours before rewarming to $37.0°C$. A comparison group of 10 neonates with NEC and multiorgan dysfunction served as a comparison group. The neonates ranged in gestational age from 26 to 30 weeks, weight of 1.0 to 1.7 kg and age of 12 to 45 days at study entry. No major adverse effects were noted; there was a relationship between target temperature and low heart rate. There was also a longer time to clot formation, slower rate of clot formation and decrease in clot strength as assessed by thromboelastography in the cooled group [35]. Additional research into this novel therapy needs to be examined as intestinal ischemic injury can occur in the animal model following mild hypothermic stress and NEC is a complication of hypothermia and cardiopulmonary bypass [36,37].

## Hypothermia for premature infants with HIE

Mild hypothermia has been shown to be effective for infants $\geq 36$ weeks' gestation. The question of a lower gestational age for cooling for HIE has not yet been answered. There is one pilot study under way to test the feasibility of the Olympic Cool Cap in infants 32–35 weeks' gestation with encephalopathy in the first 6 hours of life [NCT00620711]. Participants will be followed until 24 months of age.

## References

1. Yanamoto H, Nagata I, Nakahara I, et al. Combination of intraischemic and postischemic hypothermia provides potent and persistent neuroprotection against temporary focal ischemia in rats. *Stroke* 1999;**30**:2720–6.

2. Kollmar R, Blank T, Han JL, Georgiadis D, Schwab S. Different degrees of hypothermia after experimental stroke: short- and long-term outcome. *Stroke* 2007;**38**:1585–9.

3. Berger C, Xia F, Köhrmann M, Schwab S. Hypothermia in acute stroke – slow versus fast rewarming: an experimental study in rats. *Exp Neurol* 2007;**204**:131–7.

4. Kollmar R, Schwab S. Hypothermia in focal ischemia: implications of experiments and experience. *J Neurotrauma* 2009;**26**:377–86.

5. Krieger DW, De Georgia MA, Abou-Chebl A, et al. Cooling for acute ischemic brain damage (COOL AID): an open pilot study of induced hypothermia in acute ischemic stroke. *Stroke* 2001;**32**:1847–54.

6. De Georgia MA, Krieger DW, Abou-Chebl A, et al. Cooling for Acute Ischemic Brain Damage (COOL AID): a feasibility trial of endovascular cooling. *Neurology* 2004;**63**:312–7.

7. Hemmen TM, Lyden PD. Induced hypothermia for acute stroke. *Stroke* 2007;**38**:794–9.

8. Yenari MA, Palmer JT, Bracci PM, Steinberg GK. Thrombolysis with tissue plasminogen activator (tPA) is temperature dependent. *Thromb Res* 1995;**77**:475–81.

9. Clifton GL, Jiang JY, Lyeth BG, et al. Marked protection by moderate hypothermia after experimental traumatic brain injury. *J Cereb Blood Flow Metab* 1991;**11**:114–21.

10. Dixon CE, Markgraf CG, Angileri F. Protective effects of moderate hypothermia on behavioral deficits but not necrotic cavitation following cortical impact injury in the rat. *J Neurotrauma* 1998;**15**:95–103.

11. Clifton GL, Miller ER, Choi SC, et al. Lack of effect of induction of hypothermia after acute brain injury. *N Engl J Med* 2001;**344**:556–63.

12. Clifton GL, Drever P, Valadka A, Zygun D, Okonkwo D. Multicenter trial of early hypothermia in severe brain injury. *J Neurotrauma* 2009;**26**:393–7.

13. Povlishock JT, Wei EP. Posthypothermic rewarming considerations following traumatic brain injury. *J Neurotrauma* 2009;**26**:333–40.

14. Yu CG, Jimenez O, Marcillo AE et al. Beneficial effects of modest systemic hypothermia on locomotor function and histopathological damage following contusion-induced spinal cord injury in rats. *J Neurosurg* 2000;**93**:85–93.

15. Tetik O, Islamoglu F, Cekirdekci A, Buket S. Reduction of spinal cord injury with pentobarbital and hypothermia in the rabbit model. *Eur J Vasc Endovasc Surg* 2002;**24**:540–4.

16. Levi AD, Green BA, Wang MY, et al. Clinical application of modest hypothermia after spinal cord injury. *J Neurotrauma* 2009;**26**:407–15.

17. Jalan R, Olde Damink SW, Deutz NE, Hayes PC, Lee A. Moderate hypothermia in patients with acute liver failure and uncontrolled intracranial hypertension. *Gastroenterology* 2004;**127**:1338–46.

18. Vaquero J, Rose C, Butterworth RF. Keeping cool in acute liver failure: rationale for the use of mild hypothermia. *J Hepatol* 2005;**43**:1067–77.

19. Maeda T, Hashizume K, Tanaka T. Effect of hypothermia on kainic acid-induced limbic seizures: an electroencephalographic and 14C-deoxyglucose autoradiographic study. *Brain Res* 1999;**818**:228–35.

20. Schmitt FC, Buchheim K, Meierkord H, Holtkamp M. Anticonvulsant properties of hypothermia in experimental status epilepticus. *Neurobiol Dis* 2006;**23**:689–96.

21. Corry JJ, Dhar R, Murphy T, Diringer MN. Hypothermia for refractory status epilepticus. *Neurocrit Care* 2008;**9**:189–97.

22. Rossetti AO, Oddo M, Liaudet L, Kaplan PW. Predictors of awakening from postanoxic status epilepticus after therapeutic hypothermia. *Neurology* 2009;**72**:744–9.

23. Doherty DR, Parshuram CS, Gaboury I, et al. Hypothermia therapy after pediatric cardiac arrest. *Circulation* 2009;**119**:1492–500.

24. Meert KL, Donaldson A, Nadkarni V, et al. Multicenter cohort study of in-hospital pediatric cardiac arrest. *Pediatr Crit Care Med* 2009;**10**:544–53.

25. Moler FW, Meert K, Donaldson AE, et al. In-hospital versus out-of-hospital pediatric cardiac arrest: a multicenter cohort study. *Crit Care Med* 2009;**37**:2259–67.

26. Clark RS, Kochanek PM, Marion DW, et al. Mild posttraumatic hypothermia reduces mortality after severe controlled cortical impact in rats. *J Cereb Blood Flow Metab* 1996;**16**:253–61.

27. Hutchison JS, Ward RE, Lacroix J, et al. Hypothermia therapy after traumatic brain injury in children. *N Engl J Med* 2008;**358**:2447–56.

28. Adelson PD. Hypothermia following pediatric traumatic brain injury. *J Neurotrauma* 2009;**26**:429–36.

29. Kelly BP, Gajarski RJ, Ohye RG, Charpie JR. Intravenous induction of therapeutic hypothermia in the management of junctional ectopic tachycardia: a pilot study. *Pediatr Cardiol* 2010;**31**:11–7.

30. Nakagawa T, Fujita K, Saji Y, et al. Induced hypothermia/normothermia with general anesthesia therapy prevents neurological damage of febrile refractory status epilepticus in children. E-PAS 20103741.428.

31. Ichiba S, Killer HM, Firmin RK, et al. Pilot investigation of hypothermia in neonates receiving extracorporeal membrane oxygenation. *Arch Dis Child Fetal Neonatal Ed* 2003;**88**:F128–33.

32. Horan M, Ichiba S, Firmin RK, et al. A pilot investigation of mild hypothermia in neonates receiving extracorporeal membrane oxygenation (ECMO). *J Pediatr* 2004;**144**:301–8.

33. Field DJ, Firmin R, Azzopardi DV, et al. Neonatal ECMO Study of Temperature (NEST) – a randomized controlled trial. *BMC Pediatr* 2010;**10**:24.

34. Lichter-Knocki V, Cnaan A. A multicenter clinical trial of adjunct hypothermia treatment in hyperammonemia and encephalopathy. E-PAS20103700.18.

35. Hall NJ, Eaton S, Peters MJ, et al. Mild controlled hypothermia in preterm neonates with advanced necrotizing enterocolitis. *Pediatrics* 2010;**125**:e300–8.

36. Schneider PA, Hamilton SR, Dudgeon DL. Intestinal ischemic injury following mild hypothermic stress in the neonatal piglet. *Pediatr Res* 1987;**21**:422–5.

37. Kleinman PK, Winchester P, Brill PW. Necrotizing enterocolitis after open heart surgery employing hypothermia and cardiopulmonary bypass. *AJR Am J Roentgenol* 1976;**127**:757–60.

## Chapter 16

# Neurological follow-up of infants treated with hypothermia

Charlene M. T. Robertson and Joe M. Watt

## Introduction

The theory, timelines, measures and services for the follow-up care of high-risk infants have been well described [1–3]. Amiel-Tison's overview of the trajectory of child development after birth asphyxia in the term infant continues to give guidelines for the sequential diagnosis of abnormalities [4]. Although neural protection has been shown to lessen major disabilities among survivors [5], there is no indication that the approach to long-term follow-up should be altered. This chapter focuses on the neurological examination as a tool to assist and augment the neurodevelopmental and neurocognitive follow-up of neonates after hypothermia. Examples of assessment and rating tools are given. Many other measures would also be appropriate. Measures should be standardized for the population where the test is given and be the latest edition available. Where possible a comparison population should also be tested. Within each section, there is a discussion on early referral for intervention services to reduce adverse outcomes. The organization of this chapter is patterned after the timelines approach of Amiel-Tison [4] with less emphasis on individual disabilities than in other publications on outcome of term infants with perinatal asphyxia [6,7].

## Defining the cohort

The focus of this book is on techniques to preserve neurological function in neonates compromised by perinatal asphyxia. By extension, follow-up should not only document outcomes but provide services to reduce the impact of the insult on limitations of function, activities and participation for each child [8]. Clarity of definition of diagnosis not only of the initial insult but of associated diagnoses will assist both outcomes research and service to the child and family

[6]. For more than three decades the words hypoxic–ischaemic encephalopathy (HIE) in the term newborn suggested neonatal encephalopathy beginning within hours of intrapartum asphyxia where there was evidence of fetal distress (fetal heart rate abnormalities, meconium-stained amniotic fluid and depression at birth [4,6]. This definition did not preclude an earlier antepartum acute or chronic hypoxic event. However, reports generally excluded children with known chromosomal abnormalities, syndromes or malformations of the central nervous system and those with intracranial haemorrhage. In general, there has been little mention of excluding children from outcome studies after HIE who also had antenatal infections such as cytomegalovirus, or exposure to toxins such as maternally consumed illicit drugs. Such exclusions should be considered in the future.

The current definition of HIE mandates clinical signs of neonatal encephalopathy in the absence of other aetiologies [7]. Few studies vigorously document intrapartum asphyxia according to the Guidelines of the American College of Obstetricians and Gynecologists [7,9,10]. These guidelines include evidence of metabolic acidosis in the fetal umbilical cord arterial blood obtained at delivery (pH < 7 and base deficit of $\geq 12$ mmol/L) [10]. Confirmation of asphyxia is now often obtained by amplitude-integrated EEG and magnetic resonance imaging [7,11] (see Chapter 14).

The following includes details of the sequential neurological examinations of the term infant after hypothermia for perinatal asphyxia. References are made to underlying conditions that might be uncovered by examination over time. A similar test battery as outlined in this chapter to measure motor skills, intellectual function, attention, memory and learning, language and behaviour could be used for other children after neural rescue. Examples of other groups of children where

*Neonatal Neural Rescue*, ed. A. David Edwards, Denis V. Azzopardi and Alistair J. Gunn. Published by Cambridge University Press. © Cambridge University Press 2013.

hypothermia is often considered include neonates post-complex cardiac surgery and children post-traumatic brain injury.

# The first follow-up neurological examination at age 7 days

Before the availability of hypothermic therapy, daily neurological examinations were recommended to determine the most severe abnormal within the first week of life using the Sarnat staging system [6,12]. The most severe stage is known to be predictive of outcome [6,12]. Normality at 7 days was considered to be predictive of a normal outcome [4,13]. Hypothermia does not affect the stage of encephalopathy at 4 days of age, but hypothermia has rendered the Sarnat scoring less predictive of early childhood outcomes [14]. Similarly, continued use of sedation or anticonvulsants or their delayed clearance may alter encephalopathy staging and hence prediction [14]. It is suggested that a detailed neurological examination should be completed at age 7 days or soon thereafter as sedatives are no longer required. This examination should include a head circumference measurement and a record of this measurement from birth.

The infant should be awake and at the time of the examination, within the limits of the stage of HIE. For the term infant, this is usually approximately 2 hours after an oral feeding and an hour or more before the next feeding. The room should be warm enough for most clothing/covers to be removed. Placement of the infant perpendicular to the examiner allows for a full observation of symmetry. The focus of the examination should be alertness, muscle tone, movement patterns and primitive reflexes.

## Alertness

The level of alertness is very sensitive to insult [15]. Observation of visual fixation on the examiner's face or a red object with early bilateral horizontal tracking is an expected sign for a term infant. Optokinetic nystagmus elicited by a rotating drum suggests intactness of the subcortical ocular system, including the second cranial nerve [15]. Tropism or turning of the eyes toward a soft light is a positive sign. Failure to demonstrate visual following under optimal examination conditions likely indicates persistence of reduced awareness and ongoing encephalopathy. If the appearance of visual alertness is not accompanied by visual following full recovery is not present. This finding within the first few hours after asphyxia insult in the stage 1, hyperalert period, presents as staring, decreased blinking and widened pupils at rest suggesting a sympathomimetic manifestation. If this has occurred, it is important to consider the differential diagnosis of maternal cocaine use. For all infants, a maternal history of substance abuse, especially alcohol, is important documentation for possible future diagnoses.

Decreased visual awareness accompanying persistent lethargy with diminished arousal and reduced quantity of spontaneous movement indicates persistence of stage 2 HIE. If there is ongoing improvement at this time, there may be an increasing irritability as well. Pupils may still be small yet reactive to light, reflecting ongoing parasympathetic effects. Improving visual awareness and increasing alertness herald recovery from stage 2 HIE. If the infant with stage 2 or 3 HIE is free of sedation and presents with cortical visual impairment (no or minimal visual responses with intact pupillary responses), often associated with other defects, a referral should be made to a visual therapist in addition to a consultation with a paediatric ophthalmologist. Specially trained (often occupational or educational) therapists with government or private agencies will make home visits and counsel parents and other therapy disciplines working with the child on visual, auditory and kinaesthetic techniques to enhance development and reduce self-stimulatory activity, which often develops in visually impaired children.

Persistence of stage 3 HIE may show dilated fixed pupils associated with other evidence of brainstem failure with oculomotor disturbances and sucking and swallowing impairment.

It is suggested that a retinal examination be done by a paediatric ophthalmologist for all survivors to rule out optic nerve hypoplasia, optic atrophy and choreoretinitis. The small discs of optic nerve hypoplasia can lead to endocrinological investigation for complications of septo-optic dysplasia, although unlikely with a normal pituitary on MRI. The pale, poorly vascularized discs of optic atrophy may follow a hypoxic insult associated with oedema or raised intracranial pressure or reflect other unexpected anomalies. Choreoretinitis may occur with antenatal infections of toxoplasmosis, cytomegalovirus, rubella or herpes simplex that may coincide with a hypoxic insult and, as each requires their own diagnosis, treatment and follow-up, should not be missed.

While not specifically related to alertness, unilateral decrease in the size of a pupil that remains reactive to light may be seen with Horner's syndrome. After HIE at term, this is likely associated with a brachial plexus injury including damage to the eighth cervical root and first thoracic root, hence the cervical sympathetic ganglia. These findings necessitate referral to a paediatric physiatrist or neurologist for electrophysiological studies. If recovery is considered unlikely, an early referral to a surgeon experienced in brachial plexus surgery is needed.

An alert vigilant infant will startle to sound and be attentive to voice. However, the neurological examination cannot uncover hearing loss. The recommendation for hearing testing includes examination of the external auditory canal for debris and the tympanic membrane for evidence of middle ear fluid, as well as audiological evaluation using otoacoustic emissions to determine cochlear integrity and brainstem audiological evoked response testing to identify auditory neuropathy/dyssynchrony [16].

A return to normal sleep–wake cycle is a positive sign [15]. The presence of neonatal seizures accompanying reduced alertness increases the likelihood of neurological sequelae [6,7,13].

## Muscle tone and movement

Flexion posturing is part of a normal neurological examination of the term infant. Normal spontaneous movements show movement against gravity, good amplitude and quantity and good quality with a rhythmic movement pattern accompanying the examiner's voice modulations. Examination of passive tone should be done with the infant's head in midline to avoid any superimposed effect from an asymmetrical tonic neck reflex response.

Observed facial movement at rest or as movement begins may show low tone secondary to HIE [15]. In facial weakness of cerebral origin, the upper face is spared [15]. Low facial tone interferes with good lip closure on the nipple during bottle feeding and can be compensated for by lip/cheek closure during feeding until spontaneous improvement occurs. Severe bilateral upper and lower facial weakness with impairment of eye closure and sucking accompanying brainstem involvement of stage 3 HIE requires differentiation from Moebius syndrome.

Observation of full spontaneous movement during crying or grimacing may show pulling of the lower face toward the normal side revealing a facial palsy.

Bilateral facial weakness with ptosis and generalized hypotonia requires consideration of myasthenia gravis. Myopathies preceding asphyxia can give rise to generalized muscle weakness requiring investigation.

There is an improvement of low muscle tone during recovery after stage 2 HIE. Following prolonged, partial asphyxia and the usually associated watershed abnormality between the anterior and middle cerebral arteries, the infant demonstrates hypotonia of the trunk, shoulder girdle and upper extremities. For children without subsequent cerebral palsy, shoulder girdle tone recovery may take months. Cognitive delay with and without spastic cerebral palsy may follow this injury.

Hypotonia may be due to cerebral cortical, cerebellar cortical and/or anterior horn cell insult. Deep tendon reflexes are usually present and not increased at 7 days post-insult; however, they may be absent with spinal asphyxia and show delayed recovery. Characteristic of stage 3 HIE, general flaccidity may still persist at 7 days. Intermittent decerebrate posturing may occur in response to stimuli. At this early stage, a physical therapist may assist parents with holding the child and monitoring tone changes.

## Primitive reflexes

While many primitive reflexes have been described, it is best to become familiar with a few and apply them regularly to understand their interpretation.

### Sucking and swallowing

The most important reflex to evaluate is sucking and swallowing. Poor sucking with normal swallow is unlikely to be accompanied by an abnormal gag reflex; abnormal swallowing is often associated with reduced or absent gag reflex. At day 7, feeding of the infant that appears to have fully recovered should be observed by the examiner or by an experienced nurse or therapist. The infant should demonstrate vigorous latching, good lower face and mouth tone, effective stripping action (if bottle fed), coordinated swallow with no choking or coughing and sustained feeding that is sufficient to supply adequate nutrition. If these criteria are not present, an analysis of the sucking ability and alternatives in position or facial tone support should be made before discharge. If difficulties are due to bulbar palsy or incoordination or absent swallowing, then alternate feeding methods should be used with sensory lip and mouth stimuli therapy directed by a feeding specialist. Therapists may find an algorithm for the diagnosis and treatment of feeding or nutritional difficulties useful at this stage as well as later [17].

## Moro

The Moro reflex requires normal brainstem and reticular function with limited higher centre inhibitory control. The greatest information from the infant's Moro reflex can be obtained by eliciting the reflex in the safest and most reliable way and comparing the response to normal infants of the same age. In the wakeful, alert state, the infant is held in supine with one of the examiner's hands and forearm beneath the infant's head and shoulders and the other hand and forearm supporting the trunk and legs. The examiner's hand is straightened and the infant's head is abruptly but gently allowed to drop in extension a distance of approximately 3 cm at the crown. The full term infant's arms briskly abduct and extend. The hands open. The legs flex and hips abduct. The arms then clasp over the body. Some tremor may be present. The Moro reflex is sensitive to the alertness of the infant. A suppressed (incomplete) response is usually associated with persistent hypotonia and lethargy indicating a prolonged stage 2 HIE. An absent Moro after 1 week in the absence of heavy sedation, upper spinal cord injury, advanced anterior horn cell disease or severe myopathy, in a flaccid, stuperous infant indicates persistence of stage 3 HIE.

An asymmetrical Moro response suggests a fractured clavicle or brachial plexus injury and is unlikely to be a sign of subsequent hemiparetic cerebral palsy.

## Palmer grasp

In the normal infant, the grasp reflex is strong but releases with stroking of the dorsal surface of the hand. A grasp position is not present at all times in a normal infant whose hands open periodically. With persistent stage 2 HIE distal flexion of the fingers may continue after one week with incomplete extension of the fingers with stroking. Cortical thumbs may persist. Infants with persistent stage 3 HIE may have flaccid hands, although extension at the elbows with pronated wrists may be present. The grasp reflex is absent.

As hypothermia is used more frequently, detailed post-treatment neurological examinations over time will assist in determining which of the HIE changes in alertness, muscle tone, movement patterns, primitive reflexes and/or brainstem signs will be the best predictors of outcome.

# Follow-up planning and parental counselling

If the 7-day neurological examination, brain imaging and hearing screening are within the normal limits and assuming regular paediatric care, the next follow-up visit can be planned at 6 months of age. Parents may be reassured that major disability is unlikely. If the 7-day examination is abnormal, selective follow-up and/or treatment with specific disciplines for feeding, motor development, vision or hearing should be initiated. The pattern of brain injury on imaging will assist in focusing the interval neurological examinations [18] (see Chapter 14). In the early months, the treating physical therapist should have knowledge of the Hammersmith infant neurological examination (optimality score) [1] and the general movement assessment [1,19].

Serial head circumference measurements assist prediction of microcephaly and associated cognitive impairment. A decrease in head circumference ratio of greater than 3.1% between birth and 4 months of age has been shown to be predictive of future microcephaly [20].

Not only do we need to be aware of selective vulnerability of the neonatal brain to hypoxic–ischaemic insult, we must be aware of variations in parental vulnerability to the lack of the healthy infant they expected and the emotional trauma of their baby's illness and potential death or disability. Parent vulnerability does not always parallel the degree of illness of their child and depends on their resilience and resources. The addition of a new life-saving treatment such as hypothermia to their child's care may alter parents' responses, possibly to make their child more "special" or to make adverse outcome more difficult to accept. In all cases, the normal parent–infant bonding that relies on infant cues to the parent is altered by the illness and treatment; thus, caretakers must understand and support parents. Full disclosure of the infant's illness must be given in a way that builds upon the parent–child relationship and does not encourage parents to overprotect their child in the future. An important, often unexpected outcome of newborn illness is the change in parenting styles leading to the well-known vulnerability syndrome and its consequences on the child's social, emotional and behavioural growth [21].

Specialized multidisciplinary follow-up of infants is not innocuous and it suggests to the parents that there will likely be ongoing neurodevelopmental concerns.

However, follow-up of ill neonates is generally accepted by parents who come to understand the dual purpose of follow-up to be service for developmental concerns of their child and an audit of outcomes following new complex therapies. Most parents appreciate being part of a follow-up programme that voices the mandate of helping to improve care for future children.

It is strongly recommended that all parents of children discharged following neural rescue be referred to an early intervention programme. This community resource is often forgotten at discharge. Early intervention workers promote child development, positive parenting and family resilience. They teach parents child advocacy and build developmentally age-appropriate expectations of independence for their child.

## Follow-up at 6 months of age

Six months of age is chosen for the first multidisciplinary assessment to ensure that intervention is in place for children with developmental delays/impairment, particularly hearing or vision loss, feeding difficulties and motor delay. For other children, this visit provides parent contact with the follow-up team and assurance to the parents of normalcy of the child at this time. It is a source of support for parents should questions or concerns arise. Ideally, the follow-up team at the 6-month assessment includes an audiologist and physical therapist allowing continuity with therapy programmes as needed. Consultation with a dietician is suggested.

The neurological examination looks for visual alertness with full horizontal and vertical tracking with no strabismus, adequate head growth without premature closure of the anterior fontanelle, appropriate feeding abilities, symmetry of motor development, normal muscle tone, protective and equilibrium reactions for age and normal voice, vocalizations and social interactive abilities. For children later diagnosed with cerebral palsy, the Hammersmith Infant Neurological Examination shows good negative correlation with neurological examination and gross motor function ability at 2 years of age [22].

Delayed-onset hearing loss may occur. Sound-field testing in a soundproof room by an audiologist is recommended. Should sensorineural hearing loss or auditory neuropathy be diagnosed, a referral to an otolaryngologist for investigation of aetiology and approval for hearing amplification is the usual practice. Should profound loss be confirmed referral to a cochlear implant team for assessment is recommended. Persistent conductive hearing loss also requires referral to an otolaryngologist.

An experienced paediatric physical therapist evaluates movement patterns, muscle tone, posture, motor developmental level, primitive reflexes, protective and equilibrium reactions. The goal of this assessment should be to evaluate quality of movement, not only developmental level and provide a therapy programme to optimize motor function should that be required. Standardized evaluation is recommended. The advantage of the Alberta Infant Motor Scale (AIMS) is its ability to evaluate qualitative and quantitative abilities and its suitability to longitudinal testing and re-evaluation [23]. Widely used scales, such as the Bayley Scales of Infant and Toddler Development, Third Edition (Bayley-III), provide quantitative gross and fine motor scores [24]. While these scales are useful for outcome studies, they do not provide sufficient observational detail to be used in establishing a neuromotor therapy programme.

There should be a high suspicion for cerebral palsy and an ongoing willingness to begin occupational and physical therapy based on neuromotor/neurosensory findings, even if a diagnosis of cerebral palsy cannot yet be given with certainty. Cerebral palsy is a clinical diagnosis based on a constellation of findings and requires clinical experience. At present the term cerebral palsy describes a group of permanent disorders of the development of movement and posture, causing activity limitation, that are attributed to non-progressive disturbances that occurred in the developing fetal or infant brain [25]. The motor disorders of cerebral palsy are often accompanied by disturbances of sensation, perception, cognition, communication and behaviour, by epilepsy and by secondary musculoskeletal problems [25]. Treating therapists should have a thorough knowledge of the international classification of function [8]. They should be familiar with motor scales used to classify severity and indicate prognosis [26,27], the emerging treatments for hemiparetic cerebral palsy including constraint-induced movement therapy and hand–arm bimanual intensive therapy [28], and knowledge of the early positive results of constraint-induced therapy under one year of age [29].

At the time of diagnosis of cerebral palsy, a physician from a cerebral palsy treating team should be consulted to determine the best early therapy. The transfer of the child to that team may be delayed until the child is older when a more complete picture of developmental strengths and deficits can be established. Such a consultant will bring knowledge of expected patterns of injury [18] and understanding of the dependence of spinal cord development on cortical spinal input [30], and will focus on the spectrum of treatments available to enhance an individual child's developmental trajectory. Therapies include feeding, movement and integration of primitive reflexes, seating, standing and orthotics as well as spasticity therapy including pharmacological and surgical management [31–34]. It is recommended that a baseline hip x-ray be done at the time of diagnosis in view of possible future subluxation [35]. Children with multiple impairments require input from disciplines concerning feeding, movement, communication, sensory enhancement and early cognitive functioning. A case manager is critical for coordination of these therapies and parent support. For children with developmental concerns at 6 months, reviews with specific disciplines should recur as needed.

## Follow-up at 18 to 24 months of age

This follow-up visit is best completed as a multidisciplinary assessment and if possible should include a minimum of follow-up physician, nurse (to monitor diet, feeding, sleeping, immunization, illnesses, parental support) and a therapist trained in assessment of toddlers. A physical and occupational therapist may see the children with motor or visual concerns. Should the child's communication be inadequate, audiological assessment to rule out delayed-onset hearing loss is also indicated.

The focus of the neurological examination for children should be adequate head growth, ocular alignment, muscle tone, balance, communication and social interaction. Low tone and reduced balance for age with normal deep tendon reflexes and absent primitive reflexes usually accompany gross motor delay. Suggestions for motor activities and balance enhancement to assist children of this age are usually welcomed by the family.

With the understanding that mental ability measurements used at this age are not intelligence tests, a standardized measure of development is recommended for those free of major impairment. Results may assist in targeting early developmental intervention. Commonly used individually administered assessment measures are the Bayley Scales of Infant and Toddler Development,

Third Edition [24], giving separate cognitive, language and motor scores based on a population mean of 100 and a standard deviation of 15. The accompanying parent-completed Social-Emotional and Adaptive-Behavior Questionnaires are helpful in attaining a larger picture of the child. The latter is similar to the Adaptive Behavior Assessment System, Second Edition, (ABAS-II) [36]. This is a measure of adaptive function, that is, personal and social skills needed to live independently. It gives an overall general adaptive composite score as well as conceptual, social and practical composite scores. These scores supplement the assessed scores and if assessment is not possible due to distance, correlate well with assessed scores. The scaled scores for the 10 skill areas are very useful to review the child's profile. Of particular value is a method of determining the strengths and weaknesses for an individual child. Knowledge of this can be used in intervention programmes or for referral to specialized areas such as communication disorder therapists. Children needing intensive care, particularly those needing new technological treatments, may not be given parental expectations adequate for their developmental level and often show weaknesses on self-care. Self-care skills are necessary for independence and confidence as young children reach preschool. Poor adaptive functioning may contribute to secondary disabilities. This Adaptive-Behaviour Questionnaire can be used for monitoring throughout childhood [36] and requires fewer resources than an interview.

Delayed communication skills, particularly expressive language, have long been reported following HIE [6,7]. Referral to a speech–language pathologist is recommended if that discipline is not part of the assessment team.

For children with developmental–behaviour concerns, referral to a child psychiatrist may be indicated. Reassessment at approximately 3 years of age will assist in appropriate early education or specialized preschool placement. As for any group of at-risk children, there should be surveillance for possible Autism Spectrum Disorder followed by referral for appropriate diagnostic tests and educational programmes.

## Follow-up at 4 to 5 years of age

For all survivors, a complete multidisciplinary assessment at four to five years of age provides the basis for ongoing educational placement and specialized medical care and therapy. A classical neurological examination should be completed. For otherwise normal children, reduced hand and trunk tone along with decreased balance skills may persist. For such children fine motor/pencil skills may be difficult and coordination insufficient for adequate functioning in the playground may reduce self-confidence. The Movement Assessment Battery for Children, Second Edition, (M-ABC-2) provides items to test manual dexterity, ball skills and balance [37]. A detailed examination for athetosis/dystonia should be done as these may be of delayed onset. Behaviour should be observed.

At this age, intelligence ability can be reliably measured. A chartered psychologist with paediatric experience can administer a standardized test such as the Wechsler Preschool and Primary Scale of Intelligence, Third Edition (WPPSI-III) [38]. From 10 subtest scaled scores, composite scores are calculated for verbal performance, full-scale intelligence and processing speed quotients and a general language composite. An intelligence test should be supplemented with the results of a parent-completed questionnaire such as the ABAS-II [36] before a diagnosis of cognitive impairment is given. Cognitive scores of less than 70 define cognitive impairment as determined by the American Association for Intellectual and Developmental Disabilities [39]. In some countries, performance of less than 70 is classified as a severe learning disability. Scores of ≥ 70 through 84 define a child likely to have school learning difficulties. Observations by a psychologist should support the parent-completed behaviour questionnaire such as the Behaviour Assessment System for Children, Second Edition (BASC-2) yielding scores for externalizing, internalizing problems, adaptive skills and behavioural symptoms index [40].

Assessment by a speech–language pathologist using a measure such as the Clinical Evaluation of Language Fundamentals, Preschool, Second Edition (CELF-2) allows for detailed breakdown of comprehension and expressive language [41].

A quality of life parent completed measure such as the PEDS QL™ [42] together with an adaptive behaviour measure [36] and questions on health and growth supplement the assessment and can give a quite complete review of a child if a full assessment is not possible.

## Follow-up at school age

To assist the child and optimize school learning through psychoeducational testing, ages to 6 to 7 years may be a preferred age for this assessment. However, variance in school curricula, hence differences in teaching, and different maturational rates suggest that a better overall picture of school-related functioning post-neonatal insult can be obtained at 8 to 10 years of age. Such long-term follow-up is needed to determine the proportion of children free from adverse outcome in the post-neural rescue era. The focus of this assessment is intellectual ability, academic achievement, executive functioning (attention, inhibition, concept formation, sorting and set shifting), memory and learning, behaviour and adaptive functioning. Readers are referred to publications on outcome after HIE for more detailed information on measures [6,7,43]. Only a few examples of measures are given in this brief overview.

A neurological examination should include a test of visual depth perception and "soft" neurological signs. Motor function should be assessed [37]. A diagnosis of Developmental Coordination Disorder may need to be considered.

A full intelligence test has been recommended at 4 to 5 years to obtain as much supportive education as possible. At school age, a short form of a standardized test, such as the Wechsler Intelligence Scale for Children, Fourth Edition (WISC-IV) [44], can be used. For children with severe to profound hearing loss or poor language proficiency, a non-verbal test is suggested. As at 4 years, an adaptive-behaviour measure [36] should accompany intelligence test administration to have a parallel parental view of functioning. Having results from this measure [36] as a toddler, at preschool and during the school years allows tracking of the trajectory of adaptive function in relation to peers over time.

An achievement test, such as the Wechsler Individual Achievement Test, Second Edition (WIAT-II) gives results for reading, spelling, mathematics and total achievement and can be related to general intelligence [45]. Achievement results from the school may supplement or replace this measure.

The NEPSY II (NEuroPSYchology) is a standardized neuropsychological battery for children of ages 3 to 17 years from which subtests can be chosen to assess functioning across six domains: executive functioning and attention, memory and learning, sensorimotor functioning, social perception, language and visuospatial processing [46].

As for the preschool child, behaviour may be rated using the BASC-2 [40]. Specific school-related behaviour such as working memory, organizational and monitoring skills may be determined using the questionnaire, the Behavioural Rating Inventory of Executive Function (BRIEF-II) [47] as completed by parents or teachers. The BRIEF is also available as the BRIEF-P for the preschool child. The BRIEF is an excellent tool to assess executive functioning and complements the NEPSY-II. The Strengths and Difficulties Questionnaire (SDQ) provides a screen for mental health completed by parents or teachers and is available in many languages [48].

For children unable to attend a full assessment, the questionnaires mentioned above supplement the neurological examination and give an overview of abilities or concerns [36,40,42,47,48]. A child health questionnaire and/or quality of life measure can also be completed by the child.

## Conclusions

As with the practice of medicine, the longitudinal follow-up of children at-risk for adverse neurodevelopmental/neurocognitive outcome is a privilege. Follow-up accepts the responsibility of surveillance for adverse outcome, supplies or refers children to appropriate services as needed and informs future practice. While this approach is based upon a deficit model of care, follow-up practitioners are well aware of the importance of reporting and building on the strengths of each child.

We expect post-asphyxial neural rescue to reduce adverse outcomes. However, it will only be with extended and universal longitudinal follow-up that the full effect of this new mode of therapy will be known.

## References

1. Cioni G, Mercuri E, editors. Neurological assessment in the first two years of life: instruments for the follow-up of high-risk newborns. *Clinics in developmental medicine No. 176*. London: MacKeith Press; 2007.

2. The American Academy of Pediatrics. Follow-up care of high-risk infants. *Pediatrics* 2004;**114**:1377–97.

3. Taeusch HW, Vogman MW, editors. *Follow-up management of the high-risk infant*. Boston: Little, Brown and Company; 1987.

4. Amiel-Tison C, Ellison P. Birth asphyxia in the fullterm newborn: early assessment and outcome. *Dev Med Child Neurol* 1986;**28**:671–82.

5. Edwards AD, Brocklehurst P, Gunn AJ, et al. Neurological outcomes at 18 months of age after moderate hypothermia for perinatal hypoxic ischemic encephalopathy: Synthesis and met-analysis of trial data. *BMJ* 2010;**340**:c363.

6. Robertson CMT. Long-term follow-up of term infants with perinatal asphyxia. In: Stevenson BK, Benitz WE, Sunshine P, editors. *Fetal and neonatal brain injury: mechanisms, management and the risk of practice*. 3rd edition. Cambridge: Cambridge University Press; 2003. p. 829–58.

7. Miller SP, Latal B. Neurocognitive outcomes of term infants with perinatal asphyxia. In: Stevenson BK, Benitz WE, Sunshine P, Heintz SR, Druzin ML, editors. *Fetal and neonatal brain injury, 4th edition*. Cambridge: Cambridge University Press; 2009. p. 574–83.

8. Simeonsson RJ, Leonardi M, Lollar D, et al. Applying the International Classification of Functioning, Disability and Health (ICF) to measure childhood disability. *Disabil Rehabil* 2003;**25**:602–10.

9. Pin TW, Eldridge B, Galea MP. A review of developmental outcomes of term infants with post-asphyxia neonatal encephalopathy. *Eur J Paed Neurol* 2009;**13**:224–34.

10. American College of Obstetricians and Gynecologists. Neonatal encephalopathy and cerebral palsy: Executive Summary. *Obstet Gynecol* 2004;**103**:780–81.

11. Hallberg B, Grossman NK, Bartocci M, Blennow M. The prognostic value of early aEEG in asphyxiated infants undergoing systemic hypothermia treatment. *Acta Paediatr* 2010;**99**:531–36.

12. Sarnat HB, Sarnat MS. Neonatal encephalopathy following fetal distress: A clinical and electrocephalographic study. *Arch Neurol* 1976;**33**:696–705.

13. Volpe JJ. Hypoxic-ischemic encephalopathy: clinical aspects. In: *Neurology of the newborn*. 5th edition. Philadelphia: Sanders Elsevier; 2008. p. 400–80.

14. Gunn AJ, Wyatt JS, Whitelaw A, et al. Therapeutic hypothermia changes the prognostic value of clinical evaluation of neonatal encephalopathy. *J Pediatr* 2008;**152**:55–8.

15. Volpe JJ. Neurological examination: normal and abnormal features. In: *Neurology of the newborn*. 5th edition. Philadelphia: Sanders Elsevier; 2008. p. 121–53.

16. American Academy of Pediatrics Joint Committee on Infant Hearing. 2007 Position statement: principles and guidelines for early hearing protection and intervention programs. *Pediatrics* 2007;**120**:898–921.

17. Schwarz SM, Corredor J, Fisher-Medina J, Cohen J, Rabinowitz S. Diagnosis and treatment of feeding disorders in children with developmental disabilities. *Pediatrics* 2001;**108**:671–6.

18. Miller SP, Ramaswamy V, Michelson D, et al. Patterns of brain injury in term neonatal encephalopathy. *J Pediatr* 2005;**146**:453–60.

19. Prechlt HFR, Ferrari F, Cioni G. Predictive value of general movement in asphyxiated full term infants. *Early Hum Dev* 1993;**35**:91–120.

20. Cordes I, Roland EH, Lupton BA, Hill A. Early prediction of the development of microcephaly after hypoxic-ischemic encephalopathy in the full term newborn. *Pediatrics* 1994;**93**:703–7.

21. Thomasgard M, Metz WP. Parent-child relationship disorders: what do the Child Vulnerability Scale and the Parent Protection Scale measure? *Clin Pediatr* 1999;**38**:347–56.

22. Romeo DMM, Cioni M, Scoto M, et al. Neuromotor development of infants with cerebral palsy investigated by Hammersmith Infant Neurological Examination during the first year of age. *Eur J Pediatr Neurol* 2008;**12**:24–31.

23. Piper MC, Darrah J. *Motor assessment of the developing infant*. Philadelphia: WB Saunders Co; 1994.

24. Bayley N. *Manual for the Bayley Scales of Infant and Toddler Development*. 3rd edition. San Antonio, TX: The Psychological Corporation; 2006.

25. Rosenbaum P, Panif N, Leviton A, Rosenstein M, Max M. A report: the definition and classification of cerebral palsy, April 2006. In: *The definition and classification of cerebral palsy. Dev Med Child Neurol* 2007;**49**(Suppl 109):1–43.

26. Rosenbaum P, Walter S, Hanna S, et al. Prognosis for gross motor function in cerebral palsy: creation of motor developmental curves. *JAMA* 2002;**288**:1357–63.

27. Eliasson A-C, Krumlinde-Sundholm L, Rösbald B, et al. The Manual Ability Classification System (MACS) for children with cerebral palsy: scale development and evidence of validity and reliability. *Dev Med Child Neurol* 2006;**48**:549–54.

28. Sakzewski L, Ziviani J, Boyd R. Systematic review and meta-analyses of therapeutic management of upper-limb dysfunction in children with congenital hemiplegia. *Pediatrics* 2009;**123**:e1111–22.

29 Coker P, Labkicher C, Harris L, Snape J. The effects of constraint-induced movement therapy for a child of less than a year of age. *Neurorehabilitation* 2009;**24**:199–208.

30. Clowry GJ. The dependence of spinal cord development on cortical spinal input and its significance in understanding and treating spastic cerebral palsy. *Neural Sci Behav Rev* 2007;**31**:1114–24.

31. Rona S, Gold JT. Nonoperative management of spasticity in children. *Childs Nerv Syst* 2007;**23**:943–56.

32. Delgado MR, Hirtz D, Aisen M, et al. Practice parameter: pharmacological treatment of spasticity in children and adolescence with cerebral palsy (an evidenced based review): Report on the quality standard subcommittee of the American Academy of Neurology and the Practice Subcommittee of the Child Neurology Society. *Neurology* 2010;**74**:336–43.

33. Heinen F, Desloovere K, Schroeder AS, et al. The updated European consensus 2009 on the use of botulism toxin for children with cerebral palsy. *Eur J Pediatr Neurol* 2010;**14**:45–66.

34. Novacheck TF, Gage JR. Orthopedic management of spasticity in cerebral palsy. *Childs Nerv Syst* 2007;**23**:1015–31.

35. Australasian Academy of Cerebral Palsy and Developmental Medicine. *Consensus Statement on Hip Surveillance for Children with Cerebral Palsy*. Australian Standard of Care. 2008. www.cpaustralia. com.au/ausacpdm (Accessed, July 7, 2010.)

36. Harrison PL, Oakland T. *Manual for the adaptive behavior assessment system*. 2nd edition. San Antonio, TX: The Psychological Corporation; 2003.

37. Henderson SE, Sugden DA, Barnett AL. *Movement assessment battery for children, 2nd edition*. London: Harcourt Assessment; 2007.

38. Wechsler D. *Manual for the preschool and primary scale of intelligence*. 3rd edition. San Antonio, TX: The Psychological Corporation; 2002.

39. American Association for Intellectual and Developmental Disabilities. *Definition, classification and systems of support*. 11th edition. Washington, DC: American Association for Intellectual and Developmental Disabilities; 2010.

40. Reynolds CR, Kamphaus RW. *Manual for the behaviour assessment system for children*. 2nd edition. Circle Pines, MN: American Guidance Services, Inc; 2004.

41. The Psychological Corporation. *Clinical evaluation of language fundamentals, preschool*. 2nd edition. San Antonio, TX: The Psychological Corporation; 2004.

42. Varni JW, Seid M, Kurtin PS. The Peds QL 4.0: reliability and validity of pediatric quality of life inventory version 4.0 generic core scales in healthy and patient populations. *Med Care* 2001;**30**:800–12.

43. Marlow N, Rose AS, Rans CE, Diaper ES. Neuropsychological and educational problems at

school age associated with neonatal encephalopathy. *Arch Dis Child Fetal Neonatal Ed* 2005;**90**:F380–7.

44. Wechsler D. *Manual of the intelligence scale for children*. 4th edition. San Antonio, TX: The Psychological Corporation; 2004.

45. Wechsler D. *Manual for the Wechsler individual achievement test*. 2nd edition. San Antonio, TX: The Psychological Corporation; 2001.

46. Korkman M, Kirk U, Kemp S. *Clinical and interpretative manual for the NEPSY-II*. 2nd edition.

San Antonio, TX: The Psychological Corporation; 2007.

47. Gioia GA, Isquith PK, Guy SC, Kentworthy L. *Behaviour rating inventory of executive function*. Lutz, FL: Psychological Assessment Resources, Inc; 2001.

48. Goodman R, Ford T, Simmonds H, Gratward R, Meltzer H. Using Strengths and Difficulties Questionnaire (SDQ): to screen for child psychiatric disorders in a community sample. *Br J Psychiatry* 2000;**177**:534–9.

# Registry surveillance after neuroprotective treatment

Robert H. Pfister, Jeffrey D. Horbar and Denis V. Azzopardi

## Introduction

Clinicians worldwide are encouraged by the results of the large randomized controlled trials (RCTs) and systematic reviews that demonstrated the efficacy of hypothermia in improving neurologic and developmental outcomes in term and late preterm infants with hypoxic–ischaemic encephalopathy (HIE) [1–5]. These studies have brought an increased interest in the aetiology, recognition, management and outcome of encephalopathic infants. Based on these studies, many clinicians have started or are considering offering therapeutic hypothermia for the treatment of HIE. As more infants are receiving treatment, registries have been and are being developed that use observational study methods to gain insight and information regarding neonatal encephalopathy (NE) and therapeutic hypothermia outside of RCTs. This chapter will focus on how these registries shed light on how effective this emerging therapy will be in the real world setting and how the registry method may track adverse events that occur in frequencies too rare to be discovered in the trials that proved efficacy. One can anticipate that centres will be using this therapy for infants outside of the inclusion parameters and methods designated by the initial trials; registries will track this "therapeutic drift". The registries also document the evaluations and treatments that a typical infant receives and are ideally suited to track the dissemination of adjunctive therapies as they arise. Registries are able to obtain information on the larger cohort of infants with neonatal encephalopathy in addition to smaller subsets of those cooled. Last, this chapter will focus solely on infants receiving therapy and report on the characteristics and initial results of the two registries currently in use: the United Kingdom TOBY Cooling Register (TOBY Register) and the Vermont Oxford Network Neonatal Encephalopathy Registry (VON NER).

## Efficacy versus effectiveness

Despite the efficacy and relative safety demonstrated by the recent trials, many questions exist with regards to the safety, refinement and optimization of the procedure. Future randomized controlled trials of hypothermia versus normothermia will be difficult to perform as randomization to a normothermic control group could be construed as unethical [6]. To further study encephalopathic infants and monitor the practice of therapeutic hypothermia, research methods beyond RCTs are indicated. Although RCTs are considered the foundation by which we determine whether a given intervention is efficacious, they are ill suited to address issues such as safety monitoring and establishing effectiveness in a real world setting.

Randomized trials and systematic reviews of such trials provide the best estimate of the effects of an intervention or its efficacy. *Efficacy* describes the effects of an intervention under ideal conditions, for example in a laboratory setting or within the protocol of a randomized, controlled trial. However, when an intervention whose efficacy is proven in research studies is used in clinical practice, its actual effects may differ from those seen in the original research. *Effectiveness* is the extent to which a specific intervention does what it is intended to do for a defined population in actual practice. Efficacy is high on internal validity but at the expense of generalizability; effectiveness is high on external validity but at the expense of careful controls.

In this case, therapeutic hypothermia is proven efficacious in improving survival without adverse neurodevelopmental outcome. However, to prove that

*Neonatal Neural Rescue*, ed. A. David Edwards, Denis V. Azzopardi and Alistair J. Gunn. Published by Cambridge University Press. © Cambridge University Press 2013.

cooling is also effective in a real world setting other than those in which it was initially tested, one must answer the following questions (among others):

- Which are the patients who might benefit from cooling?
- What is the optimal temperature for cooling?
- Which cooling method should be used?
- Which centres should administer the treatment?
- What is the optimal timing of treatment?
- What adjuvant treatments are beneficial?
- Were rare adverse events unrecognized in the RCTs?

Observational studies like registries are increasingly being used to begin to address these issues. Registries are organized systems that use observational study methods to collect uniform data to evaluate specified outcomes for a population defined by a particular disease, condition, or exposure and that serves a predetermined scientific, clinical or policy purpose. The registry approach is ideal for monitoring practices, clinical patterns and patient outcomes of a heterogeneous group of individually rare disorders such as those that underlie the syndrome of NE. In particular, registries are ideal for the study of actual standard medical practice and "real world" dissemination of a novel therapy, such as therapeutic hypothermia, outside the narrow confines of a clinical trial.

## Therapeutic drift

The initial studies that demonstrated efficacy detailed strict exclusion criteria: preterm infants, growth restricted infants and infants unable to receive cooling therapy by 6 hours of age. As this novel therapy disseminates into the real world setting outside the confines of trials, centres are cooling infants that would have been unable to receive cooling through one of the trials. In addition, the manner in which the cooling is being performed likely varies from what was proven efficacious in the original studies. The lack of alternative interventions will create substantial pressure to offer hypothermic therapy and perhaps to broaden the selection criteria beyond those used in the trials. Significant differences exist in the neurologic outcomes between different centres. The local practices of individual neonatal intensive care units (NICUs) may play a significant role in determining outcome of infants with brain injury [7]. A retrospective chart review in the United Kingdom found that suboptimal care deemed significant or major occurred in 64% of the cases of documented neonatal encephalopathy [7]. An average of 2.5 episodes were reported for each encephalopathy case. The emergence of hypothermic therapy in the treatment of infants with neonatal encephalopathy has created numerous opportunities for variation in care. Although the treatment protocols used in the trials are published and available, translating these into the context of daily practice will require adaptation and interpretation.

As therapeutic hypothermia becomes embraced by more and more centres and enters routine practice it is anticipated that there will be significant gaps between the conditions for implementation of this therapy within clinical trials and what occurs in clinical practice. Whether or not this "therapeutic drift" will impact the effectiveness (as opposed to efficacy) or safety profile of this novel procedure is unknown. Noticing the inevitable "therapeutic drift" that is occurring, both the National Institute of Child Health and Human Development and the American Academy of Pediatrics Committee on Fetus and Newborn have cautioned that if therapeutic hypothermia is to be implemented outside of a trial, clinicians should follow published trial protocols, ensure systematic follow-up of survivors and submit patient data to registries [8,9].

## Adverse events/safety monitoring

The care of preterm infants is concentrated in specialized facilities often staffed and equipped for highly technical care or research. In contrast, the births of term and late preterm infants are scattered over a broad range of facilities, many of which care for relatively few infants each year with NE. HIE is a relatively uncommon condition. Accordingly, the study of these larger, older and rarer infants is more challenging. Diseases of term infants have, therefore, received much less systematic investigation; their perinatal and subsequent courses are not well studied compared to those of the premature infant. Tracking these infants for rare adverse events has proven difficult and as such hypothermic therapy currently lacks long-term safety data. Safety of a new treatment such as therapeutic hypothermia can be studied by following typical patients *in situ* who receive the new treatment to evaluate whether any untoward events occur. One of the chief aims of any registry for hypothermia is to identify complications that may be associated with the introduction of the novel intervention into routine clinical practice. Many of the clinical complications described in these observational types of studies could be due to asphyxia or a cause other than moderate hypothermia; as such, one should be careful when attributing causation.

Vigilance for safety of infants treated with hypothermia for HIE was a component of the initial pilot studies, large RCTs and meta-analyses of cooling. The early studies of whole body cooling and head cooling were not designed or powered to detect uncommon adverse events. Although the original RCTs were well powered to prove efficacy of therapeutic hypothermia and did not demonstrate any major adverse events, even systematic reviews of the RCTs reporting on adverse events are not adequate to truly assess the frequency of adverse outcomes or safety [5]. Caution and vigilance are warranted; uncontrolled hypothermia in newborns can cause neurodevelopmental disturbances in survivors [10]. Among the other potential complications of therapeutic hypothermia are sclerema, multisystem organ damage (especially pulmonary haemorrhage, renal failure and disseminated intravascular coagulopathy), hypovolamia, glucose instability and pulmonary hypertension [11]. Anticonvulsants and sedatives, which are often co-administered to infants receiving cooling therapy, may exacerbate pulmonary hypertension and cause untoward cardiovascular changes [12]; and metabolism of common medications may be altered in the face of therapeutic hypothermia [13]. The RCTs have consistently demonstrated reversible cardiovascular effects, specifically sinus bradycardia and hypotension [2–4]. In the Cochrane Systematic Review of Cooling for Newborns with HIE, more cooled infants had significant thrombocytopenia and the incidence of hypotension requiring treatment with inotropes in cooled infants was of borderline significance [5]. However, despite these pooling methods, rare adverse events might still not have been evident. The method of cooling may play a role in the manifestation of adverse events. Selective brain cooling is associated with requiring a more modest degree of systemic hypothermia compared to whole body cooling; this may translate to fewer adverse events related to hypothermia. However, selective cooling is also associated with creation of less uniform temperature gradients across the brain, the significance of which is currently unknown. In the large RCTs of cooling, pyrexia was consistently noted to occur in some instances among infants in the "normothermia group" [2,3,14] and an association between pyrexia and adverse outcome has been observed [15,16]. Since the frequency of cooling is low, a registry with potential for many enrolled infants is needed to have adequate power to detect and monitor for these types of unsuspected events. As the number of patients in the registries expands, we will have larger numbers of adverse events which will allow identification of risk to patient safety and examination for variation of rare adverse events among centres and infants.

Unlike new drugs that require a substantial amount of research and assessment before licensing, new procedures often find their way into clinical practice with incomplete or non-existent evidence. RCTs demonstrating efficacy may report adverse events inadequately [17] and are limited by their inability to adequately blind procedures or control for variation in operators' competency [18]. Information from registries regarding safety may also be used by regulatory agencies to make decisions regarding safety and compensation of these novel interventions. For instance, recently in the United States, data from a registry led the Centers for Medicare and Medicaid Services to expand its coverage for positron emission tomography [19]. The UK National Institute of Health and Clinical Excellence has used registry data to evaluate other interventional procedures [20]. Following the results of the large study of selective head cooling (the Coolcap trial), in 2006 the Food and Drug Administration (FDA) approved the Natus Cool-Cap to provide selective head cooling in infants with clinical evidence of moderate to severe HIE. Natus Corporation contracted with the Vermont Oxford Network to provide de-identified reports for those infants enrolled in the Registry to participating hospitals that have given permission to be included in the reports which may be submitted to the U.S. Food and Drug Administration (FDA) for post-marketing surveillance. Despite FDA approval, selective head cooling with the Coolcap device is rare [21,22]; most centres elect to use whole body cooling methods. The devices used in the published whole body cooling have been commercially available for many years and are already available in many if not most hospitals. However, these devices are not FDA approved for cooling for HIE and do not come with a detailed step-by-step cooling protocol. Nonetheless, many of the common treatments used in neonatology are "off-label" and safety and efficacy of these whole body cooling methods have been demonstrated in RCTs. An ideal cooling register will allow collection of data for all patients undergoing any version of this novel procedure and will enable generation of valuable evidence about both efficacy and safety, complementing and enhancing evidence from randomized trials.

## Registries may help refine the cooling procedure

There remain several unanswered questions about hypothermia for neonates with HIE. Further RCTs are essential; however, given the small effect sizes that could be anticipated, RCT testing of different inclusion criteria, cooling methods or technical protocols of cooling treatment will require exponentially more patients than the initial RCTs that demonstrated efficacy and will be difficult if not impractical to perform. A registry approach could enable examination of progressive modifications to the existing treatment protocols and generate hypotheses for future trials. There are several examples worthy of discussion.

What is the role of cooling for premature infants with suspected HIE? The studies that proved efficacy excluded more premature infants. However, clinicians will be tempted to provide therapeutic hypothermia to late preterm infants. It is currently unknown at what gestational age the benefits of cooling are outweighed by the risks. Registries could track short-term outcomes and adverse event rates of infants cooled more prematurely than those in the RCTs.

What is the role of cooling for infants after 6 hours of age? Given that it is difficult to identify and provide hypothermic therapy to outborn infants within 6 hours of life and given that the severity of the hypoxic–ischaemic insult is inversely proportional to the length of the therapeutic window, whether initiation of cooling outside of 6 hours of age is effective is an important question. Currently one study, funded by the NICHD, is enrolling infants that meet all inclusion criteria for cooling but do not present until greater than 6 hours of age with normothermia versus whole body hypothermia (ClinicalTrials.gov, CT00614744). However, registries of cooling already contain valuable information on infants that were cooled at greater than 6 hours of age and may give additional insights.

What is the role of hypothermia for known postnatal insults? Infants receiving care may suffer severe ischaemic insults while in the intensive care setting. Given the rarity of there events, randomized controlled trials studying these infants are not feasible. However, infants receiving postnatal cooling could be tracked using registry methods.

Other questions include the ideal temperature to aim for, the duration of cooling and whether selective head or systemic methods of hypothermia are more effective in terms of limitation of adverse neurodevelopmental outcomes. Another concern with the application of therapeutic hypothermia is with regards to how the severity of injury impacts the usefulness of cooling. Injury severity was used to stratify infants using clinical assessment or amplitude-integrated EEG (or both) in the RCTs that demonstrated efficacy. Although an overall reduction in mortality was accompanied by a reduction in disability among survivors, meta-analysis of the largest trials has showed that, although moderate and severely affected infants benefit, the relative risk for the combined outcome of death or severe disability was lower in infants with moderate than in those with severe encephalopathy [23]. Registries will be important to identify whether there are identifiable subgroups that are not responsive or are less responsive to cooling [6,9]. These questions should not require comparison with normothermia as a control and are ideal for study within the registries of hypothermia by allowing incremental refinement of techniques and improvements in outcome analogous to the strategy used to develop paediatric cancer therapy.

Other novel treatment agents and modalities for encephalopathic neonates are being developed. Several possible strategies include combinations of potentially neuroprotective drugs with hypothermia. One potential way of improving neuroprotective treatment would be to combine cooling with an existing medication. There are some data supporting additive effects of drugs with hypothermia, including some already FDA-approved anticonvulsant drugs (topiramate, phenobarbital) [24,25], anti-oxidants (N-acetylcysteine) [26], diuretics (Bumetanide) [27] and human recombinant erythropoietin [28,29]. Other promising novel therapies being studied in animal models include the inert gas xenon [30,31]. As these therapies are tested in human newborns, it is inevitable that some will be adopted. Registries tracking NE and novel cooling therapies are ideally situated to morph into neurocritical care registries once these adjunctive therapies reach the bedside [32].

# Registries document variation in care of routine evaluations and treatments

The optimal routine care of infants with neonatal encephalopathy is unknown. Registries identify and document important variation between the evaluations and medical treatments these infants receive. For example, although it is agreed that magnetic resonance imaging (MRI) is preferred over other imaging techniques, acquisition and optimal timing of these studies are not uniformly obtained in infants being evaluated with encephalopathy [33]. Seizures are a common complication of HIE and HIE is the most common cause of seizures in term neonates. The routine aggressive or prophylactic use of anticonvulsants for infants with suspected HIE is an important unresolved question for neonatal clinicians, particularly because the aetiology of seizures is invariably a significant determinant of neurodevelopmental outcome and animal studies suggest potential neurotoxicity of anticonvulsant drugs in neonates [34,35]. More recently, high-resolution MRI studies suggest that clinical neonatal seizures in the setting of HIE are associated with worse neurodevelopmental outcome and in animal models suggest that administration of phenobarbital may augment the neuroprotective efficacy of therapeutic hypothermia [24,36]. Registries will reflect clinician variation in management and give valuable information for randomized controlled trials to determine whether differences in seizure management can improve outcome. The impact of routine sedation and continuous brain monitoring when undergoing therapeutic hypothermia on outcomes also remains unclear. Registries will help evaluate these and other variations in current practice of providing hypothermic therapy to identify areas for improvement.

To maximize the neuroprotective effect among infants with HIE, initiation of hypothermia at outlying referring hospitals and during transport is an attractive proposition. Community hospitals are already getting involved and providing cooling in transport; clearly there are many systems issues involved in the delivery of this therapy. Tied to the question of cooling while on transport is the issue of regionalization. There are no clear guidelines on what constitutes a sufficient volume of cases to merit development of a neonatal cooling programme. Several reports indicate that cooling can be performed on transport but the safety of the procedure remains a concern [37–39]. As such, it is important that centres providing this therapy have enough practical experience and this will need to be balanced against geographical isolation. Registries will shed additional light on the safety and complex systems issues that hospitals must overcome with regards to neonatal transport.

# Vermont Oxford Network Neonatal Encephalopathy Registry

The Vermont Oxford Network (VON) has created a registry for encephalopathic infants. VON is a nonprofit voluntary collaboration of health care professionals dedicated to improving the quality and safety of medical care for newborn infants and their families. The Network comprises of over 800 Neonatal Intensive Care Units around the world. Data from VON have been used in numerous research studies assessing the associations between infant and hospital characteristics, variations in care and neonatal intensive care unit (NICU) patient outcomes [40–43]. VON maintains one of the world's largest databases regarding the care and outcomes of very low birth weight (VLBW) infants treated in NICUs around the world. Vermont Oxford Members receive confidential quarterly and annual reports that include information for NICU infants at their centre compared to infants at all centres participating in the VLBW Database and Expanded Database. VON established a Registry for NE (NER) that began enrolling patients in 2006 with the primary objective of characterizing infants born with NE. Secondary objectives included the identification of the antenatal and perinatal factors associated with encephalopathy; description of the evaluations and medical treatments that these infants receive and how treatment varies among centres; identification of the co-morbidities and outcomes of these infants; monitoring the introduction and dissemination of hypothermic therapy (HT) and other emerging novel therapies. Ultimately, these data will help define clinical research questions and identify opportunities for improved care of infants with encephalopathy.

The VON NER is intended to capture data on term and near-term infants with NE and a subset of these infants treated with therapeutic hypothermia (Figure 17.1). Historically, the presence of NE has

## Registry Eligibility and Infact Characteristics

Infants who are admitted to a VON neonatal intensive care unit (NICU) within the first 28 days of life, or who die at a VON NICU within the first 28 days of life, are eligible for the Registry if:

- The infant received hypothermic therapy.

**OR**

- Gestational age was 36 completed weeks or more.

**AND**

- No central nervous system birth defect was present

  **AND** one or more of the following conditions was present:

  - Stupor or coma within the first 72 hours of life

  - Seizures within the first 72 hours of life

  - 5-minute APGAR score of 3 or less

  - Neuro-muscular blockade within 4–72 hours of life

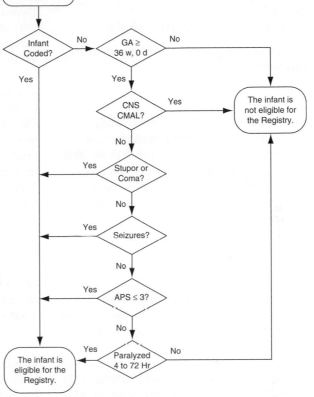

**Figure 17.1.** Criteria for eligibility to the Vermont Oxford Neonatal Encephalopathy Registry.

been considered *sine qua non* of hypoxic–ischaemic injury or birth asphyxia. However, the aetiology of NE is not limited to hypoxic–ischaemic injury and displays considerable diversity [44]. To ensure that all encephalopathic infants regardless of aetiology are included in the Registry, the working definition used is the presence of seizures and/or altered consciousness (stupor, coma) during the first 72 hours of life. Additional inclusion parameters were set to capture all potentially encephalopathic infants treated with hypothermia independent of their neurologic status, and infants whose neurologic status might be difficult to assess (i.e., paralyzed, mechanically ventilated, or sedated infants). Utilizing a registry is a method well suited to the study of the broad and heterogeneous population of infants with

NE, as well as to evaluating how an intervention such as HT is implemented in clinical practice.

The purpose of any registry is to provide information about a specific patient population to whom all study results are meant to apply. The VON NER populations of interest are infants born with NE and infants exposed to HT. A purposive non-probability sampling strategy is used in which these two predefined groups are deliberately sampled.

There are essentially two paths of entry into the VON NER:

- Any infant born at 36 weeks' gestation or more displaying evidence of NE within 3 days of birth is eligible. Infants born with central nervous system birth defects are excluded. NE is defined as presence of seizures and/or altered consciousness (stupor, coma) during the first 72 hours of life. To capture all infants potentially affected by NE, infants with a 5-minute APGAR score of ≤3 or that receive neuromuscular blockade extending through the first 72 hours of life are also eligible.

- Any infant that has received HT is eligible.

All infants with known central nervous system anomalies are excluded.

## VON NER results

Participation in the VON NER has grown steadily since its inception. In 2006, 41 centres participated in the Registry and identified 433 infants with NE. By 2008, there were 67 participating centres that had screened 88,527 infants to identify 1,775 cases of neonatal encephalopathy. Of those infants identified as encephalopathic, 495 received therapeutic hypothermia from 2006 to 2008. However, as evidence that centres are cooling more frequently, 547 infants were cooled in 2009 alone.

The typical infant in the VON NER that received cooling weighed 3265 grams (interquartile range: 2880 grams to 3670 grams), was 39 weeks gestation (interquartile range: 37.0 weeks to 40.0 weeks) and received cooling 4.7 hours after delivery (interquartile range 3.1 hours to 5.8 hours).

Among the 88,527 infants screened, 1,144 infants in the VON NER had seizures before discharge [45]. Conventional EEG (cEEG) was performed in 85%, while amplitude-integrated EEG (aEEG) was performed in 37% of infants with NS; 35% of NS cases underwent both types of EEG. 48% had EEG confirmation of clinically recognized seizures, while 4% had electrographic seizures only (cEEG or aEEG). Of the remaining cases, nearly half (48%) of infants with NS were diagnosed solely by clinical assessment. Nearly half of those infants identified as having seizures did not have electrophysiological confirmation of the diagnosis. Relatively few infants were diagnosed with NS based on EEG results only. These results suggest that the decision of when and how to implement electrophysiologic tests remains a significant area for improvement in the care of infants with NS, especially considering the inaccuracy of clinical diagnosis and the regularity with which these patients receive medication. Of NS cases surviving to discharge, 62% were receiving seizure medication at discharge.

The VON NER recorded data on the imaging modalities obtained and results in all infants with encephalopathy [46]. A total of 1,453 of 1,775 (83%) infants received neuroimaging evaluation. Seven hundred fifty-one (43%) underwent a cranial ultrasound, 493 (28%) underwent cranial tomography (CT) scanning and 1,098 (63%) underwent magnetic resonance imaging (MRI) studies. Although CT scanning showed abnormalities in 57% of infants, half of these were extra-axial haemorrhages. Ventriculomegaly and vascular lesions were noted to occur in approximately 4% of infants. Cerebral dysgenesis was noted in 5% of NE infants. MRI revealed the highest frequency of abnormalities, particularly in relation to white matter (WM) and deep nuclear grey matter injury (DNGM). One in five infants with NE did not receive any neuroimaging. CT scanning remains commonly used in practice despite its low detection of prognostically important parenchymal cerebral lesions and the risk from radiation exposure, signifying significant room for improvement. In the VON NER, a wide range of cerebral lesions is found in NE and the preferred imaging modality (MRI) is inconsistently used.

The frequency of recorded antecedent factors in mother and fetus/infant is captured by the VON NER [47]. Of the 1,775 infants with NE, 24.3% had one or more maternal risk factors for NE that pre-dated the onset of labour, such as hypothyroidism (2.4%), diabetes (9.4%), hypertension (13.7%) or lack of prenatal care (2.9%). Twenty-five percent of encephalopathic infants had one or more antenatal risk factors such as birth defect (8.1%) or smallness for dates (16.4%). Intrapartum asphyxial factors, of which the most common were maternal haemorrhage (10.4%) and cord prolapse (2.8%), were observed in 14.4% of infants. Inflammatory factors including maternal fever in labour ≥ 38°C (17.9%) and chorioamnionitis (9.9%) were noted in 21.3% of cases. Of infants with NE, 66.1% had neither asphyxial nor inflammatory risk factors, 19.5% had inflammatory factors only, 12.8% had asphyxial factors only and 1.6% had both. These observations from the VON NER are in agreement with previous studies in finding that intrapartum factors appear to account for only a minority of NE, that inflammatory factors are at least as common and that much or most of NE remains unexplained.

Among the 495 infants that received therapeutic hypothermia in the VON NER, 75% were cooled using whole body methods and 49% were cooled using selective head methods [22]. Of these infants, 12 (2.4%) were born at < 36 weeks' gestation and only four received HT as part of a RCT. HT was started > 6 hours of birth in 89 (18%) treated infants. The majority (77%) of cooled infants were born at referral hospitals and were transported during their initial hospital stay. HT was provided to 9% of infants while at a referral hospital before transport and to 36% during transport. HT as introduced into routine care deviates from the protocols used in the original RCTs in several ways including treatment of infants < 36 weeks' gestation, initiation of HT > 6 hours after birth and use of HT before and during transport. The impact of these differences is unknown. Adverse events within 7 days of birth for infants receiving HT included: arrhythmia 24%, thrombosis 1%, hypotension 33%, seizure during rewarming 10%, scalp oedema 34%, skin breakdown 5%, sclerema 1% and thrombocytopenia 33% [22]. Survival through to ultimate hospital discharge occurred in 83% of infants treated with HT.

## VON NER link to quality improvement

The NER is one key part of a larger coordinated campaign to improve the quality and care provided to newborns by joining evidence to outcomes through quality improvement (QI) methods. As such, in alignment with the VON NER are VON sponsored and supported coordinated systems of quality improvement. The NER provides valuable information that serves as benchmarking data that members use while participating in two types of multicentre quality improvement collaboratives, called NICQ and iNICQ. The data from the NER are used to identify opportunities for improvement and constitute a link between making change, measurement and action. The NICQ programme allows for more intensive, face-to-face collaboration while our iNICQ programme allows centres to participate with others over the Internet by means of Web-based conferences.

All centres that submitted data to the VON NER were encouraged to participate in a recent iNICQ Quality Improvement Collaborative regarding NE. iNICQ collaboratives are a series of 90-minute live multicentre interactive Web conferences that include plenary presentations by expert faculty, case studies from real NICU teams and a dedicated e-mail discussion list open to all participants. The iNICQ collaborative, entitled Improving Care for Neonatal Encephalopathy, was designed for multidisciplinary NICU teams to improve participating hospitals' ability to identify infants with NE reliably, diagnose and treat neonatal seizures appropriately, use brain monitoring and neuroimaging effectively,

understand whether and how to use hypothermia in the NICU and address the needs of families with NE and facilitate follow-up of affected infants. The series comprised five Web conferences led by experts in the field on high-impact topics of encephalopathy. The iNICQ series all have an audio component as well as slides and is freely available. It may be found at the following Web address: http://www.vtoxford.org/research/enceph/enceph.aspx# NERMMedia. (Note: These presentations require Internet Explorer 5.0 or later, Netscape Navigator 7.0 or later, or Internet Explorer 5.2.2 or later for Mac.)

The recent NICQ collaborative also focused on the care of NE infants. The NICQ Neurointensive Care Group is led by a "faculty trio" including an expert, a quality improvement facilitator and a member of a participating team serving as a clinical leader. NICQ participants attend two meetings annually where they participate in plenary sessions, group work and poster sessions. These meetings serve as a forum for networking, social interaction and direct collaboration with teams from other NICUs. NICQ teams continue their QI work between meetings by means of regular local team meetings, interest group conference calls and a dedicated email listserver. The overall goal of the NICQ Neurointensive Care Group is to improve the outcomes and decrease the variability of care provided to encephalopathic infants. A neonatal encephalopathy Quality Improvement Starter Kit (QIK) that identifies evidenced based Potentially Better Practices (PBPs) specific to improvement in outcomes of NE infants is provided to the group to jump start their improvement work. Centres implement the PBPs to make changes and track their work over 2-year cycles. Participating centres are encouraged to track neurodevelopmental follow-up at 18–24 months in NE infants with participation in a registry such as the VON NER. However, short-term goals are also established to track improvement since long-term follow-up by definition takes time. To track progress in terms of rapid cycle quality improvement, one of the most recent NICQ Neurointensive Care Group participating hospitals, DeVos Hospital, strove to implement the following PBP: "Implement a system that coordinates care with referring hospitals to ensure hypothermic therapy will be initiated on 100% of the eligible transported infants within 6 hours of birth". This unit used VON NER data to document the time from birth to the start of cooling and was able to implement change ideas that demonstrated significant reduction in delay in initiation of cooling. Since implementation at this hospital, 100% of eligible infants were able to receive cooling within 6 hours.

VON has also developed NICQpedia, a Web-based repository for our Quality Improvement work. NICQ participants have access to and are expected to contribute to NICQpedia. The Neurointensive Care Group QIKs reside on NICQpedia wiki pages and will be continually refined by NICQ members during the course of the future collaboratives. Improvement Stories, tools and other resources developed by teams and shared as posters at the NICQ meetings, are being posted to NICQpedia to provide valuable practice improvement implementation stories. NICQpedia enhances collaboration between centres on improvement in the care of NE infants as well as archiving the tremendous work of this group. NICQpedia is available to all VON centres.

## VON NER compared to TOBY register

One other registry, called the UK TOBY Cooling Register, captures data on neonatal hypothermia [48,49]. The TOBY trial of therapeutic hypothermia was a randomized controlled trial that completed enrollment in November 2006 [4,14]. The TOBY Register was designed after enrollment of the very large and well-conducted TOBY trial was completed but before cooling was accepted as the standard of care upon recognition that many physicians were offering HT out of the context of any trial. The TOBY investigators, therefore, created guidelines, informational material and Register forms to monitor the spread of HT in the United Kingdom [49].

The VON NER was conceived as a study of all late preterm and term infants with NE, including but not limited to infants treated with therapeutic hypothermia. Accordingly the entry criteria of the VON NER are intentionally very broad to study the full spectrum of patients with NE. The TOBY Register, by contrast, is a phase 4 study of the specific methods of the TOBY randomized hypothermia trial. It has a more specific set of inclusion criteria, limited to infants receiving therapeutic hypothermia following standards that followed the TOBY randomized trial. The TOBY Register does not provide data on aetiologies of NE other than in those who receive HT; however, the TOBY Register design allows for very accurate monitoring of the adoption of this intervention within the United Kingdom. Comparison of information in the VON and the TOBY registries will be useful in understanding dissemination of this therapy when implemented strictly in accordance with a trial (TOBY) versus in a more broad clinical setting (VON).

## Implementation of therapeutic hypothermia in the United Kingdom: data from the UK TOBY Cooling Register

Data from the UK TOBY Cooling Register provide the opportunity to examine how a new effective therapy for newborn infants suspected of suffering asphyxial encephalopathy – therapeutic hypothermia – was implemented in the United Kingdom. Data forms from 1,384 (67%) of the 2,069 infants notified to the Register from inception in December 2006 to mid 2011 were analysed [50]. The monthly rate of notifications increased from median {IQR} 18 {15–31} to 33 {30–39} after the announcement of the results of the TOBY trial and to 50 {36–55} after their publication. This rate further increased to 70 {64–83} following official endorsement of the therapy and is now close to the expected numbers of eligible infants in the United Kingdom.

In the United Kingdom, cooling was started at 3.3 {1.5–5.5} hours after birth and the time taken to achieve the target 33–34°C rectal temperature was 1 {0–3} hours. The rectal temperature was in the target range in 83% of measurements. From 2006 to 2011, there was evidence of extension of treatment to slightly less severely affected infants. The proportion of infants with suspected clinical seizures before cooling decreased over the time period of the Register. Similarly, the proportion of infants with a severely abnormal aEEG grade decreased over time. There was also an improvement in Apgar scores at 10 minutes and first blood base excess from 2007 to 2011.

Several adverse events were reported to the Register, including: sepsis (17%), hypoglycaemia (25%), hypotension (40%), coagulopathy (31%) and arrhythmias (9%). Subcutaneous fat necrosis was reported in 1–2% of cases [51].

Twenty percent of the infants reported to the Register died at 2.9 {1.4–4.1} days of age; the rates of death fell slightly over the period of the Register. At 2 years of age, cerebral palsy was diagnosed in 22% of survivors; half of these were spastic bilateral. Factors independently associated with adverse outcome were clinical seizures before cooling and severely abnormal amplitude-integrated EEG.

The UK Toby Register enables national surveillance of changing practice and outcomes of infants treated with cooling. The data suggest that therapeutic hypothermia was implemented widely within the UK, which may be due in part to participation by neonatal units in clinical trials, the establishment of the national Register and its endorsement by advisory bodies.

## Limitations of the registry method

Since participating in any registry is voluntary, concerns exist as to whether or not participating centres are representative of all NICUs caring for encephalopathic infants. Vermont Oxford has over 750 participating centres and is the largest network tracking outcomes on infants treated in NICUs in the world. The VON currently has over 75 centres contributing data to the NER. Flexibility regarding data items to maximize the usefulness of the information is ongoing and intended to be of maximal usefulness to participating centres. The TOBY UK Register has participation from over 60 centres and captures patient records for essentially all infants treated with therapeutic hypothermia in the United Kingdom.

As with all registries, careful analysis and interpretation of the data are necessary and sources of bias may be difficult to identify. Registries are more susceptible to bias, identified and unidentified, than randomized trials [52]. Bias refers to a systematic, unintended influence in the way in which patients are selected, outcomes are measured, or data are analyzed. Selection biases can lead to the wrong group of patients receiving experimental treatments, or to misinterpretation of results. As an example, if more severely affected patients receive therapeutic hypothermia within the registry data and if these patients have worse outcomes due to their underlying disease severity, findings may be misinterpreted as a failed treatment effect. Alternately, if less severely affected infants are preferentially cooled, it may create an overestimation of effect.

An intrinsic limitation of studies testing interventions such as hypothermia and observational research is the inability to perform blinding in a meaningful way.

Any unblinded trial risks bias since severely affected infants frequently die secondary to withdrawal of care. Accordingly, the unblinded provider has a very real potential influence on whether and when infants die. This type of bias might lead to an increase in severe morbidity in survivors; however, this finding was not observed in any of the large RCTs of hypothermia [53]. In fact, therapeutic hypothermia significantly reduced the combined rate of death and severe disability and increased survival with normal neurological function and in survivors reduced the rates of severe disability [23]. However, when utilizing registries of hypothermia, researchers must be careful when interpreting data from unblinded studies, given their inherent susceptibility to risk of bias, when in the process of establishing outcome events.

Although careful analysis and execution can improve interpretation and minimize confounding due to recognized factors, this limitation further restricts clinicians from applying registry data to clinical decision-making. Conversely, awareness and recognition of bias in registry data may add to their heuristic value for planning clinical research, or guiding NICUs' policies.

## References

1. Edwards AD, Brocklehurst P, Gunn AJ, et al. Neurological outcomes at 18 months of age after moderate hypothermia for perinatal hypoxic ischaemic encephalopathy: synthesis and meta-analysis of trial data. *Br Med J* 2010;**340**:c363.

2. Gluckman PD, Wyatt JS, Azzopardi D, et al. Selective head cooling with mild systemic hypothermia after neonatal encephalopathy: multicentre randomised trial. *Lancet* 2005;**365**(9460):663–70.

3. Shankaran S, Laptook AR, Ehrenkranz RA, et al. Whole-body hypothermia for neonates with hypoxic-ischemic encephalopathy. *N Engl J Med* 2005;**353**:1574–84.

4. Azzopardi DV, Strohm B, Edwards AD, et al. Moderate hypothermia to treat perinatal asphyxial encephalopathy. *N Engl J Med* 2009;**361**:1349–58.

5. Jacobs S, Hunt R, Tarnow-Mordi W, Inder T, Davis P. Cooling for newborns with hypoxic ischaemic encephalopathy. *Cochrane Database Syst Rev* 2007(4): CD003311.

6. Wilkinson DJ. Cool heads: ethical issues associated with therapeutic hypothermia for newborns. *Acta Paediatr* 2009;**98**:217–20.

7. Draper ES, Kurinczuk JJ, Lamming CR, et al. A confidential enquiry into cases of neonatal encephalopathy. *Arch Dis Child Fetal Neonatal Ed* 2002;**87**:F176–80.

8. Blackmon LR, Stark AR. Hypothermia: a neuroprotective therapy for neonatal hypoxic-ischemic encephalopathy. *Pediatrics* 2006;**117**:942–8.

9. Higgins RD, Raju TN, Perlman J, et al. Hypothermia and perinatal asphyxia: executive summary of the National Institute of Child Health and Human Development workshop. *J Pediatr* 2006;**148**:170–5.

10. Culic S. Cold injury syndrome and neurodevelopmental changes in survivors. *Arch Med Res* 2005;**36**:532–8.

11. Bower BD, Jones LF, Weeks MM. Cold injury in the newborn. A study of 70 cases. *Br Med J* 1960;**1**:303–9.

12. Thoresen M, Whitelaw A. Cardiovascular changes during mild therapeutic hypothermia and rewarming in infants with hypoxic-ischemic encephalopathy. *Pediatrics* 2000;**106**(Pt 1):92–9.

13. Roka A, Melinda KT, Vasarhelyi B, et al. Elevated morphine concentrations in neonates treated with morphine and prolonged hypothermia for hypoxic ischemic encephalopathy. *Pediatrics* 2008;**121**:e844–9.

14. Azzopardi DV, Strohm B, Edwards AD, et al. TOBY Study Group. *N Engl J Med* 2009;**361**:1349–58. Erratum in: *N Engl J Med* 2010;362:1056.

15. Wyatt JS, Gluckman PD, Liu PY, et al. Determinants of outcomes after head cooling for neonatal encephalopathy. *Pediatrics* 2007;**119**:912–21.

16. Laptook A, Tyson J, Shankaran S, et al. Elevated temperature after hypoxic-ischemic encephalopathy: risk factor for adverse outcomes. *Pediatrics* 2008;**122**:491–9.

17. Ioannidis JP, Lau J. Improving safety reporting from randomised trials. *Drug Saf* 2002;**25**:77–84.

18. Campbell WB, Barnes SJ, Kirby RA, et al. Association of study type, sample size and follow-up length with type of recommendation produced by the National Institute for Health and Clinical Excellence Interventional Procedures Programme. *Int J Technol Assess Health Care* 2007;**23**:101–7.

19. Hillner BE, Siegel BA, Liu D, et al. Impact of positron emission tomography/computed tomography and positron emission tomography (PET) alone on expected management of patients with cancer: initial results from the National Oncologic PET Registry. *J Clin Oncol* 2008;**26**:2155–61.

20. Lyratzopoulos G, Patrick H, Campbell B. Registers needed for new interventional procedures. *Lancet* 2008;**371**:1734–6.

21. Kapetanakis A, Azzopardi D, Wyatt J, Robertson NJ. Therapeutic hypothermia for neonatal encephalopathy: a UK survey of opinion, practice and neuro-investigation at the end of 2007. *Acta Paediatr* 2009;**98**:631–5.

22. Pfister RH, Bingham P, Carpenter JH, et al. Hypothermia in practice: initial observations from the Vermont Oxford Network. In: Society PA, editor. 2010 *PAS Annual Meeting*. Vancouver, British Columbia; 2010.

23. Edwards AD, Brocklehurst P, Gunn AJ, et al. Neurological outcomes at 18 months of age after moderate hypothermia for perinatal hypoxic ischaemic encephalopathy: synthesis and meta-analysis of trial data. *BMJ* 2010;**340**:c363.

24. Barks JD, Liu YQ, Shangguan Y, Silverstein FS. Phenobarbital augments hypothermic neuroprotection. *Pediatr Res* 2010;**67**:532–7.

25. Liu Y, Barks JD, Xu G, Silverstein FS. Topiramate extends the therapeutic window for hypothermia-mediated neuroprotection after stroke in neonatal rats. *Stroke* 2004;**35**:1460–5.

26. Jatana M, Singh I, Singh AK, Jenkins D. Combination of systemic hypothermia and N-acetylcysteine attenuates hypoxic-ischemic brain injury in neonatal rats. *Pediatr Res* 2006;**59**:684–9.

27. Chen H, Luo J, Kintner DB, Shull GE, Sun D. Na(+)-dependent chloride transporter (NKCC1)-null mice exhibit less gray and white matter damage after focal cerebral ischemia. *J Cereb Blood Flow Metab* 2005;**25**:54–66.

28. Elmahdy H, El-Mashad AR, El-Bahrawy H, El-Gohary T, El-Barbary A, Aly H. Human recombinant erythropoietin in asphyxia neonatorum: pilot trial. *Pediatrics* 2010;**125**:e1135–42.

29. Zhu C, Kang W, Xu F, et al. Erythropoietin improved neurologic outcomes in newborns with hypoxic-ischemic encephalopathy. *Pediatrics* 2009;**124**:e218–26.

30. Chakkarapani E, Dingley J, Liu X, et al. Xenon enhances hypothermic neuroprotection in asphyxiated newborn pigs. *Ann Neurol* 2010;**68**:330–41.

31. Ma D, Hossain M, Chow A, et al. Xenon and hypothermia combine to provide neuroprotection from neonatal asphyxia. *Ann Neurol* 2005;**58**:182–93.

32. Glass HC, Bonifacio SL, Peloquin S, et al. Neurocritical care for neonates. *Neurocrit Care* 12: 421–9.

33. Rutherford M, Malamateniou C, McGuinness A, et al. Magnetic resonance imaging in hypoxic-ischaemic encephalopathy. *Early Hum Dev* 2010;**86**:351–60.

34. Silverstein FS. Do seizures contribute to neonatal hypoxic-ischemic brain injury? *J Pediatr* 2009;**155**:305–6.

35. Bittigau P, Sifringer M, Genz K, et al. Antiepileptic drugs and apoptotic neurodegeneration in the developing brain. *Proc Natl Acad Sci U S A* 2002;**99**:15089–94.

36. Glass HC, Glidden D, Jeremy RJ, et al. Clinical neonatal seizures are independently associated with outcome in infants at risk for hypoxic-ischemic brain injury. *J Pediatr* 2009;**155**:318–23.

37. Fairchild K, Sokora D, Scott J, Zanelli S. Therapeutic hypothermia on neonatal transport: 4-year experience in a single NICU. *J Perinatol* 2010;**30**:324–9.

38. Anderson ME, Longhofer TA, Phillips W, McRay DE. Passive cooling to initiate hypothermia for transported encephalopathic newborns. *J Perinatol* 2007;**27**:592–3.

39. Zanelli SA, Naylor M, Dobbins N, et al. Implementation of a 'Hypothermia for HIE' program: 2-year experience in a single NICU. *J Perinatol* 2008;**28**:171–5.

40. Horbar JD, Badger GJ, Lewit EM, Rogowski J, Shiono PH. Hospital and patient characteristics associated with variation in 28-day mortality rates for very low birth weight infants. Vermont Oxford Network. *Pediatrics* 1997;**99**:149–56.

41. Rogowski JA, Horbar JD, Staiger DO, et al. Indirect vs direct hospital quality indicators for very low-birth-weight infants. *JAMA* 2004;**291**:202–9.

42. Morales LS, Staiger D, Horbar JD, et al. Mortality among very low-birthweight infants in hospitals serving minority populations. *Am J Public Health* 2005;**95**:2206–12.

43. Zupancic JA, Richardson DK, Horbar JD, et al. Revalidation of the score for neonatal acute physiology in the Vermont Oxford Network. *Pediatrics* 2007;**119**:e156–63.

44. Edwards AD, Nelson KB. Neonatal encephalopathies. Time to reconsider the cause of encephalopathies. *BMJ* 1998;**317**:1537–8.

45. Bingham PM, Carpenter JH, Horbar JD, et al. Diagnosis and treatment of neonatal seizures in a neonatal encephalopathy registry. In: Society PA, editor. 2010 *PAS Annual Meeting*. Vancouver, British Columbia; 2010.

46. Inder TE, Bingham P, Carpenter JH, et al. Neuroimaging in the Vermont Oxford Network. In:

Society PA, editor. 2010 *PAS Annual Meeting*. Vancouver, British Columbia; 2010.

47. Nelson KB, Bingham P, Carpenter J, et al. Antecedents of neonatal encephalopathy in the Vermont Oxford Network. In: Society PA, editor. 2010 *PAS Annual Meeting*. Vancouver, British Columbia; 2010.

48. Azzopardi D, Strohm B, Edwards AD, et al. Treatment of asphyxiated newborns with moderate hypothermia in routine clinical practice: how cooling is managed in the UK outside a clinical trial. *Arch Dis Child* 2009;**94**:F260–4.

49. www.npeu.ox.ac.uk/tobyregister

50. Azzopardi D, Strohm B, Linsell L, Hobson A, Juszczak E, Kurinczuk JJ, Brocklehurst P, Edwards AD; UK TOBY Cooling Register. Implementation and conduct of therapeutic hypothermia for perinatal asphyxial encephalopathy in the UK – analysis of national data. *PLoS One.* 2012;7:e38504.

51. Luepker RV. Observational studies in clinical research. *J Lab Clin Med* 2005;**146**:9–12.

52. Kirpalani H, Barks J, Thorlund K, Guyatt G. Cooling for neonatal hypoxic ischemic encephalopathy: do we have the answer? *Pediatrics* 2007;**120**:1126–30.

53. Strohm B, Hobson A, Brocklehurst P, Edwards AD, Azzopardi D; UK TOBY Cooling Register. Subcutaneous fat necrosis after moderate therapeutic hypothermia in neonates. *Pediatrics* 2011;**128**:e450–2.

# Novel neuroprotective therapies

Sandra E. Juul, Donna M. Ferriero and Mervyn Maze

## Introduction

This chapter will review the evidence for selected novel neuroprotective therapies, providing background information, *in vitro* and *in vivo* data for safety, efficacy, clinical feasibility and where available, a review of clinical studies. Examples of growth factors (erythropoietin), cell-based therapies and inhaled agents (xenon) will be discussed. We aim to give an overview of therapies that may be added to our armamentarium in the next decade. Ideally, in the future, the approach to neuroprotection will be integrated, with combined therapies timed to target specific mechanisms of injury and repair.

## Erythropoietin

### Introduction

Erythropoietin (Epo) is a 34-kDa glycoprotein originally identified for its role in erythropoiesis, but which has since been found to have other functions. During embryologic and fetal development, Epo receptors (EpoR) are widespread [1] and Epo appears to have trophic effects on the vascular and nervous systems among others [2,3]. As the fetus develops, EpoR become increasingly regionally and cell-specific [4]. The non-haematopoietic function of Epo as it interacts with these receptors has been the subject of extensive investigation over the past 15 years. In particular, the neuroprotective effects of Epo and the mechanisms by which these effects occur have been researched in experimental paradigms ranging from cell culture to knockout mice, to small and large animal models of brain injury.

### Erythropoietic effects of Epo

The safety and efficacy of Epo as an erythropoietic agent has been tested in both adults and children, although Epo is not approved for use in neonates.

Epo is now widely used to treat or prevent anaemia due to a variety of causes. Neonates require higher doses of Epo, with more frequent dosing to achieve an equivalent haematopoietic response to adults, due to their greater plasma clearance, high volume of distribution and short fractional elimination time.

### *In vitro* Epo effects

EpoR are present on multiple cell types within the central nervous system. These include neuron progenitor cells [5], select populations of mature neurons [6], astrocytes [7], oligodendrocytes [8], microglia [9] and endothelial cells [5]. Epo has direct neuroprotective effects: it binds to cell surface EpoRs, which dimerize to activate anti-apoptotic pathways by means of phosphorylation of Janus kinase 2 (JAK2), phosphorylation and activation of the mitogen-activated protein kinase (MAPK), extracellular signal-regulated kinase (ERK1/2) as well as the phosphatidylinositol 3-kinase (PI3K)/Akt (protein kinase B) pathway and signal transducer and activator of transcription 5 (STAT5), which are critical in cell survival [10]. Epo improves viability of neurons cultured in varied noxious conditions, including oxygen glucose deprivation, glutamate toxicity and nitric oxide toxicity [10]. Epo also has direct effects on oligodendrocytes, the cells hypothesized to have critical vulnerability in the development of white matter injury seen so commonly in preterm infants. Epo promotes the maturation and differentiation of oligodendrocytes in culture [7], protects these cells from interferon-γ and LPS toxicity [11] and improves white matter survival *in vivo* [12].

### *In vivo* Epo effects

Early *in vivo* experiments were done using intraventricular injections of Epo, because Epo was not thought to

*Neonatal Neural Rescue*, ed. A. David Edwards, Denis V. Azzopardi and Alistair J. Gunn. Published by Cambridge University Press. © Cambridge University Press 2013.

cross the blood–brain barrier. This approach changed after Brines *et al* demonstrated neuroprotection using high-dose Epo (5,000 U/kg i.p.) in adult models of brain injury [13]. Further studies in animals and humans demonstrated that high doses of Epo could be systemically administered and result in detectable increases in Epo concentrations in spinal fluid and brain extract which, based on *in vitro* work, could be within a neuroprotective range [14,15]. The minimum effective dose has not yet been established and may depend on whether the blood–brain barrier is intact or not. Thus, the mechanism of brain injury may dictate the dose of Epo required for neuroprotection.

To date, hundreds of Epo neuroprotection studies have been published using adult and neonatal models of brain injury. Mechanisms of brain injury include stroke, trauma, kainate-induced seizures, hypoxia–ischaemia and subarachnoid haemorrhage. Epo doses tested range from 300 U/kg/dose to 30,000 U/Kg [16]. The highest doses (20–30,000 U/kg) lose protective properties, may cause harm and are not recommended [17]. When tested *in vivo*, protective effects important for reducing acute brain injury include a decrease in excitotoxicity [18], glutamate toxicity [19], neuronal apoptosis [10] and inflammation [20]. Another mechanism which seems to be important in Epo neuroprotection is its stimulation of, and interaction with, other protective factors such as brain-derived neurotrophic factor (BDNF) and glial cell-derived neurotrophic factor (GDNF) [5,21]. Epo is directly involved in prevention of oxidative stress with generation of anti-oxidant enzymes, inhibition of nitric oxide production and decrease of lipid peroxidation. It also provides benefit though its role in angiogenesis, which may be necessary for long-term survival of injured or newly generated cells. Epo has angiogenic properties itself, but also promotes angiogenesis and repair together with vascular endothelial growth factor (VEGF) [22,23]. Epo treatment also increases migration of neural progenitor cells by stimulating secretion of metalloproteinase 2 and 9 by endothelial cells by means of PI3K/Akt and ERK1/2 signaling pathways [24]. Thus, some protective effects of Epo are the result of direct neuronal receptor-mediated interaction and others are indirect. In fact, a recent study shows there to be neuroprotective effects of Epo in the absence of neural EpoR [25].

Multiple Epo doses following brain injury in rodent models provides more sustained neuroprotection using lower doses than when a single-dose strategy is pursued [16,26], possibly because Epo continues

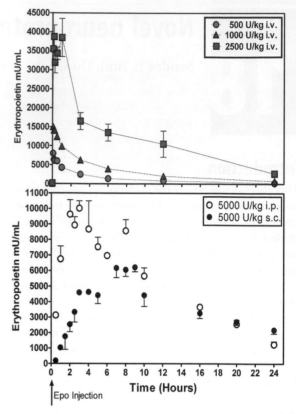

**Figure 18.1.** A comparison of pharmacokinetics from rats (lower figure) given 5,000 U/kg by intraperitoneal (i.p.) or subcutaneous (s.c.) injection [15] with human preterm infants (upper figure) given either 500, 1,000, or 2,500 U/kg [30].

to decrease late apoptosis and may stimulate processes involved in repair such as neurogenesis, angiogenesis and migration of regenerating neurons [27]. Further studies are ongoing in larger animal models such as sheep [28] and non-human primates [29].

The optimal dose for neuroprotection in humans is not yet known, nor is the optimal dosing interval or timing of administration. Figure 18.1 shows a comparison of pharmacokinetics from rats given 5000 U/kg by intraperitoneal (i.p.) or subcutaneous (s.c.) injection [15] with human preterm infants given either 500, 1,000 or 2,500 U/kg [30]. Peak Epo plasma concentrations in rat pups given 5,000 U/kg are comparable to those in preterm human infants given 500 U/kg i.v.; however, clearance is more rapid after the i.v. dose [16,30]. The 1,000 U/kg dose provided a more sustained plasma level of drug in the preterm humans. Based on these data, effective Epo dosing in humans might include more frequent but lower dosing (500 U/kg), or higher doses such as 1,000 U/kg given daily.

# Clinical trials of Epo neonatal neuroprotection

Clinical translation of the basic science research on Epo as a neuroprotectant has begun. Four clinical trials examining the safety and efficacy of high-dose Epo as a potential therapy for neonatal brain injury have been published: two in preterm infants and two in term infants with hypoxic–ischaemic encephalopathy (HIE) [30–33]. The pilot studies done in preterm infants tested a range of doses from 500 to 3,000 U/kg, with daily doses given for the first 3 days of life. The pharmacokinetics of doses up to 2500 U/kg are shown in Figure 18.1 (upper panel) [30]. Of the 60 infants treated in these two studies, no Epo-related adverse events were noted. A multicentre randomized controlled study of Epo neuroprophylaxis in very low birth weight (VLBW) babies is ongoing in Switzerland. Another trial targeting extremely low birth weight (ELBW) infants is in the planning stage in the United States.

Term infants with hypoxia–ischaemia were studied in a prospective case-control study of 45 infants, 15 of whom received Epo (2,500 IU/kg, s.c., daily for 5 days), 15 were HIE controls and 15 were normal term infants [33]. EEG backgrounds improved significantly ($P = 0.01$) and NO concentrations decreased ($P < 0.001$) in the HIE-Epo group compared with the HIE-control group. At 6 months, infants in the HIE-Epo group had fewer neurologic ($P < 0.05$) and developmental ($P < 0.05$) abnormalities. In the second study of term infants, 167 infants with moderate to severe HIE were randomized to either Epo (n = 83) or conventional treatment (n = 84). Epo-treated babies received either 300 U/kg (n = 52) or 500 U/kg (n = 31), every other day for 2 weeks. Death or disability occurred in 43.8% of controls compared to 24.6% in the Epo groups ($P = 0.017$) at 18 months, with no discernable difference between Epo doses. No adverse effects of Epo were reported [32]. Another phase 1 trial (NEAT trial) is ongoing and will provide pharmacokinetic data for term infants.

Two retrospective reports support the thesis that Epo is neuroprotective. In a study designed to test the effects of Epo on erythropoiesis, infants ≤ 1250 g birth weight were randomized to Epo or control treatment from day 4 of life until 35 weeks corrected gestational age [34]. Infants < 1,000 g with serum Epo concentrations > 500 U/mL had higher Mental Development Index (MDI) scores than infants with Epo concentrations < 500 mU/mL when tested at 18 to 22 months corrected age [35]. Similarly, a retrospective cohort study of 82 infants < 1,500 g and ≤ 30 weeks of gestation at birth were evaluated at 2 years. Higher MDI scores were associated with higher cumulative doses of Epo, among other factors [36].

## Epo-mimetic peptides

The possibility of developing Epo-mimetic peptides that have specific subsets of Epo characteristics has been of great interest, because these molecules might circumvent unwanted clinical effects or provide improved permeability with the ability to cross the placenta or blood–brain barrier. The tissue protective functions of Epo can be separated from its stimulatory action on haematopoiesis and novel Epo derivatives such as asialo-Epo [37] and carbamylated Epo [38,39] have been developed. Epotris is an Epo-mimetic peptide which corresponds to the C alpha-helix region (amino-acid residues 92–111) of human Epo and which has neuroprotective properties [40]. No studies have been done to assess safety or efficacy of these compounds as prenatal treatments.

## Potential risks of high-dose erythropoietin

In adults, complications of Epo treatment include polycythaemia, rash, seizures, hypertension, shortened time to death, myocardial infarction, congestive heart failure, progression of tumours and stroke. None of these adverse effects have been reported in Epo-treated neonates. In addition, no prospective studies of Epo treatment of neonates have reported group differences in the incidence of neonatal morbidities, including intraventricular haemorrhage, retinopathy of prematurity (ROP), necrotizing enterocolitis, chronic lung disease or late-onset sepsis [41].

Epo is a potent erythropoietic growth factor. Thus, high doses of Epo given for neuroprotective treatment might be expected to increase erythropoiesis and possibly megakaryocytopoiesis. In neonatal rats, there is a transient increase in haematocrit following high-dose Epo [42] but in preterm infants, while three doses of Epo increased reticulocytosis, they did not affect haematocrit, likely due to early phlebotomy losses [30]. The effect of brief treatments of high-dose Epo on iron balance is not known.

The potential contribution of Epo to the development of ROP in preterm populations is controversial. ROP occurs in two phases, the first involving a loss of retinal vasculature following birth and the second involving uncontrolled proliferation of retinal vessels. EpoR are present on endothelial cells and Epo stimulation increases their angiogenic expression [43]. Early high-dose Epo might theoretically have a protective effect on the retina by ameliorating the first stage of ROP. Alternatively, the angiogenic properties of Epo may prevail, resulting in an increase in ROP. The Cochrane meta-analyses of prospective studies of Epo (for which ROP was not a primary outcome measure) showed an increase risk of ROP after early Epo exposure [44]. This analysis could not separate out the potential effects of anaemia or iron treatment as confounders [45]. Animal data suggest timing of Epo exposure might be very important. In a mouse model of ROP, early Epo treatment decreased the development of ROP, while late treatment given during the proliferative stage contributed to neovascularization and disease [45]. In contrast, using a rat model of ROP, no beneficial or harmful effects of repeated high-dose Epo administration (5,000 U/kg × 3 doses) on retinal vascularization were observed [46].

## Summary

Epo has great potential as a neuroprotective therapy in both preterm and term infants. It is easy to administer, FDA approved (although not for neuroprotective indications and not in neonates), relatively inexpensive, accessible and has been safe in all neonatal studies. More data are needed to define the optimal dose, number of doses and timing of treatment. Given what we know about the process of brain injury and repair from injury and what we know about mechanisms of Epo function, combined early and late treatment may provide optimal benefit. Early apoptosis and inflammation may be best treated with early doses, while stimulation of repair through angiogenesis and neurogenesis might best be accomplished using later doses. The ideal dosing schedule may vary with the mechanism of injury. Thus, a dosing regimen that is optimal for neuroprotection to reduce HIE sequelae may not be ideal for prophylaxis of white matter disease in ELBW preterm infants. Future possibilities include the use of Epo with other treatment modalities such as hypothermia. The possibility of improving protection by combining hypothermia with Epo is being investigated in adult populations [47,48].

## Cell-based therapy

Multiple types of cell-based therapy have been developed and tested over the past decade and have led to some interesting and promising avenues for therapy of neonatal hypoxic–ischaemic encephalopathy (HIE) (for review see [49]). Although stem cells have been widely tested for certain neurodegenerative conditions such as Parkinson's disease, this form of therapy is still at an early preclinical stage for treatment of neonatal HIE. Cells tested preclinically have ranged from those derived from human umbilical cord blood (HUCBC) and human adult bone marrow (MAPCS) to rodent derived cells such as mouse embryonic stem cells (ES), rodent mesenchymal stem cells (MSC) and neurally derived stem (NSC) and progenitor cells (NPC). Despite limited preclinical data, HUCBC are now in clinical trial for newborns with HIE (ClinicalTrials. gov, Identifier: NCT00593242, Fisher). This is a pilot study to evaluate the safety and feasibility of infusions of autologous umbilical cord blood cells in term newborn infants with moderate to severe HIE within 14 days of life.

The preclinical evidence for cell-based therapy will be reviewed in this section of the chapter.

## Fetal grafts

For neonatal HIE, cell-based therapy really began with studies using fetal neocortical grafts in adult rodents [50]. These investigators showed that injured cortical neurons sprouted fibres into surviving fetal grafts. Later, others showed in neonatal models of rodent hypoxia–ischaemia (HI) that fetal grafts could "take" [51], but the grafts did not assume normal cortical architecture or alter the extent of injury. However, using fetal cell suspensions, investigators demonstrated some benefit in functional outcome in the neonatal HI model [52]. These studies charted the path for the elegant studies of this decade.

## Neural stem cells

Multipotent precursors such as neural stem cells self-renew and retain the ability to differentiate into a variety of neuronal and non-neuronal cell types throughout the brain. These cells reside in neurogenic zones throughout life, including the subventricular zone lining the ventricles and the subgranular layer of the hippocampal dentate gyrus in rodents. They seem to be primarily responsible for maintaining baseline turnover of cells, as well as replacing injured cells through migration to tissue after ischaemic injury. NSC transplantation has shown potential as a therapeutic strategy in adult animal models of brain injury. Implanted cells integrate into injured tissue [53], decrease volume loss [54–56] and improve behavioural outcomes [57,58] in adult models of stroke and ischaemia. In neonatal models, intraventricular implantation of NSCs after HI results in their migration to injured areas [55,56] and differentiation into neurons, astrocytes, oligodendrocytes and undifferentiated progenitors [56]. These cells promote regeneration, angiogenesis and neuronal cell survival in both rodent and primate models, while non-neuronal progeny inhibit inflammation and scar formation [59,60]. However, it appears that for some multipotent stem cells, like the astrocytic stem cell, injury must be present in order for the cells to differentiate into neuronal phenotypes in the neonatal brain [61]. Better success with transplantation has occurred in the neonatal model when NSCs are transplanted with factors that can modulate the endogenous environment, such as NSCs co-injected with chondroitinase (ChABC) that may trigger the release of endogenous neurotrophic factors [62].

Although complications of implantation have not been noted in these models, efficacy does depend on timing of implantation and the therapeutic window is not known. More recent technology enables labelling of stem cells, which can then be tracked from the site of implantation through their migratory path into the ischaemic tissue [63–66], making their identification in humans possible.

# Human umbilical cord blood cells

The value of human umbilical cord blood cells lies in their ability to be given systemically, with the potential to migrate to the brain. The key population of cells in HUCB is the mesenchymal stem cells that are able to differentiate not only into cells of mesodermal lineage, but into neurons as well. MSCs also migrate to the ischaemic brain, and cells derived from bone marrow MSCs possess neuronal properties that allow them to hone to ischaemic tissue. Robust growth of MSCs after intracranial injection is seen better in the neonatal than the adult brain [67]. Cord blood MSCs may also have effects on the innate and adaptive immunity of the recipient [68], providing neuroprotection in adult models of stroke through modulation of regulatory T

cells. In keeping with this theory, intraperitoneal transplantation of HUCB 3 hours after an HI insult in P7 rat pups resulted in functional improvement early after the injury. This improvement was associated with a decrease in the number of activated microglial cells in the cerebral cortex of treated animals [49], suggesting an impact on neuro-inflammation.

One of the difficulties with using peripheral cord blood cells is delivery into the ischaemic brain. When HUCB cells were given intravenously 1 day after the HI insult in P7 rats no benefit either structurally or functionally was seen 3 weeks later and only a few HUCB cells were located in the brain [69]. However, when HUCB therapy is combined with mannitol to open the blood–brain barrier 7 days after an HI insult, improvement is seen. Behavioural tests at post-transplantation days 7 and 14 showed that these HI animals had improved function. In addition, elevated levels of GDNF, NGF and BDNF in those that received HUCB cells alone or when combined with mannitol were observed. However, there were very few HUCB cells detected, suggesting that it was the upregulation of trophic factors, rather than cell replacement itself, that contributed to the functional improvement [70].

# Mesenchymal stem cells

Human MSCs have been delivered intracardiac to neonatal rats 3 days after the hypoxic–ischaemic insult. Although brain volume was not restored by MSC, nor were cell types different, neurologic performance was significantly improved on the cylinder test at 14 and 21, but not 40 days after therapy [71].

One of the most exciting recent studies showing potential efficacy of cell-based therapy used repeated intracranial treatments with MSCs to induce repair in a neonatal rodent model of perinatal asphyxia [72]. The investigators demonstrated that a single treatment 3 days after the injury improved sensorimotor function and reduced the lesion anatomically. An additional intracranial dose 10 days after injury further improved function and with this double therapy, there was also axonal remodelling in the spinal cord as well. While the single therapy at 3 days revealed an increase in newly born neurons and oligodendrocytes, the second dose 10 days later did not increase numbers of these cells. These studies suggest that mesenchymal stem cells adapt their growth and differentiation factor production according to the environment at the time of injection. This study supports the role for the injured brain milieu in controlling the reaction to exogenous therapy and highlights the importance of timing of therapy after injury.

When adult multipotent progenitor cells (MAPCS) derived from human bone marrow are given either intracerebrally or intravenously to the neonatal ischaemic brain 1 week after the insult, cell preservation can be seen 14 days after transplantation [73].

## ES cell-derived precursors

Using a mouse ES cell line, investigators injected stem cell grafts 2 days after HI injury in C57/Bl6 rat pups intracerebroventricularly after they were induced to neurally differentiate *in vitro* [74]. This procedure appeared to increase the number of neurons in the CA1 region of the hippocampus in lesioned animals receiving the graft and using a LacZ reporter, engrafted cells were found in the hippocampus up to 8 months after placement. Functional improvement using the Morris water maze was also realized in the engrafted group of mice. This is the first report that transplanted cells migrate and alter functional recovery favourably. Importantly, no tumour cells were observed in any of the transplanted mice with the differentiated ES cell-derived cells.

## Growth factors by means of cell-based therapy

Some of the growth factors cited above in this chapter can boost the endogenous neurogenetic response to neonatal ischaemic injury in rodents, such as Epo, basic fibroblast growth factor (bFGF) and granulocyte-colony stimulating factor (G-CSF) [75–77].

Grafting of encapsulated glial cell line-derived cells to deliver growth factors is another method to boost the endogenous neurogenic response. In a series of studies, baby hamster kidney cells were transfected with human GDNF, implanted into the 12-day-old Wistar rats and then 2 days later the pups received a hypoxic/ischaemic stress. One week later, brain damage was measured and appeared to be less in implanted brains [78]. A follow-up study showed sustained structural and functional improvement after 18 weeks [79].

## Summary

Accumulating evidence suggests that cell-based therapies may provide benefit to the newborn brain after a sustained hypoxic–ischaemic insult. Further data are needed in larger animal models to understand the mechanisms, timing and selection of cell-based therapies. The clinical feasibility trial ongoing at Duke may provide necessary safety data for the human newborn with HIE, but caution and additional data should be realized before a randomized clinical trial can be executed.

# Anaesthetics and neuronal injury during development

## Introduction

The initiation of general anaesthetics for treatment of brain injury was predicated upon their ability to profoundly suppress neuronal activity and thereby reduce the brain's metabolic rate. Based upon the fact that failure of energetics is a pathogenic step in many types of brain injury, including HIE [80], the goal of decreasing energy requirements with anaesthetics was actively pursued and spawned use of barbiturate coma [81]. What has become evident is that the putative salubrious effects of general anaesthetics for brain injury are based upon their ability to interact with and modulate specific protein targets that play a pivotal role in neuronal injury and repair [82]. Notwithstanding the undoubted neuroprotective efficacy of anaesthetics in many injury paradigms, these powerful drugs are also capable of disrupting neurodevelopment and hence their safety in the early postnatal period is the subject of intense investigation.

Based upon molecular targets, as well as clinical and electroencephalographic effects, anaesthetics may be classified as follows:

1. Intravenous drugs, such as propofol, etomidate and barbiturates, which act primarily on $GABA_A$ receptors (GABAergic) and produce unconsciousness more effectively than immobilization
2. Xenon, nitrous oxide, cyclopropane and ketamine, which act primarily on N-methyl-D-aspartate (NMDA) receptors and are most effective as analgesics
3. Potent volatile anaesthetics that possess properties of unconsciousness, immobilization and analgesia to about the same degree. These agents are pleiotropic in their targets with none qualifying as a unitary mechanism of their anaesthetic properties

4. Intravenous highly selective agonists at specific receptors of which there is a single example – the $\alpha_2$ adrenoceptor agonist dexmedetomidine which is a general anaesthetic only at very high doses.

In this section of the chapter, we detail the mechanisms and uses of the more promising anaesthetic candidates for possible prevention and treatment of HIE: xenon and the potent volatile anaesthetic agents as well as those anaesthetic and sedative agents that are likely to cause developmental complications (barbiturates are dealt with in Chapter 11). Why anaesthetics are both helpful and harmful to the injured and developing nervous system respectively is not completely resolved but we will attempt to provide insights into possible mechanisms for this paradox in the setting of HIE.

# Neuroprotective effects of anaesthetics

## Xenon

This noble gas has all the features of the ideal anaesthetic agent apart from the high cost of extracting it from the atmosphere where it is present at an extremely low concentration (0.09 parts per billion). This expense precludes its routine use for surgeries. Following the revelation that xenon is an antagonist of the NMDA subtype of the glutamate receptor [83], a series of *in vitro* studies established that xenon reduced injury in a mouse neuronal-glial cell culture induced by excitotoxins, oxygen deprivation or oxygen–glucose deprivation (OGD) [84]. Subsequently, the neuroprotective

effects of xenon have been demonstrated by several groups using *in vivo* models of acute neuronal injury involving administration of excitotoxins to rats [85], cardiopulmonary bypass in rats [86], middle cerebral artery occlusion in mice [87] and rats [88], and cardiac arrest in pigs [89]. As a neuroprotectant xenon is more efficacious than other NMDA antagonists (including either gavestinel or dizolcipine that have been clinically tested) and does not share the psychotomimetic side-effects that characterize this class of neuroprotectant. Xenon's enhanced efficacy and lack of toxicity resulted in a broadening of the search for possible neuroprotective mechanisms. Xenon lacks the dopamine-releasing properties that are present in other NMDA antagonists and this probably accounts for the absence of the "Olney lesion" [90]. Regarding xenon's enhanced efficacy three other mechanisms have been identified. Xenon activates two species of potassium channels including the inwardly rectifying $K_{ATP}$ [91] and the two pore domain leak current [92], both of which have been linked to neuroprotection. However, it is the fact that xenon increases the translational efficiency of HIF-1$\alpha$ through an mTOR pathway [93] that has resulted in its potential application in HIE for both post-injury treatment and as a preconditioner. The prolonged increase in expression of HIF-1$\alpha$ by xenon causes upregulation of cytoprotective proteins such as erythropoietin (dealt with elsewhere in this chapter), VEGF and glucose transporter 1 protein [93] (Figure 18.2).

The possible utility of xenon for HIE was first evaluated in 2005 in the Vannucci model; xenon was shown to be effective in reducing infarct volume when

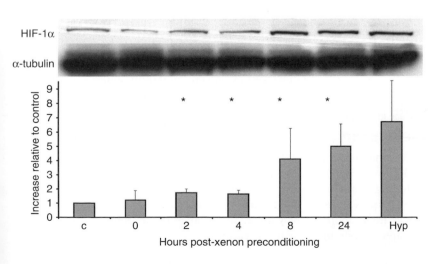

**Figure 18.2.** Effect of xenon exposure on expression of HIF-1$\alpha$ in mouse brains. Exposure to 75% xenon and 25% oxygen for 2 hours increased HIF-1$\alpha$ protein expression in the mouse brain after 2 hours (*$P < 0.05$). By comparison exposure to 8% hypoxia (hyp) caused an acute increase in mouse brains within 10 minutes. N = 3/group.

administered up to 6 hours post-injury [94]. Independently, this finding was subsequently corroborated [95]. Thereafter, the preconditioning effect of xenon was also demonstrated in the Vannucci model [96]; in this paradigm it was demonstrated that xenon activated the anti-apoptotic effectors Bcl-XL and Bcl-2 possibly by increasing phosphorylation of the transcription factor cyclic-AMP response element binding protein [96]. It is not known which of xenon's known neuroprotective molecular targets is required for this property.

More recently, supplementing moderate hypothermia strategies with xenon has been explored in several preclinical models of HIE; the nature of the interaction may well be synergistic [96]. Further elaboration of studies investigating the combination of xenon with hypothermia for HIE can be found in Chapter 2.

## Other noble gases

The utility of other noble gases in neuronal injury settings has recently been explored, not because of their anaesthetic properties but because these elements are chemically inert with a full outer shell of electrons [97]. Argon appears to be most promising in this regard, although its efficacy is much lower than that of xenon and it lacks anaesthetic properties under isobaric condition (i.e. at one atmosphere).

### Potent volatile anaesthetics

Each of isoflurane, sevoflurane and desflurane has been shown to exhibit neuroprotection in several neuronal injury models. The mechanisms include activation of KATP channels and PI3K-AKT pathways as well as modulation of pathways that give rise to reactive oxygen species. To date, only sevoflurane has been tested in a model that is relevant to HIE; it was found to be effective in a preconditioning paradigm at analgesic doses [98].

## Neuroapoptotic and injurious effects of anaesthetics during development

Prolonged exposure to potent volatile anaesthetics (including isoflurane [99], sevoflurane [100]), intravenous GABAergic agents (including propofol [101], midazolam [102], diazepam [99]) and NMDA antagonists (ketamine [102]) produces neuroapoptosis during the period of rapid synaptogenesis in several species ranging from rodents to non-human primate models. Deficits in learning and memory have followed neonatal exposure to these anaesthetics when tested weeks to months later. Apart from the neuroapoptotic properties, anaesthetics are also capable of interfering with dendritic arbour development [103].

## Mechanisms

Several mechanisms have been proposed for the development of anaesthetic-induced apoptotic neurodegeneration. It appears unlikely that a physiological derangement accompanying the anaesthetic state is the cause since neither xenon [104] nor dexmedetomidine [105] anaesthesia induces neuroapoptosis; in fact both of these drugs are capable of preventing neuroapoptosis induced by other anaesthetic agents. Moreover, anaesthetic neurotoxicity has also been demonstrated *in vitro* in hippocampal slice preparations in which physiologic parameters were carefully controlled [104]. Another mechanism that has been advanced is "synaptic silencing" that prevents expression of trophic factors (BDNF) required to sustain neurons forming a synapse [106]. It is noteworthy that both xenon and dexmedetomidine *increase* expression of trophic factors especially BDNF and are also two anaesthetics that do not produce neuroapoptosis. It has been conjectured that while xenon is an NMDA antagonist, it may have selectivity for the extrasynaptic NMDA receptors, leaving neurotransmission at glutamatergic synapses intact. The "excitotoxicity" theory for the neuroapoptic properties of anaesthetics is based upon the fact that the GABA-A receptor is excitatory during early neurodevelopment. Also, antagonism of the NMDA receptors can result in upregulation of the NR1 subunit resulting in excessive calcium influx. It remains to be clarified how NMDA antagonism, GABA-A agonism, an imbalance between excitation and inhibition and modulation of neurotrophin activity can lead to the activation of apoptotic pathways. Also, apoptosis may be triggered through specific targets including IP3 or ryanodine receptors as well as specific mitochondrial targets. Because *in vitro* studies revealed that volatile anaesthetic agents reduce the proliferation of neuronal progenitor cells [107], the inability of the brain to compensate for injury may also play a role in the anaesthetic-induced injury during neurodevelopment.

## Human studies

Direct extrapolation of data from animal models (even those involving non-human primates) to humans is highly speculative because of the differences in brain development, anatomy, pharmacokinetics and pharmacodynamics as well as the duration of exposure required to produce injury [108,109]. Furthermore, animal models have not examined the impact of the surgery-requiring illnesses, postoperative morbidity and the use of analgesics which occur in the clinical setting. Notwithstanding these differences, the demonstration of neuronal death in animal models during neurodevelopment is of significant concern [110,111] and the US Food and Drug Administration (FDA) has called for further research into the subject.

The FDA and the IARS have created SmartTots (Strategies for Mitigating Anesthesia-Related Toxicity in Tots) to support clinical investigation in this area (www.smartots.org). Retrospective studies have linked two or more operations before the age of 4 to increased risk of learning disability [112], although a retrospective study of twins failed to detect a causal relationship [113]. As with the animal models, appropriate controls for the presence of the surgical condition as well as for co-morbidities has been lacking in these epidemiologic studies.

## Future

Given the multiple means by which anaesthetics both protect and injure the brain, it is highly unlikely that a unifying mechanism can explain both these processes. Clinical trials seeking to identify the utility of anaesthetics for the treatment of HIE (in combination with moderate therapeutic hypothermia) are now ongoing albeit with a surrogate outcome.

There are also ongoing prospective human studies on anaesthetic-induced neurotoxicity, but these are unlikely to shed further light for some years to come because of the length of follow-up required (5 years). Until then it would seem prudent that the future use of anaesthetics as an adjunct to hypothermia in the management of HIE should be confined to those in which neurotoxicity has not been demonstrated, i.e. xenon and dexmedetomidine. Furthermore, critical review of available databases need to be undertaken to examine the possible adverse impact of sedatives during hypothermic therapy for HIE.

## References

1. Juul SE, Yachnis AT, Christensen RD. Tissue distribution of erythropoietin and erythropoietin receptor in the developing human fetus. *Early Hum Dev* 1998;**52**:235–49.

2. Yu X, Shacka JJ, Eells JB, et al. Erythropoietin receptor signalling is required for normal brain development. *Development* 2002;**129**:505–16.

3. Chen ZY, Asavaritikrai P, Prchal JT, Noguchi CT. Endogenous erythropoietin signaling is required for normal neural progenitor cell proliferation. *J Biol Chem* 2007;**282**:25875–83.

4. Juul SE, Yachnis AT, Rojiani AM, Christensen RD. Immunohistochemical localization of erythropoietin and its receptor in the developing human brain. *Pediatr Dev Pathol* 1999;**2**:148–58.

5. Wang L, Zhang Z, Wang Y, Zhang R, Chopp M. Treatment of stroke with erythropoietin enhances neurogenesis and angiogenesis and improves neurological function in rats. *Stroke* 2004;**35**:1732–7.

6. Wallach I, Zhang J, Hartmann A, et al. Erythropoietin-receptor gene regulation in neuronal cells. *Pediatr Res* 2009;**65**:619–24.

7. Sugawa M, Sakurai Y, Ishikawa-Ieda Y, Suzuki H, Asou H. Effects of erythropoietin on glial cell development; oligodendrocyte maturation and astrocyte proliferation. *Neurosci Res* 2002;**44**:391–403.

8. Nagai A, Nakagawa E, Choi HB, et al. Erythropoietin and erythropoietin receptors in human CNS neurons, astrocytes, microglia and oligodendrocytes grown in culture. *J Neuropathol Exp Neurol* 2001;**60**:386–92.

9. Chong ZZ, Kang JQ, Maiese K. Erythropoietin fosters both intrinsic and extrinsic neuronal protection through modulation of microglia, Akt1, Bad and caspase-mediated pathways. *Br J Pharmacol* 2003;**138**:1107–18.

10. Digicaylioglu M, Lipton SA. Erythropoietin-mediated neuroprotection involves cross-talk between Jak2 and NF-kappaB signalling cascades. *Nature* 2001;**412**:641–7.

11. Genc K, Genc S, Baskin H, Semin I. Erythropoietin decreases cytotoxicity and nitric oxide formation induced by inflammatory stimuli in rat oligodendrocytes. *Physiol Res* 2006;**55**:33–8.

12. Vitellaro-Zuccarello L, Mazzetti S, Madaschi L, et al. Chronic erythropoietin-mediated effects on the expression of astrocyte markers in a rat model of contusive spinal cord injury. *Neuroscience* 2008;**151**:452–66.

13. Brines ML, Ghezzi P, Keenan S, et al. Erythropoietin crosses the blood-brain barrier to protect against

experimental brain injury. *Proc Natl Acad Sci U S A* 2000;**97**:10526–31.

14. Juul SE, McPherson RJ, Farrell FX, et al. Erythropoietin concentrations in cerebrospinal fluid of nonhuman primates and fetal sheep following high-dose recombinant erythropoietin. *Biol Neonate* 2004;**85**:138–44.

15. Statler PA, McPherson RJ, Bauer LA, Kellert BA, Juul SE. Pharmacokinetics of high-dose recombinant erythropoietin in plasma and brain of neonatal rats. *Pediatr Res* 2007;**61**:671–5.

16. Kellert BA, McPherson RJ, Juul SE. A comparison of high-dose recombinant erythropoietin treatment regimens in brain-injured neonatal rats. *Pediatr Res* 2007;**61**:451–5.

17. Weber A, Dzietko M, Berns M, et al. Neuronal damage after moderate hypoxia and erythropoietin. *Neurobiol Dis* 2005;**20**:594–600.

18. Keller M, Yang J, Griesmaier E, et al. Erythropoietin is neuroprotective against NMDA-receptor-mediated excitotoxic brain injury in newborn mice. *Neurobiol Dis* 2006;**24**:357–66.

19. Kawakami M, Iwasaki S, Sato K, Takahashi M. Erythropoietin inhibits calcium-induced neurotransmitter release from clonal neuronal cells. *Biochem Biophys Res Commun* 2000;**279**:293–7.

20. Sun Y, Calvert JW, Zhang JH. Neonatal hypoxia/ischemia is associated with decreased inflammatory mediators after erythropoietin administration. *Stroke* 2005;**36**:1672–8.

21. Dzietko M, Felderhoff-Mueser U, Sifringer M, et al. Erythropoietin protects the developing brain against N-methyl-D-aspartate receptor antagonist neurotoxicity. *Neurobiol Dis* 2004;**15**:177–87.

22. Wang L, Chopp M, Gregg SR, et al. Neural progenitor cells treated with EPO induce angiogenesis through the production of VEGF. *J Cereb Blood Flow Metab* 2008;**28**:1361–8.

23. Bocker-Meffert S, Rosenstiel P, Rohl C, et al. Erythropoietin and VEGF promote neural outgrowth from retinal explants in postnatal rats. *Invest Ophthalmol Vis Sci* 2002;**43**:2021–6.

24. Wang L, Zhang ZG, Zhang RL, et al. Matrix metalloproteinase 2 (MMP2) and MMP9 secreted by erythropoietin-activated endothelial cells promote neural progenitor cell migration. *J Neurosci* 2006;**26**:5996–6003.

25. Xiong Y, Mahmood A, Qu C, et al. Erythropoietin improves histological and functional outcomes after traumatic brain injury in mice in the absence of the neural erythropoietin receptor. *J Neurotrauma* 2010;**27**:205–15.

26. Gonzalez FF, Abel R, Almli CR, et al. Erythropoietin sustains cognitive function and brain volume after neonatal stroke. *Dev Neurosci* 2009;**31**:403–11.

27. Tsai PT, Ohab JJ, Kertesz N, et al. A critical role of erythropoietin receptor in neurogenesis and post-stroke recovery. *J Neurosci* 2006;**26**:1269–74.

28. Rees S, Hale N, De Matteo R, et al. Erythropoietin is neuroprotective in a preterm ovine model of endotoxin-induced brain injury. *J Neuropathol Exp Neurol* 2010;**69**:306–19.

29. Juul SE, Aylward E, Richards T, et al. Prenatal cord clamping in newborn Macaca nemestrina: a model of perinatal asphyxia. *Dev Neurosci* 2007;**29**:311–20.

30. Juul SE, McPherson RJ, Bauer LA, et al. A phase I/II trial of high-dose erythropoietin in extremely low birth weight infants: pharmacokinetics and safety. *Pediatrics* 2008;**122**:383–91.

31. Fauchere JC, Dame C, Vonthein R, et al. An approach to using recombinant erythropoietin for neuroprotection in very preterm infants. *Pediatrics* 2008;**122**:375–82.

32. Zhu C, Kang W, Xu F, et al. Erythropoietin improved neurologic outcomes in newborns with hypoxic-ischemic encephalopathy. *Pediatrics* 2009;**124**: e218–26.

33. Elmahdy H, El-Mashad AR, El-Bahrawy H, et al. Human recombinant erythropoietin in asphyxia neonatorum: pilot trial. *Pediatrics* 2010;**125**:e1135–42.

34. Ohls RK, Ehrenkranz RA, Das A, et al. Neurodevelopmental outcome and growth at 18 to 22 months' corrected age in extremely low birth weight infants treated with early erythropoietin and iron. *Pediatrics* 2004;**114**:1287–91.

35. Bierer R, Peceny MC, Hartenberger CH, Ohls RK. Erythropoietin concentrations and neurodevelopmental outcome in preterm infants. *Pediatrics* 2006;**118**:e635–40.

36. Brown MS, Eichorst D, Lala-Black B, Gonzalez R. Higher cumulative doses of erythropoietin and developmental outcomes in preterm infants. *Pediatrics* 2009;**124**:e681–7.

37. Mennini T, De Paola M, Bigini P, et al. Nonhematopoietic erythropoietin derivatives prevent motoneuron degeneration in vitro and in vivo. *Mol Med* 2006;**12**:153–60.

38. Sturm B, Helminger M, Steinkellner H, et al. Carbamylated erythropoietin increases frataxin independent from the erythropoietin receptor. *Eur J Clin Invest* 2010;**40**:561–5.

39. Wang L, Zhang ZG, Gregg SR, et al. The Sonic hedgehog pathway mediates carbamylated erythropoietin-enhanced proliferation and

differentiation of adult neural progenitor cells. *J Biol Chem* 2007;**282**:32462–70.

40. Pankratova S, Kiryushko D, Sonn K, et al. Neuroprotective properties of a novel, non-haematopoietic agonist of the erythropoietin receptor. *Brain* 2010;**133**:2281–94.

41. Ohls RK. The use of erythropoietin in neonates. *Clin Perinatol* 2000;**27**:681–96.

42. McPherson RJ, Demers EJ, Juul SE. Safety of high-dose recombinant erythropoietin in a neonatal rat model. *Neonatology* 2007;**91**:36–43.

43. Ribatti D, Presta M, Vacca A, et al. Human erythropoietin induces a pro-angiogenic phenotype in cultured endothelial cells and stimulates neovascularization in vivo. *Blood* 1999;**93**:2627–36.

44. Ohlsson A, Aher SM. Early erythropoietin for preventing red blood cell transfusion in preterm and/or low birth weight infants. *Cochrane Database Syst Rev* 2006;**3**:CD004863.

45. Chen J, Smith LE. A double-edged sword: erythropoietin eyed in retinopathy of prematurity. *J AAPOS* 2008;**12**:221–2.

46. Slusarski JD, McPherson RJ, Wallace GN, Juul SE. High-dose erythropoietin does not exacerbate retinopathy of prematurity in rats. *Pediatr Res* 2009;**66**:625–30.

47. Cariou A, Claessens YE, Pene F, et al. Early high-dose erythropoietin therapy and hypothermia after out-of-hospital cardiac arrest: a matched control study. *Resuscitation* 2008;**76**:397–404.

48. Tseng MY, Hutchinson PJ, Richards HK, et al. Acute systemic erythropoietin therapy to reduce delayed ischemic deficits following aneurysmal subarachnoid hemorrhage: a Phase II randomized, double-blind, placebo-controlled trial. Clinical article. *J Neurosurg* 2009;**111**:171–80.

49. Pimentel-Coelho PM, Mendez-Otero R. Cell therapy for neonatal hypoxic-ischemic encephalopathy. *Stem Cells Dev* 2010;**19**:299–310.

50. Sharp FR, Gonzalez MF, Ferriero DM, Sagar SM. Injured adult neocortical neurons sprout fibers into surviving fetal frontal cortex transplants: evidence using NADPH-diaphorase staining. *Neurosci Lett* 1986;**65**:204–8.

51. Elsayed MH, Hogan TP, Shaw PL, Castro AJ. Use of fetal cortical grafts in hypoxic-ischemic brain injury in neonatal rats. *Exp Neurol* 1996;**137**:127–41.

52. Jansen EM, Solberg L, Underhill S, et al. Transplantation of fetal neocortex ameliorates sensorimotor and locomotor deficits following neonatal ischemic-hypoxic brain injury in rats. *Exp Neurol* 1997;**147**:487–97.

53. Park KI, Teng YD, Snyder EY. The injured brain interacts reciprocally with neural stem cells supported by scaffolds to reconstitute lost tissue. *Nat Biotechnol* 2002;**20**:1111–7.

54. Hoehn M, Kustermann E, Blunk J, et al. Monitoring of implanted stem cell migration in vivo: a highly resolved in vivo magnetic resonance imaging investigation of experimental stroke in rat. *Proc Natl Acad Sci U S A* 2002;**99**:16267–72.

55. Park KI, Himes BT, Stieg PE, et al. Neural stem cells may be uniquely suited for combined gene therapy and cell replacement: evidence from engraftment of Neurotrophin-3-expressing stem cells in hypoxic-ischemic brain injury. *Exp Neurol* 2006;**199**:179–90.

56. Park KI, Hack MA, Ourednik J, et al. Acute injury directs the migration, proliferation and differentiation of solid organ stem cells: evidence from the effect of hypoxia-ischemia in the CNS on clonal "reporter" neural stem cells. *Exp Neurol* 2006;**199**:156–78.

57. Capone C, Frigerio S, Fumagalli S, et al. Neurosphere-derived cells exert a neuroprotective action by changing the ischemic microenvironment. *PLoS One* 2007;**2**:e373.

58. Hicks AU, Hewlett K, Windle V, et al. Enriched environment enhances transplanted subventricular zone stem cell migration and functional recovery after stroke. *Neuroscience* 2007;**146**:31–40.

59. Imitola J, Raddassi K, Park KI, et al. Directed migration of neural stem cells to sites of CNS injury by the stromal cell-derived factor 1alpha/CXC chemokine receptor 4 pathway. *Proc Natl Acad Sci U S A* 2004;**101**:18117–22.

60. Mueller FJ, Serobyan N, Schraufstatter IU, et al. Adhesive interactions between human neural stem cells and inflamed human vascular endothelium are mediated by integrins. *Stem Cells* 2006;**24**:2367–72.

61. Zheng T, Rossignol C, Leibovici A, et al. Transplantation of multipotent astrocytic stem cells into a rat model of neonatal hypoxic-ischemic encephalopathy. *Brain Res* 2006;**1112**:99–105.

62. Sato Y, Nakanishi K, Hayakawa M, et al. Reduction of brain injury in neonatal hypoxic-ischemic rats by intracerebroventricular injection of neural stem/progenitor cells together with chondroitinase ABC. *Reprod Sci* 2008;**15**:613–20.

63. Modo M, Mellodew K, Cash D, et al. Mapping transplanted stem cell migration after a stroke: a serial, in vivo magnetic resonance imaging study. *Neuroimage* 2004;**21**:311–7.

64. Guzman R, Uchida N, Bliss TM, et al. Long-term monitoring of transplanted human neural stem cells in developmental and pathological contexts with MRI. *Proc Natl Acad Sci U S A* 2007;**104**:10211–6.

65. Rice HE, Hsu EW, Sheng H, et al. Superparamagnetic iron oxide labeling and transplantation of adipose-derived stem cells in middle cerebral artery occlusion-injured mice. *AJR Am J Roentgenol* 2007;**188**:1101–8.

66. Obenaus A, Robbins M, Blanco G, et al. Multi-modal magnetic resonance imaging alterations in two rat models of mild neurotrauma. *J Neurotrauma* 2007;**24**:1147–60.

67. Phinney DG, Baddoo M, Dutreil M, et al. Murine mesenchymal stem cells transplanted to the central nervous system of neonatal versus adult mice exhibit distinct engraftment kinetics and express receptors that guide neuronal cell migration. *Stem Cells Dev* 2006;**15**:437–7.

68. Liesz A, Suri-Payer E, Veltkamp C, et al. Regulatory T cells are key cerebroprotective immunomodulators in acute experimental stroke. *Nat Med* 2009;**15**:192–9.

69. de Paula S, Vitola AS, Greggio S, et al. Hemispheric brain injury and behavioral deficits induced by severe neonatal hypoxia-ischemia in rats are not attenuated by intravenous administration of human umbilical cord blood cells. *Pediatr Res* 2009;**65**:631–5.

70. Yasuhara T, Hara K, Maki M, et al. Mannitol facilitates neurotrophic factor up-regulation and behavioural recovery in neonatal hypoxic-ischaemic rats with human umbilical cord blood grafts. *J Cell Mol Med* 2010;**14**:914–21.

71. Lee JA, Kim BI, Jo CH, et al. Mesenchymal stem-cell transplantation for hypoxic-ischemic brain injury in neonatal rat model. *Pediatr Res* 2010;**67**:42–6.

72. van Velthoven CT, Kavelaars A, van Bel F, Heijnen CJ. Repeated mesenchymal stem cell treatment after neonatal hypoxia-ischemia has distinct effects on formation and maturation of new neurons and oligodendrocytes leading to restoration of damage, corticospinal motor tract activity and sensorimotor function. *J Neurosci* 2010;**30**:9603–11.

73. Yasuhara T, Hara K, Maki M, et al. Intravenous grafts recapitulate the neurorestoration afforded by intracerebrally delivered multipotent adult progenitor cells in neonatal hypoxic-ischemic rats. *J Cereb Blood Flow Metab* 2008;**28**:1804–10.

74. Ma J, Wang Y, Yang J, et al. Treatment of hypoxic-ischemic encephalopathy in mouse by transplantation of embryonic stem cell-derived cells. *Neurochem Int* 2007;**51**:57–65.

75. Gonzalez FF, McQuillen P, Mu D, et al. Erythropoietin enhances long-term neuroprotection and neurogenesis in neonatal stroke. *Dev Neurosci* 2007;**29**:321–30.

76. Jin-qiao S, Bin S, Wen-hao Z, Yi Y. Basic fibroblast growth factor stimulates the proliferation and differentiation of neural stem cells in neonatal rats after ischemic brain injury. *Brain Dev* 2009;**31**:331–40.

77. Yata K, Matchett GA, Tsubokawa T, et al. Granulocyte-colony stimulating factor inhibits apoptotic neuron loss after neonatal hypoxia-ischemia in rats. *Brain Res* 2007;**1145**:227–38.

78. Katsuragi S, Ikeda T, Date I, et al. Grafting of glial cell line-derived neurotrophic factor secreting cells for hypoxic-ischemic encephalopathy in neonatal rats. *Am J Obstet Gynecol* 2005;**192**:1137–45.

79. Katsuragi S, Ikeda T, Date I, et al. Implantation of encapsulated glial cell line-derived neurotrophic factor-secreting cells prevents long-lasting learning impairment following neonatal hypoxic-ischemic brain insult in rats. *Am J Obstet Gynecol* 2005;**192**:1028–37.

80. Lorek A, Takei Y, Cady EB, et al. Delayed ("secondary") cerebral energy failure after acute hypoxia-ischemia in the newborn piglet: continuous 48-hour studies by phosphorus magnetic resonance spectroscopy. *Pediatr Res* 1994;**36**:699–706.

81. Todd MM, Chadwick HS, Shapiro HM, et al. The neurologic effects of thiopental therapy following experimental cardiac arrest in cats. *Anesthesiology* 1982;**57**:76.

82. Franks NP. General anaesthesia: from molecular targets to neuronal pathways of sleep and arousal. *Nat Rev Neurosci* 2008;**9**:370–86.

83. Franks NP, Dickinson R, de Sousa SL, Hall AC, Lieb WR. How does xenon produce anaesthesia? *Nature* 1998;**396**:324.

84. Wilhelm S, Ma D, Maze M, Franks NP. Effects of xenon on in vitro and in vivo models of neuronal injury. *Anesthesiology* 2002;**96**:1485–91.

85. Ma D, Wilhelm S, Maze M, Franks NP. Neuroprotective and neurotoxic properties of the 'inert' gas, xenon. *Br J Anaesth* 2002;**89**:739–46.

86. Ma D, Yang H, Lynch J, et al. Xenon attenuates cardiopulmonary bypass-induced neurologic and neurocognitive dysfunction in the rat. *Anesthesiology* 2003;**98**:690–8.

87. Homi HM, Yokoo N, Ma D, et al. The neuroprotective effect of xenon administration during transient middle cerebral artery occlusion in mice. *Anesthesiology* 2003;**99**:876–81.

88. David HN, Leveille F, Chazalviel L, et al. Reduction of ischemic brain damage by nitrous oxide and xenon. *J Cereb Blood Flow Metab* 2003;**23**:1168–73.

89. Schmidt M, Marx T, Gloggl E, Reinelt H, Schirmer U. Xenon attenuates cerebral damage after ischemia in pigs. *Anesthesiology* 2005;**102**:929–36.

90. Sakamoto S, Nakao S, Masuzawa M, et al. The differential effects of nitrous oxide and xenon on extracellular dopamine levels in the rat nucleus

accumbens: a microdialysis study. *Anesth Analg* 2006;**103**:1459–63.

91. Bantel C, Maze M, Trapp S. Noble gas xenon is a novel adenosine triphosphate-sensitive potassium channel opener. *Anesthesiology* 2010;**112**:623–30.

92. Gruss M, Bushell TJ, Bright DP, et al. Two-pore-domain K+ channels are a novel target for the anesthetic gases xenon, nitrous oxide and cyclopropane. *Mol Pharmacol* 2004;**65**:443–52.

93. Ma D, Lim T, Xu J, et al. Xenon preconditioning protects against renal ischemic-reperfusion injury via HIF-1alpha activation. *J Am Soc Nephrol* 2009;**20**:713–20.

94. Ma D, Hossain M, Chow A, et al. Xenon and hypothermia combine to provide neuroprotection from neonatal asphyxia. *Ann Neurol* 2005;**58**:182–93.

95. Dingley J, Tooley J, Porter H, Thoresen M. Xenon provides short-term neuroprotection in neonatal rats when administered after hypoxia-ischemia. *Stroke* 2006;**37**:501–6.

96. Ma D, Hossain M, Pettet GK, et al. Xenon preconditioning reduces brain damage from neonatal asphyxia in rats. *J Cereb Blood Flow Metab* 2006;**26**:199–208.

97. Jawad N, Rizvi M, Gu J, et al. Neuroprotection (and lack of neuroprotection) afforded by a series of noble gases in an in vitro model of neuronal injury. *Neurosci Lett* 2009;**460**:232–36.

98. Luo Y, Ma D, Ieong E, et al. Xenon and sevoflurane protect against brain injury in a neonatal asphyxia model. *Anesthesiology* 2008;**109**:782–9.

99. Jevtovic-Todorovic V, Hartman RE, Izumi Y, et al. Early exposure to common anesthetic agents causes widespread neurodegeneration in the developing rat brain and persistent learning deficits. *J Neurosci* 2003;**23**:876–82.

100. Liang G, Ward C, Peng J, et al. Isoflurane causes greater neurodegeneration than an equivalent exposure of sevoflurane in the developing brain of neonatal mice. *Anesthesiology* 2010;**112**:1325–34.

101. Cattano D, Young C, Straiko MM, Olney JW. Subanesthetic doses of propofol induce neuroapoptosis in the infant mouse brain. *Anesth Analg* 2008;**106**:1712–4.

102. Young C, Jevtovic-Todorovic V, Qin YQ, et al. Potential of ketamine and midazolam, individually or in combination, to induce apoptotic neurodegeneration in the infant mouse brain. *Br J Pharmacol* 2005;**146**:189–97.

103. Vutskits L, Gascon E, Tassonyi E, Kiss JZ. Effect of ketamine on dendritic arbor development and survival of immature GABAergic neurons in vitro. *Toxicol Sci* 2006;**91**:540–9.

104. Ma D, Williamson P, Januszewski A, et al. Xenon mitigates isoflurane-induced neuronal apoptosis in the developing rodent brain. *Anesthesiology* 2007;**106**:746–53.

105. Sanders RD, Xu J, Shu Y, et al. Dexmedetomidine attenuates isoflurane-induced neurocognitive impairment in neonatal rats. *Anesthesiology* 2009;**110**:1077–85.

106. Lu LX, Yon JH, Carter LB, Jevtovic-Todorovic V. General anesthesia activates BDNF-dependent neuroapoptosis in the developing rat brain. *Apoptosis* 2006;**11**:1603–15.

107. Sall JW, Stratmann G, Leong J, et al. Isoflurane inhibits growth but does not cause cell death in hippocampal neural precursor cells grown in culture. *Anesthesiology* 2009;**110**:826–33.

108. Loepke AW, Soriano SG. An assessment of the effects of general anesthetics on developing brain structure and neurocognitive function. *Anesth Analg* 2008;**106**:1681–707.

109. Loepke AW, McGowan FX Jr, Soriano SG. CON: the toxic effects of anesthetics in the developing brain: the clinical perspective. *Anesth Analg* 2008;**106**:1664–9.

110. Olney JW, Young C, Wozniak DF, Ikonomidou C, Jevtovic-Todorovic V. Anesthesia-induced developmental neuroapoptosis. Does it happen in humans? *Anesthesiology* 2004;**101**:273–5.

111. Todd MM. Anesthetic neurotoxicity: the collision between laboratory neuroscience and clinical medicine. *Anesthesiology* 2004;**101**:272–3.

112. Wilder RT, Flick RP, Sprung J, et al. Early exposure to anesthesia and learning disabilities in a population-based birth cohort. *Anesthesiology* 2009;**110**:796–804.

113. Bartels M, Althoff RR, Boomsma DI. Anesthesia and cognitive performance in children: no evidence for a causal relationship. *Twin Res Hum Genet* 2009;**12**:246–53.

## Chapter 19

# Combining hypothermia with other therapies for neonatal neuroprotection

Faye S. Silverstein and John D. Barks

## Introduction

There is compelling evidence that therapeutic hypothermia confers significant benefit in term neonates with post-asphyxial encephalopathy. Yet, over 40% of treated infants have poor neurodevelopmental outcomes and there is an urgent need to identify treatments that effectively supplement the beneficial effects of hypothermia. This chapter focuses on discussion of clinically available therapeutic agents that could be administered in conjunction with hypothermia and that have the potential to augment the neuroprotective efficacy of cooling. Target populations for combination therapies include both infants who have poor outcomes with current treatments and also infants who are ultimately classified as having "good" outcomes, but who could have the potential for better long-term neurobehavioural function.

There is an inevitable delay period before therapeutic hypothermia can be started. Since time to onset of cooling is a major determinant of neuroprotective efficacy experimentally, agents that extended the duration of the therapeutic window for initiation of hypothermia would be desirable. Supplemental therapies could conceivably be administered prenatally, intrapartum, in conjunction with resuscitation, during post-resuscitation stabilization, or during transport to a neonatal intensive care unit. For any treatment administered more broadly to "at risk" neonates, before a diagnosis of encephalopathy, safety would be a critical pre-requisite and adequate documentation of safety in this population would inevitably be very challenging. For agents administered to symptomatic neonates, concurrently with onset of cooling, it would be essential to analyze drug/hypothermia interactions and take into account the impact of acute kidney or liver injury on drug pharmacokinetics. As more is understood both about endogenous mechanisms of

brain repair and the mechanisms that underlie the beneficial effects of hypothermia, it may also become feasible to target therapies specifically to replicate or strengthen these mechanisms to enhance recovery after the end of hypothermia.

In considering strategies for neonatal neuroprotection, there are important developmental issues that merit consideration. Maturational stage can influence mechanisms of brain injury (apoptosis vs. necrosis vs. continuum cell death pathways), regional and/or cellular selective vulnerability (e.g., heightened susceptibility of immature oligodendroglia) and mechanisms of brain repair (endogenous stem cells and trophic factors). There is experimental evidence that maturational stage influences susceptibility to adverse effects of specific neuroactive drugs (such as anaesthetics and anticonvulsants).

Hypothermia influences multiple molecular cascades that occur after reperfusion and its beneficial effects are likely mediated not only by limiting deleterious pathways, but also by selectively upregulating protective signalling. Targeted drug development to simulate or amplify hypothermia remains challenging when the mechanisms underlying its neuroprotective efficacy remain uncertain. Combination therapies have potential to interfere with some of the intrinsic protective effects of hypothermia. Thus, it will be essential to ensure that any combination therapy does not attenuate the efficacy of hypothermia.

The scientific underpinnings of the chapter are provided primarily by experimental animal data. Yet, as hypothermia is more widely used as a therapeutic modality, important complementary clinical data should emerge and these observations will provide opportunities to accelerate progress – by identifying treatment combinations that should be prioritized for clinical trial evaluation or alternatively that have unanticipated adverse effects when administered in conjunction with cooling.

The next four sections of this chapter discuss the preclinical evidence to support specific combination therapies and the final section highlights some of the complex issues that will influence the design and implementation of future clinical trials to evaluate any of these combination therapies.

## Antiepileptic drugs and hypothermia

Neonates with hypoxic–ischaemic encephalopathy frequently have seizures in the first 3 days of life. Typically, seizures are recognized 6–12 hours after resuscitation and persist for several days. Clinicians commonly treat seizures with a loading dose of an antiepileptic drug and phenobarbital is used most frequently, although uncertainty persists with regard to optimal treatment of neonatal seizures. The clinical diagnosis of neonatal seizures is imprecise and particularly after administration of phenobarbital, dissociation between clinically apparent and electrographically detected seizures (with disappearance of clinical seizures) is frequent. There is now widespread acceptance of the principle that electrophysiological monitoring (simplified and/or conventional electroencephalography [EEG]) is required to accurately diagnose neonatal seizures and amplitude-integrated EEG devices (aEEGs) that allow viewing of "raw" EEG tracings are becoming widely integrated into neonatal intensive care unit practice. However, whether aggressive treatment of electrographic seizures will influence long-term neurodevelopmental outcomes remains uncertain [1–3].

There has been some degree of therapeutic nihilism with regard to neonatal antiepileptic drug therapy. This clinical perspective stemmed from multiple factors, including the limited efficacy of conventional antiepileptic drugs, the view that seizures were primarily a reflection of antecedent brain injury and the absence of evidence that treatment of seizures improved outcome of neonatal encephalopathy. This view was reinforced by experimental data which indicated that the neonatal brain was resistant to seizure-induced neuronal damage. Moreover, concerns were raised for many years that the developing brain could be at heightened risk for antiepileptic-drug related neurotoxicity [4]; in the past decade, these concerns were amplified by reports that many antiepileptic drugs induced neuroapoptosis in neonatal animals [5,6]. Yet, it is important to emphasize

that antiepileptic drug toxicity studies have been performed in healthy young animals (or *in vitro*) and the balance of risk versus benefit of antiepileptic drug therapy and specific toxicity mechanisms could well differ between normal and acutely injured brains.

Perspectives are changing and multiple lines of investigation have yielded evidence that neonatal seizures can have long-lasting adverse effects (reviewed in Holmes [7]). Seizures in early life can disrupt neural developmental programmes; in animal models, neonatal seizures can result in changes in neuronal signalling properties. Many variables influence the impact of seizures on brain integrity and these factors are not yet well-characterized. Experimental studies to evaluate whether or not seizures amplify neonatal hypoxic–ischaemic brain injury have yielded contradictory results and available models are imperfect. One frequently cited supportive study was performed in 10-day-old rats; a very mild hypoxic–ischaemic insult, which did not result in overt neuronal damage, was followed by infusion of the glutamate agonist kainate and this combination resulted in prolonged seizures and hippocampal neuronal injury [8]. Of interest in the context of this chapter, fever prevention blocked the deleterious effects of seizures in this model [9]. A complementary finding emerged from experiments in the fetal asphyxia sheep model, which provided a foundation for clinical trials of hypothermia neuroprotection; in this model, hypothermia lost its protective efficacy if initiation of cooling was delayed until after seizure onset [10].

Clinical evidence that neonatal seizures amplify ischaemic brain injury has been difficult to collect. Rigorous analysis of this question would need to take into account an accurate measure of electrographic seizure burden over a prolonged period of observation, a detailed analysis of antiepileptic drug therapy and an independent sensitive and accurate quantitative measure of ischaemic brain injury. To date, this level of rigour has not been attained. Yet, meaningful trends are emerging. Miller *et al* analyzed brain magnetic resonance spectroscopy in infants with asphyxia and seizures; they found that seizure severity (scored clinically) contributed to abnormal metabolism (increased lactate: choline ratio) and the magnitude of brain injury (decreased N-acetyl-aspartate: choline ratio), when controlling for severity of structural injury on conventional MR imaging and for extent of initial resuscitation [11]. Glass *et al* [12] subsequently compared cognitive and motor outcomes at age 4 years in 77 children who were born at term, who were at risk for hypoxic–ischaemic brain injury and who had brain magnetic resonance imaging (MRI) in the newborn period; 25/77 had clinically detected neonatal seizures. Neonatal MRIs were classified with respect to anatomic distribution and severity of acute injury. Neonatal seizure severity and MRI injury severity were scored and multivariate regression was applied to examine the effect of seizures on outcome, controlling for the severity of MRI-documented neonatal injury. The major findings were that seizure severity was associated with worse neurodevelopmental outcomes, independent of severity of MRI-scored brain injury. Van Rooij et al reported complementary findings; they incorporated continuous electrophysiological monitoring and evaluated the predictive power of the duration of neonatal status epilepticus and found that longer durations were predictive of poor outcome only with hypoxic-ischaemic encephalopathy (HIE) (all 10 infants with HIE and drug-resistant status epilepticus died) [13]. Conversely, absence of seizures was an independent predictor of better outcome in a *post-hoc* analysis of results from the Cool-Cap hypothermia trial, but whether this trend reflected less severe underlying injury could not be discerned [14].

There are many mechanisms whereby seizures could amplify ischaemic brain injury [2,3]. Increased neuronal firing results in increased release of the excitatory amino acid neurotransmitter glutamate; synaptic glutamate is removed from the synaptic cleft by ATP-dependent re-uptake transporters. Prolonged seizures could increase brain temperature and thereby increase metabolic demands throughout the brain. Seizures increase local cerebral blood flow and brain regions with borderline perfusion may be relatively compromised. All these mechanisms could limit the glucose and oxygen supply that is available to sustain endogenous protective and repair mechanisms in injured tissue. Prolonged seizures may stimulate production of diffusible neurotoxic molecules (e.g. cytokines, reactive oxygen species) to which injured cells are particularly vulnerable.

Together, these findings prompted our laboratory to undertake experiments to evaluate whether anticonvulsants could augment the efficacy of hypothermia for neonatal neuroprotection. Our initial goal was to determine if administration of an antiepileptic drug could prolong the therapeutic window for initiation of cooling. Our studies have been performed in a widely used, well-characterized animal model in 7-day-old (P7) rats. To elicit hypoxic–ischaemic injury, one carotid artery is tied off and cut ("ligated") under anaesthesia, animals subsequently recover and then they are exposed to moderate hypoxia (8% oxygen) for 90 minutes; only the combination of artery ligation plus hypoxia results in brain damage (forebrain infarction on the side of the artery ligation) [15]. Strengths of the model include relative simplicity and reproducibility, low mortality and high long-term survival and ability to integrate functional and pathological outcome measures. Weaknesses include variability in outcome, limited behavioural repertoire of rodents and uncertainty with regard to translation of many elements of experimental protocols to clinical settings. In our protocol to evaluate combination therapies, the test drug or an equal volume of saline is injected 15 minutes after the end of hypoxia exposure (i.e. modelling the time period of a resuscitation). Hypothermia (3 hours at 30°C) is delayed for 1 or 3 hours (modelling clinical delays that would be encountered before initiation of cooling); this delayed cooling intervention, alone, confers no benefit. The rationales for our hypothermia protocols are detailed in cited publications [16,17].

The first antiepileptic drug that we evaluated was topiramate, which has intrinsic neuroprotective properties, attributed to its actions as a glutamate antagonist. We found that a single high dose of topiramate (30 mg/kg), which alone conferred no benefit, when combined with mild hypothermia, initiated 3 hours later, resulted in improved sensorimotor function and sustained neuroprotection [16]. No parenteral formulation of topiramate is available currently and its use in neonates has been limited. We initially interpreted the beneficial effects of topiramate as attributable primarily to its intrinsic neuroprotective properties rather than anticonvulsant mechanisms. However, prompted both by interest from clinicians and also the study by Hall et al [18] which reported better outcomes in asphyxiated neonates who received phenobarbital, we then evaluated phenobarbital in the same protocol. Administration of phenobarbital (40 mg/kg), in combination with cooling, initiated after a 1-hour or 3-hour delay, resulted in sustained improvements in sensorimotor function and a greater than 50% reduction in the extent of brain damage, in comparison with saline-injected, hypothermia-treated controls [17].

Recently, we evaluated the antiepileptic drug levetiracetam in this paradigm [19]. Levetiracetam, which is now widely used for treatment of epilepsy in children, has a distinctive mechanism of action and does not directly alter glutamate or GABA synaptic activity or neuronal excitability [20]. We evaluated a dose of levetiracetam (60 mg/kg) that does not induce neuroapoptosis in P7 rats [21], in conjunction with onset of cooling after a 1-hour delay period. We found that this combination therapy resulted in: sustained marked sensorimotor improvement, subtle improvement in cognitive performance and sustained attenuation of brain damage, in comparison with controls that received injections of saline and then underwent the same hypothermia treatment.

Thus, in this neonatal rodent model, three anticonvulsant drug therapies with different modes of action each improved the neuroprotective efficacy of hypothermia, compared with saline-injected hypothermia controls. All three treatment combinations conferred functional benefits and reduced the severity of brain damage. Although the dosing schedule suggests that treatment prevented or attenuated post-ischaemic seizures, we could not directly test this hypothesis because of the technical challenges inherent in performing and analyzing EEGs in P7 rats. It is relevant to note that antiepileptic drugs have neuroprotective properties that are independent of their anticonvulsant actions [22].

Our results prompt us to hypothesize that prophylactic antiepileptic drug therapy (i.e. drug administration before clinical recognition of seizures) could augment hypothermic neuroprotection in neonates with HIE. It could be feasible to administer such treatment acutely, either intra-partum in a high-risk situation, or in the early postnatal period, after resuscitation and before, or concurrently with initiation of hypothermia, in neonates who meet criteria for this intervention. It is intriguing to note that a clinical trial to evaluate antenatal therapy to attempt to reduce birth asphyxia-induced brain damage with allopurinol has been implemented (ALLO-Trial) [23] and a similar scenario could be envisaged for evaluation of an antiepileptic drug. Although there are no precedents for long-term benefits of prophylactic antiepileptic drug therapy in other clinical settings, the potential benefits for combination therapies that incorporate hypothermia have not yet been explored.

Of the three drugs that we have studied, each may ultimately warrant evaluation in clinical trials in combination with hypothermia. Phenobarbital is an attractive candidate because neonatologists have substantial experience in using this drug to treat critically ill infants. Topiramate is infrequently used in intensive care units currently, since no parenteral formulation is available; preliminary studies of combination therapy with hypothermia and the oral formulation have been reported [24,25]. A parenteral formulation of levetiracetam is available and this antiepileptic drug is also being used to treat neonatal seizures [26]; however, long-term safety and efficacy data in this age group are lacking.

## Xenon and hypothermia

The preceding chapter included a discussion of the neuroprotective properties of xenon. Here, we highlight some of the experimental data that support combination therapy of xenon with hypothermia.

In 2005, Ma and colleagues reported that in the same P7 rat hypoxia–ischaemia model described in the preceding section, delayed initiation of brief, concurrent low-dose xenon (20%) and mild hypothermia (35°C) resulted in synergistic benefits with preservation of neurologic function, attenuation of hemisphere volume loss and reduction of apoptosis [27]; neither treatment alone affected outcome. A subsequent report in the same model demonstrated that sequential administration of hypothermia, followed 1 or 5 hours later by xenon inhalation (20%) conferred some neuroprotection [28]. A complementary study by Thoresen and colleagues in the same P7 rat hypoxia–ischaemia model incorporated a different treatment protocol, with immediate initiation of xenon (50%), hypothermia (32°C) or both for 3 hours after hypoxia–ischaemia; they found that both xenon and hypothermia resulted in some improvement and the combination conferred the greatest benefit, with preservation of long-term neurologic function, which suggested additive effects [29]. These investigators subsequently reported that a shorter duration of xenon treatment (1 hour), when combined with the same duration of hypothermia, also potentiated brain protection, compared to hypothermia alone [30]; of clinical relevance, the beneficial effects of xenon were equivalent whether the brief xenon course was initiated immediately or 2 hours after the end of hypoxia exposure. Most recently, results of experiments, in which xenon plus hypothermia were tested in a piglet model of global cerebral hypoxia–ischaemia, provided more evidence that combination therapy yielded additive benefits [31]. Although the underlying mechanisms that mediate xenon neuroprotection remain uncertain, these studies provide a strong rationale for the implementation of clinical trials to evaluate the safety and efficacy of xenon administration in combination with therapeutic hypothermia in neonates with acute hypoxic–ischaemic brain injury. There are many unanswered questions about the optimal dose, duration and timing of xenon administration, as well as the most effective protocol for integration of this intervention with therapeutic cooling. Phase 1 and 2 [clinicaltrials.gov; NCT00934700] trials of xenon in combination with hypothermia for infants with hypoxic–ischaemic encephalopathy are under way in the United Kingdom.

## Anti-oxidants and hypothermia

Oxidative stress is strongly implicated as a major mechanism of ischaemia–reperfusion injury. There is considerable interest in the neuroprotective properties of anti-oxidants/free radical scavengers, and an added potential benefit of these agents is the opportunity to concurrently protect multiple end-organs (kidney, liver, heart, etc.) that are susceptible to ischaemic injury. Furthermore, there is substantial evidence that inflammation, initiated by infection and/or directly by ischaemia, exacerbates perinatal brain injury and that anti-oxidants may attenuate these deleterious effects. Hypothermia itself may suppress physiologically important inflammation (and thereby increase risk of infection); thus, in critically ill infants who are at substantial risk for infection, it may be safer to combine anti-oxidants rather than anti-inflammatory drugs with hypothermia.

The two clinically available drugs that have been most extensively studied in this context are N-acetylcysteine (NAC) and allopurinol. Both drugs are considered safe and both are already in clinical trials in relevant populations. Melatonin, which has free radical scavenging properties, as well as other modes of action, is discussed in the next section.

## N-Acetylcysteine

Jenkins and colleagues [32] investigated the impact of combining hypothermia and N-acetylcysteine (NAC) on outcome after neonatal hypoxia–ischaemia. Again, 7-day-old (P7) rats that underwent right common carotid artery ligation and timed 8% oxygen exposure were studied. In their protocol, mild systemic hypothermia was induced immediately after hypoxia–ischaemia and was maintained for only 2 hours. NAC (50 mg/kg) was injected daily until sacrifice. Combination treatment resulted in preserved brain volumes and myelination 4 weeks later. Similarly, a study that evaluated hypothermia in combination with another anti-oxidant, N-tert-butyl-(2-sulphophenyl)-nitrone (S-PBN) in the same neonatal rat model, yielded evidence of treatment benefit [33]. Wang et al. reported interesting complementary findings. Hypoxic–ischaemic brain injury was elicited by injecting lipopolysaccharide (LPS) before a very mild hypoxic–ischaemic insult (that would not result in injury without preceding LPS exposure; "LPS-sensitized HI brain injury") in P8 rats [34]. Multiple doses of NAC were administered (without adjuvant hypothermia) and brain injury was evaluated a week later. NAC provided marked neuroprotection if treatment was started before hypoxia–ischaemia and lesser benefit for treatment started immediately afterwards. Of note, all three cited studies included repeated NAC administration; this suggests that timing and dosage will be critical elements for clinical neuroprotection applications.

## Allopurinol

Allopurinol is a xanthine oxidase inhibitor and free-radical scavenger with modest, but well-characterized neuroprotective properties. Allopurinol reduces brain damage in the P7 rat hypoxic–ischaemic injury model, described earlier, if it is administered before hypoxia [35]. No publications (as of March 2012) have evaluated its efficacy in combination with hypothermia in this model.

Its neuroprotective efficacy has been studied in several small clinical trials that were evaluated in a recent Cochrane review [36]. The authors examined the evidence from three trials that assessed the effects of allopurinol on mortality and morbidity in neonates with suspected hypoxic–ischaemic encephalopathy. These studies were viewed to be of good methodological quality, but they were underpowered and meta-analysis did not reveal significant treatment effects. The authors concluded that available data were not sufficient to determine whether allopurinol has clinically important benefits for newborn infants with HIE and also suggested that future clinical trials could assess allopurinol as an adjunct to therapeutic hypothermia. They raised an important theme that must be considered in the design of any combination therapy trial, specifically that not only beneficial effects but also adverse effects of combination therapies should be sought.

Both NAC and allopurinol are being evaluated in clinical trials that target high-risk pregnancies. A pilot clinical trial is designed to determine the safety of NAC in women who present with chorioamnionitis (clinicaltrials.gov; NCT00724594). NAC will be administered both antenatally and postnatally; safety and pharmacokinetics in mothers and infants will be evaluated. A more ambitious randomized double blind placebo controlled multicentre study will evaluate the impact of antenatal treatment with allopurinol or placebo when fetal hypoxia is suspected (based on standardized clinical criteria or an abnormal fetal blood scalp sampling) in women with term pregnancies. Primary outcome measures are umbilical cord blood levels of S100B (as a marker for brain damage) and of oxidative stress indices; secondary outcome measures are neonatal mortality, composite neonatal morbidity and long-term neurological outcome (NCT00189007) [37]. Both studies will include treatment of infants who are low risk for adverse outcomes and safety data will be particularly important to accrue. Neither protocol comments on inclusion/exclusion of postnatal hypothermia therapy.

# Hypothermia in combination with other therapies

## Magnesium sulphate

Several investigators have advocated for evaluation of combination therapy with magnesium and hypothermia after cerebral ischaemia in adults [38]. Although concerns have been raised about the risks of magnesium sulphate therapy for treatment of neonatal hypoxic–ischaemic encephalopathy (in particular, treatment induced hypotension), there have also been reports of benefit [39]. Additional preclinical studies to evaluate the combination of magnesium infusion with hypothermia are warranted to assess interactions of these treatment modalities; these experiments should be performed in large animal models where rigorous physiological monitoring is feasible.

## Alpha2-adrenergic agonists

Alpha2-adrenergic receptor agonists exert potent analgesic and sedative/hypnotic effects and variable potency neuroprotective effects in animal models. The molecular mechanisms underlying neuroprotection are uncertain and may, at least in part, be independent of alpha2-adrenergic receptor mechanisms [40]. Dexmedetomidine, a centrally acting alpha2-adrenergic agonist, provides potent neuroprotection in a model of perinatal excitotoxic brain damage [41]; it is already quite widely used for sedation in critically ill adult and paediatric patients. Occasional adverse haemodynamic effects including bradycardia and hypotension have been reported and these adverse effects may be exacerbated with hypothermia. Tobias [42] reported two paediatric patients with traumatic brain injury who developed clinically significant bradycardia when therapeutic hypothermia was added to a sedation regimen that included dexmedetomidine and remifentanil. Whether or not adverse systemic effects represent a limiting factor in wider clinical application of this treatment combination remains to be determined.

## Melatonin

Melatonin, a naturally occurring compound, secreted primarily by the pineal gland, is very widely used to regulate circadian rhythms and promote sleep in children and adults. It has diverse modes of action and neuroprotection has been ascribed to its free radical scavenging and antioxidant properties. In the neonatal rat hypoxia–ischaemia model cited earlier in this chapter, several melatonin treatment regimens were reported to confer sustained neuroprotection [43]. However, the investigators did not directly evaluate the impact of melatonin therapy on body temperature in lesioned animals and there is evidence that melatonin, itself, can induce hypothermia [44]. Thus, whether or not this agent could represent an effective complement to conventionally induced therapeutic hypothermia remains unknown.

## Anaesthetics

In animal brain injury models, use of anaesthesia can substantially influence the efficacy of other neuroprotective therapies, including hypothermia [45]. There has long been interest in their brain-protecting properties during planned cerebral ischaemia periods intra-operatively, often together with induced hypothermia. In neonatal medicine this is most relevant in the setting of intra-operative repair of severe congenital heart disease. There are multiple challenges in extrapolating from this population to treatment of neonatal encephalopathy, including not only differences in mechanisms and timing of brain injury and systemic complications, but also depth and duration of hypothermia and concurrent administration of multiple central nervous system–active drugs intra- and post-operatively. In fact, widespread usage of potent sedative and analgesic drugs (including opioids and benzodiazepines) in neonatal ICUs represents an important variable that should be considered in the analysis of all neonatal neurodevelopmental outcome studies.

Olney and colleagues have raised concerns about developmental-stage specific risks of anaesthetics in neonates, based on findings of increased neuronal apoptosis in both immature rodents and primates after exposure to several anaesthetics with different modes of action. These findings and their interpretation have been highly controversial. In the context of this chapter, it is interesting to note that this group recently reported that induction of hypothermia reduced both anaesthesia-mediated and constitutive neuroapoptosis [46]. These findings provide important evidence of the potent, complex and incompletely characterized mechanisms of action of hypothermia on the developing brain, which remain to be elucidated.

## Growth factors

Erythropoietin has garnered substantial enthusiasm as a possible therapy to enhance recovery after neonatal brain injury. Unlike other neurotrophic factors that have been studied experimentally, this biological agent has a substantial usage track record in neonatal clinical practice. Its complex modes of action were discussed in the preceding chapter. Several clinical trials of erythropoietin are under way in neonatal populations (preterm and term); in one trial in term infants with hypoxic–ischaemic encephalopathy treatment with erythropoietin for 2 weeks resulted in a reduction in death or moderate/severe disability at 18 months [47,48]. There is little information about potential risks and benefits of combining erythropoietin with hypothermia, or regarding the optimal timing of adjunctive erythropoietin administration. Hypothermia could prolong the therapeutic window for implementation of trophic factor therapy [49]. A small study performed in adults who were resuscitated after cardiac arrest found that the combination of erythropoietin with cooling had no effect on survival or early neurological outcome [50], but these findings cannot be extrapolated to asphyxiated neonates and additional studies are warranted in this population.

## Nutritional factors

There is recognition that pre- and postnatal maternal and infant nutrition may influence susceptibility to and recovery after brain injury, yet relatively little is known about these potentially remediable factors. Whether there are any nutritional deficiencies that could attenuate the efficacy or safety of therapeutic hypothermia and whether these could be readily corrected remain uncertain. Similarly, little is known about the optimal composition of parenteral nutrition during hypothermia and subsequent recovery periods in neonates with post-asphyxial encephalopathy. Nutritional interventions could represent clinically important adjuncts for hypothermia when these gaps in knowledge are addressed.

# Hypothermia pharmacology

## Scientific background

The pivotal mechanisms underlying post-ischaemia hypothermia-mediated neuroprotection are uncertain. Hypothermia likely regulates multiple molecular and cellular cascades that are activated after reperfusion, including those associated with necrotic and apoptotic cell death. Yet, it is important to recognize that hypothermia not only blocks multiple damaging cascades but, perhaps equally important, this treatment may also selectively upregulate endogenous protective pathways. In experimental models of reperfusion injury after cardiac arrest, hypothermia increases production of the potent neurotrophin brain-derived growth factor [51]. Hypothermia may exert direct effects on neurons [52]; for example, in an *in vitro* study (that used brain slices), hypothermia stimulated neurite outgrowth and this was independent of neurotrophin signaling. Any drug used in combination with hypothermia could either amplify or attenuate its therapeutic properties [53].

Conversely, there could be circumstances in which hypothermia could mitigate adverse drug effects. There is some experimental evidence of this unanticipated benefit; moderate hypothermia suppressed anaesthesia-induced neuroapoptosis in neonatal rodents [46]. Whether these intriguing observations are relevant to clinical applications is unknown. Future clinical trials of combination therapies must be designed and powered to enable investigators to discern both positive and negative therapeutic interactions.

In one of the first studies that demonstrated a neuroprotective effect of post-ischaemic hypothermia in a neonatal animal model, Bona *et al* found that in P7 rats, post-ischaemic hypothermia differentially affected males and females and sustained improvements in sensorimotor function were limited to females [54]. In neonatal clinical trials, no differences in efficacy of hypothermia were observed. Nor has gender been reported to influence responsiveness to any of the combination therapies cited earlier in this chapter. Yet, there is accumulating evidence that sex hormone exposure early in development, effects mediated by the sex chromosomes themselves and epigenetic modifications of developmental genes that influence sexual differentiation, all contribute to sex differences in disease expression and possibly also responses to treatment [55]. Clinical observations in diverse neonatal populations suggest that male infants are at greater risk for central nervous system dysfunction. As more is learned about the underlying mechanisms for this disparity, it may become feasible to formulate gender-specific treatment combinations to optimize neonatal neuroprotection.

## Clinical translation

From a practical perspective, it is essential to consider the effects of hypothermia on the pharmacokinetics of each drug administered in conjunction with cooling. In neonates with post-asphyxial encephalopathy, interpretation of such data may be confounded by renal and/or hepatic dysfunction (i.e., depending on how each drug is metabolized and excreted). Filippi *et al* [24,25] recently reported their study of topiramate pharmacokinetics in asphyxiated neonates treated with prolonged whole body hypothermia and topiramate. Values of topiramate maximal and minimal concentration, half-life, average concentration and area under the time–concentration curve resulted in considerably higher values than those reported in normothermic infants.

One of the major challenges that will face investigators as efforts are made to translate the experimental data highlighted in this chapter into the design of future clinical trials will be the selection of optimal dosages, frequency and timing of each test agent in combination with hypothermia. There are no robust models to facilitate extrapolation of experimental animal data pharmacological measures to human infants. Even though this chapter focused on combination therapies with clinically available drugs, for most of these drugs even basic pharmacokinetic data for neonates are typically lacking. It must be acknowledged that there is a substantial risk that any combination treatment trial could fail, not only because of intrinsic lack of efficacy of the test drug, but also because the treatment protocol selected did not adequately replicate that achieved experimentally.

In this chapter, data demonstrating benefits of multiple combination treatments were presented. Yet, none of the studies cited (including those from our laboratory) provided any comparative efficacy data. Multiple factors are likely to influence decisions regarding prioritization of specific drugs for clinical trial assessment from among a broad range of attractive candidates. These factors will include safety considerations, availability of confirmatory data from additional large animal models, greater understanding of the pathophysiology of neonatal brain injury and repair, results of neuroprotection studies in other age groups and in related disorders, and investigator advocacy.

## Future directions

Implementation of future combination therapy neuroprotection clinical trials will be difficult and expensive. To discern incremental benefits in comparison with hypothermia-treated control groups, it will be essential to include large sample sizes. Moreover, the benefits of any drug could well be modest, although clinically important, in comparison with the benefit of hypothermia. Together these factors will necessitate inclusion of much larger sample sizes than were recruited in each of the initial neonatal hypothermia trials.

Another important consideration in the design of future studies is selection of optimal outcome measures. These measures should not only be sensitive for the detection of a reduced number of "poor" neurodevelopmental outcomes, but also should enable investigators to discern better outcomes in infants currently classified as having "good" neurodevelopmental outcomes. There is substantial enthusiasm for incorporation of surrogate biomarkers as the primary outcome measures in the design of future neonatal neuroprotection studies. Major advantages of surrogate measures would include more rapid assessment of efficacy and opportunities to incorporate adaptive design strategies (which reduce sample size requirements). However, validation of surrogate measures (such as magnetic resonance spectroscopy in the neonatal period) is primarily based on neurodevelopmental outcomes at 18 months and these outcomes themselves may not be sufficiently sensitive to distinguish subtle, but significant effects (particularly for cognitive function). It will be difficult to balance these conflicting factors.

The success attained in completion of the seminal neonatal hypothermia clinical trials documents the outstanding track record of collaborative research in neonatal medicine. Integration of data from future neonatal neuroprotection studies would be greatly enhanced if investigators were able to achieve consensus in the selection of common data elements and harmonization of protocol design and selection of outcome measures. The data presented in this chapter highlight the wide-ranging therapeutic options that may become available and neonatologists will hope for comparative efficacy data to guide best clinical practice.

## Acknowledgement

Funding from NICHD (HD 60348), NHLBI (HL 94345) and the Gorgeffen Fund.

## References

1. Evans DJ, Levene MI, Tsakmakis M. Anticonvulsants for preventing mortality and morbidity in full term newborns with perinatal asphyxia. *Cochrane Database Syst Rev* 2007;**18**;(3):CD001240.

2. Silverstein FS, Jensen FE. Neonatal seizures. *Ann Neurol* 2007;**62**:112–20.

3. Silverstein FS. Do seizures contribute to neonatal hypoxic-ischemic brain injury? *J Pediatr* 2009;**155**:305–6.

4. Bergey GK, Swaiman KF, Schrier BK, et al. Adverse effects of phenobarbital on morphological and biochemical development of fetal mouse spinal cord neurons in culture. *Ann Neurol* 1981;**9**:584–9.

5. Bittigau P, Sifringer M, Genz K, et al. Antiepileptic drugs and apoptotic neurodegeneration in the developing brain. *Proc Natl Acad Sci U S A* 2002;**99**:15089–94.

6. Stefovska VG, Uckermann O, Czuczwar M, et al. Sedative and anticonvulsant drugs suppress postnatal neurogenesis. *Ann Neurol* 2008;**64**:434–45.

7. Holmes GL. The long-term effects of neonatal seizures. *Clin Perinatol* 2009;**36**:901–14.

8. Wirrell EC, Armstrong EA, Osman LD, et al. Prolonged seizures exacerbate perinatal hypoxic-ischemic brain damage. *Pediatr Res* 2001;**50**:445–54.

9. Yager JY, Armstrong EA, Jaharus C, et al. Preventing hyperthermia decreases brain damage following neonatal hypoxic-ischemic seizures. *Brain Res* 2004;**1011**:48–57.

10. Gunn AJ, Bennet L, Gunning MI, et al. Cerebral hypothermia is not neuroprotective when started after postischemic seizures in fetal sheep. *Pediatr Res* 1999;**46**:274–80.

11. Miller SP, Weiss J, Barnwell A, et al. Seizure-associated brain injury in term newborns with perinatal asphyxia. *Neurology* 2002;**58**:542–8.

12. Glass HC, Glidden D, Jeremy RJ, et al. Clinical neonatal seizures are independently associated with outcome in infants at risk for hypoxic-ischemic brain injury. *J Pediatr* 2009;**155**:318–23.

13. van Rooij LGM, de Vries LS, Handryastuti S, et al. Neurodevelopmental outcome in term infants with status epilepticus detected with amplitude-integrated electroencephalography. *Pediatrics* 2007;**120**:e354–63.

14. Wyatt JS, Gluckman PD, Liu PY, et al. Determinants of outcomes after headcooling for neonatal encephalopathy. *Pediatrics* 2007;**119**:912–21.

15. Rice JE, Vannucci RC, Brierley JB. The influence of immaturity on hypoxic-ischemic brain damage in the rat. *Ann Neurol* 1981;**9**:131–41.

16. Liu YQ, Barks JDE, Xu G, et al. Topiramate extends the therapeutic window for hypothermia-mediated neuroprotection after stroke in neonatal rats. *Stroke* 2004;**35**:1460–5.

17. Barks JD, Liu YQ, Shangguan Y, et al. Phenobarbital augments hypothermic neuroprotection. *Pediatr Res* 2010;**67**:532–7.

18. Hall RT, Hall FK, Daily DK. High-dose phenobarbital therapy in term newborn infants with severe perinatal asphyxia: a randomized, prospective study with three-year follow-up. *J Pediatr* 1998;**132**:345–8.

19. Liu YQ, Shangguan Y, Barks JD, et al. Levetiracetam and brief hypothermia confer sustained neuroprotection in a neonatal rat model of hypoxic-ischemic brain injury. *Society for Pediatric Research Annual Meeting, Abstract 1365.3, May 1, 2010.*

20. Lynch BA, Lambeng N, Nocka K, et al. The synaptic vesicle protein SV2A is the binding site for the antiepileptic drug levetiracetam. *Proc Natl Acad Sci U S A* 2004;**101**:9861–6.

21. Manthey D, Asimiadou S, Stefovska V, et al. Sulthiame but not levetiracetam exerts neurotoxic effect in the developing rat brain. *Exp Neurol* 2005;**193**:497–503.

22. Calabresi P, Cupini LM, Centonze D, et al. Antiepileptic drugs as a possible neuroprotective strategy in brain ischemia. *Ann Neurol* 2003;**53**:693–702.

23. Kaandorp JJ, Benders MJ, Rademaker CM, et al. Antenatal allopurinol for reduction of birth asphyxia induced brain damage (ALLO-Trial); a randomized double blind placebo controlled multicenter study. *BMC Pregnancy Childbirth* 2010;**10**:8.

24. Filippi L, la Marca G, Fiorini P, et al. Topiramate concentrations in neonates treated with prolonged whole body hypothermia for hypoxic ischemic encephalopathy. *Epilepsia* 2009;**50**:2355–61.

25. Filippi L, Poggi C, la Marca G, et al. Oral topiramate in neonates with hypoxic ischemic encephalopathy treated with hypothermia: a safety study. *J Pediatr* 2010;**157**:361–6.

26. Silverstein FS, Ferriero DM. Off-label use of anticonvulsants for treatment of neonatal seizures. *Ped Neurol* 2008;**39**:77–9.

27. Ma D, Hossain M, Chow A, et al. Xenon and hypothermia combine to provide neuroprotection from neonatal asphyxia. *Ann Neurol* 2005;**58**:182–93.

28. Martin JL, Ma D, Hossain M, et al. Asynchronous administration of xenon and hypothermia significantly reduces brain infarction in the neonatal rat. *Br J Anaesth* 2007;**98**:236–40.

29. Hobbs C, Thoresen M, Tucker A, et al. Xenon and hypothermia combine additively, offering long-term functional and histopathologic neuroprotection after neonatal hypoxia/ischemia. *Stroke* 2008;**39**:1307–13.

30. Thoresen M, Hobbs CE, Wood T, et al. Cooling combined with immediate or delayed xenon inhalation provides equivalent long-term neuroprotection after neonatal hypoxia–ischemia. *J Cereb Blood Flow Metab* 2009;**29**:707–14.

31. Chakkarapani E, Dingley J, Liu X, et al. Xenon enhances hypothermic neuroprotection in asphyxiated newborn pigs. *Ann Neurol* 2010;**68**:330–41.

32. Jatana M, Singh I, Singh AK, Jenkins D. Combination of systemic hypothermia and N-acetylcysteine attenuates hypoxic-ischemic brain injury in neonatal rats. *Pediatr Res* 2006;**59**:684–9.

33. Hobbs CE, Oorschot DE. Neonatal rat hypoxia-ischemia: long-term rescue of striatal neurons and motor skills by combined antioxidant-hypothermia treatment. *Brain Pathol* 2008;**18**:443–54.

34. Wang X, Svedin P, Nie C, et al. N-acetylcysteine reduces lipopolysaccharide-sensitized hypoxic-ischemic brain injury. *Ann Neurol* 2007;**61**:263–71.

35. Palmer C, Vannucci RC, Towfighi J. Reduction of perinatal hypoxic-ischemic brain damage with allopurinol. *Pediatr Res* 1990;**27**:332–6.

36. Chaudhari T, McGuire W. Allopurinol for preventing mortality and morbidity in newborn infants with suspected hypoxic-ischaemic encephalopathy. *Cochrane Database Syst Rev* 2008;**16**;(2):CD006817.

37. Torrance HL, Benders MJ, Derks JB, et al. Maternal allopurinol during fetal hypoxia lowers cord blood levels of the brain injury marker S-100B. *Pediatrics* 2009;**124**:350–7.

38. Meloni BP, Campbell K, Zhu H, Knuckey NW. In search of clinical neuroprotection after brain ischemia: the case for mild hypothermia (35 degrees C) and magnesium. *Stroke* 2009;**40**:2236–40.

39. Bhat MA, Charoo BA, Bhat JI, et al. Magnesium sulfate in severe perinatal asphyxia: a randomized, placebo-controlled trial. *Pediatrics* 2009;**123**:e764–9.

40. Ma D, Rajakumaraswamy N, Maze M. alpha2A-adrenoceptor agonists: shedding light on neuroprotection? *Br Med Bull* 2005;**71**:77–92.

41. Paris A, Mantz J, Tonner PH, et al. The effects of dexmedetomidine on perinatal excitotoxic brain injury are mediated by the alpha2A-adrenoceptor subtype. *Anesth Analg* 2006;**102**:456–61.

42. Tobias JD. Bradycardia during dexmedetomidine and therapeutic hypothermia. *J Intensive Care Med* 2008;**23**:403–8.

43. Carloni S, Perrone S, Buonocore G, et al. Melatonin protects from the long-term consequences of a neonatal hypoxic-ischemic brain injury in rats. *J Pineal Res* 2008;**44**:157–64.

44. Lin MT, Chuang JI. Melatonin potentiates 5-HT(1A) receptor activation in rat hypothalamus and results in hypothermia. *J Pineal Res* 2002;**33**:14–9.

45. Tooley JR, Satas S, Porter H, et al. Head cooling with mild systemic hypothermia in anesthetized piglets is neuroprotective. *Ann Neurol* 2003;**53**:65–72.

46. Creeley CE, Olney JW. The young: neuroapoptosis induced by anesthetics and what to do about it. *Anesth Analg* 2010;**110**:442–8.

47. McPherson RJ, Juul SE. Erythropoietin for infants with hypoxic-ischemic encephalopathy. *Curr Opin Pediatr* 2010;**22**:139–45.

48. Zhu C, Kang W, Xu F, et al. Erythropoietin improved neurologic outcomes in newborns with hypoxic-ischemic encephalopathy. *Pediatrics* 2009;**124**:e218-e226.

49. Guan J, Gunn AJ, Sirimanne ES, et al. The window of opportunity for neuronal rescue with insulin-like growth factor-1 after hypoxia-ischemia in rats is critically

modulated by cerebral temperature during recovery. *J Cereb Blood Flow Metab* 2000;**20**:513–9.

50. Cariou A, Claessens YE, Pène F, et al. High-dose erythropoietin therapy and hypothermia after out-of-hospital cardiac arrest: a matched control study. *Resuscitation* 2008;**76**:397–404.

51. D'Cruz BJ, Fertig KC, Filiano AJ, et al. Hypothermic reperfusion after cardiac arrest augments brain-derived neurotrophic factor activation. *J Cereb Blood Flow Metab* 2002;**22**:843–51.

52. Schmitt KR, Boato F, Diestel A, et al. Hypothermia-induced neurite outgrowth is mediated by tumor necrosis factor-alpha. *Brain Pathol* 2010;**20**:771–9.

53. Tang XN, Liu L, Yenari MA. Combination therapy with hypothermia for treatment of cerebral ischemia. *J Neurotrauma* 2009;**26**:325–31.

54. Bona E, Hagberg H, Løberg EM, et al. Protective effects of moderate hypothermia after neonatal hypoxia-ischemia: short- and long-term outcome. *Pediatr Res* 1998;**43**:738–45.

55. Siegel C, Turtzo C, McCullough LD. Sex differences in cerebral ischemia: possible molecular mechanisms. *J Neurosci Res* 2010;**88**:2765–74.

## Chapter 20

# Biomarkers for studies of neuroprotection in infants with hypoxic–ischaemic encephalopathy

Denis V. Azzopardi and A. David Edwards

## Introduction

Trials of mild hypothermia have recently proved in principle that neuroprotective therapy after delivery is possible but the protection is only partial and additional therapies are needed [1–3]. There are several candidate treatments suitable for trial (see Chapter 18) and the challenge is how to test several therapies efficiently so that only those with a high chance of success progress to pragmatic phase 3 trials. The major costs of large randomized trials mean that it is essential that only treatments with a high chance of success are studied; indeed while the financial costs are often obvious, the opportunity cost is equally if not more important. Every patient enrolled in a trial of a useless therapy is excluded from a trial of one that might work, so ill-advised major trials are a significant drag on progress in the field. It is notable that 11 years elapsed between the first demonstration that post-asphyxial hypothermia modified perinatal hypoxic-ischaemic encephalopathy in animals and the first evidence of a clinical benefit in newborn infants.

This is a familiar problem in drug development which is usually solved by testing an agent in small and rapid phase 2 studies which employ biological markers or surrogate outcomes to define a biological effect and provide evidence to support and plan pragmatic studies. However, these intermediary endpoints have to be used with circumspection as they are not substitutes for proof of clinical benefit, merely an experimental tool for efficient study of new treatments [4].

A National Institutes of Health working group recommended the following definitions [5]:

*Clinical endpoint*: A characteristic or variable that reflects how a patient feels or functions, or how long a patient survives.

*Surrogate endpoint*: A biomarker intended to substitute for a clinical endpoint.

*Biological marker (biomarker)*: A characteristic that is objectively measured and evaluated as an indicator of normal biologic processes, pathogenic processes or pharmacologic responses to a therapeutic intervention.

A biomarker needs to be "qualified" by firm evidence that it can detect a particular effect. Biomarkers might be qualified as markers of disease if they detect that a particular condition is present, or markers of effect if they detect the modification of a disease process by a treatment. Qualification is not necessarily transferable between diseases or subject groups, but "bridging" biomarkers which detect an effect in both animals and humans are particularly valuable because they allow the transfer of information from experimental to human studies.

## Sentinel biomarkers

Biomarkers for selecting infants for trials of neuroprotective treatments must satisfy two key requirements: first, they must be applicable very soon after birth, since treatment needs to be started within 6–8 hours of birth or earlier; second, they need to identify those infants who are most likely to benefit from the intervention. Those infants who most likely will make a complete recovery or conversely have little prospect of response to treatment because of the severity or timing of the injury need to be identified and excluded. Unfortunately, clinical indicators of the severity of hypoxic ischaemic injury, such as the fetal/cord blood pH, base deficit and lactate, the Apgar score and clinical scoring of the severity of HIE, whilst strong markers of hypoxic ischaemic injury, have a

*Neonatal Neural Rescue*, ed. A. David Edwards, Denis V. Azzopardi and Alistair J. Gunn. Published by Cambridge University Press. © Cambridge University Press 2013.

low positive predictive value for presence of hypoxic ischaemic injury and neurological outcome and so are imprecise for selection of infants into trials of neuroprotective treatments [6,7]. This is evident in the clinical trials of cooling where despite strict clinical, biochemical and, in some trials, cerebral electrocortical activity criteria, treatment with cooling was unnecessary or futile in 30–40% of infants (derived from the proportion of infants in the control non-cooled groups who had a good outcome) [1–3]. When a new treatment becomes part of standard clinical care, as is now the case with therapeutic hypothermia, treatment selection criteria should have a high sensitivity and a low false negative rate so that all infants who might benefit receive the therapy. The case is different in early-phase clinical trials of candidate therapies where a high specificity and low false positive rate is more important so as to minimize risk and increase study power.

Several possible sentinel biochemical markers have been evaluated, mostly in single studies: urine lactate, first urine S100, cord blood interleukin-6, serum non–protein-bound iron, serum CD14 cell NFkB activation, serum interleukin-8, serum ionized calcium, cerebrospinal fluid (CSF) neuron specific enolase, CSF/serum interleukin-1b and serum interleukin-6 are potential predictors of death or abnormal outcomes following asphyxia (Table 20.1) [8–10]. However, there are several unresolved issues: None of the markers are specific for hypoxia ischaemia, the time course of elevation following hypoxia–ischaemia is uncertain and there have been few long-term follow-up studies. In addition, the influence of therapeutic hypothermia on these markers is uncertain, which further complicates matters. On the other hand, therapeutic hypothermia may extend the "therapeutic window" by several hours, providing an opportunity for a longer period of assessment with suitable biomarkers. In summary, although several potential biochemical/inflammatory markers show promise as markers of disease, none have been evaluated as possible biomarkers of treatment effect and further prospective studies are needed.

The combination of the standard clinical markers of asphyxia together with clinical assessment of encephalopathy was an accurate marker of hypoxic ischaemic injury in the cooling trials: very few infants were subsequently found to have a diagnosis other than HIE and the neuroimaging findings were consistent with asphyxia in almost all cases [11]. In the absence of precise prognostic markers, the best method for identifying infants for neuroprotective therapy or trials probably remains the criteria used in the cooling trials, perhaps with a reassessment of the infant's condition at 6–12 hours of age; those infants who have a normal aEEG and no or mild encephalopathy only at reassessment are likely to have a low risk of adverse outcome and so would not be suitable candidates for therapeutic trials. This approach may improve selection accuracy by excluding cases where intervention probably is unnecessary or futile, but could introduce selection or treatment bias if the investigators are not masked to the intervention.

**Table 20.1.** Biomarkers of brain injury in infants with hypoxic ischaemic encephalopathy

| Marker | Outcome measure | Standardized mean difference (95% confidence intervals) | Significance (P value) |
| --- | --- | --- | --- |
| CSF Neuron specific enolase | Normal vs. Abnormal/Dead | 1.22 (0.32–2.12) | 0.008 |
| CSF Serum IL-1b | Normal vs. Abnormal/Dead | 1.19 (0.43–1.94) | 0.002 |
| Serum IL-1b | Normal vs. Abnormal | 0.60 (0.03–1.16) | 0.04 |
| Serum IL-6 | Normal vs. Abnormal/Dead | 0.58 (0.09–1.08) | 0.02 |

Note: Only biomarkers identified as significant on meta-analysis are shown. Outcome was assessed at 12–48 months. The standardised mean difference is the mean (95% confidence interval) difference in standardized values between normal and death/abnormal groups. Data are from Ramaswamy et al [8].

# Cerebral electrocortical activity as a marker of disease severity

In experimental models of hypoxic ischaemic injury there are characteristic temporal changes in cerebral electrocortical activity during and following asphyxia: an initial variably lasting phase of absent electrocortical activity is followed by increasing paroxysmal activity that subsides over the next 24–96 hours. The duration of electrocortical silence following asphyxia is related to the duration and severity of the asphyxia and the paroxysmal activity that subsequently develops is accompanied by changes in cerebral haemodynamics and impaired cell membrane function, signalling a further phase of cerebral injury. Neuroprotective intervention is unlikely to be effective once this point is reached.

These observations suggest that continuous monitoring of cerebral electrocortical activity could be an important method for identifying the onset of the secondary phase of injury (when paroxysmal/ictal activity occurs) and could be a marker of a lack or loss of response to therapy. However, in clinical practice, the aetiology of hypoxic–ischaemic injury is heterogeneous and the experimental paradigm described above may only apply in specific situations such as following a sentinel obstetric event like placental abruption or uterine rupture. These events only occur in approximately 10–20% of cases of HIE. However, several clinical studies have confirmed the strong association of abnormal cerebral electrocortical activity during the first 72 hours after birth and subsequent neurodevelopmental outcome [12].

In the clinical trials and in the cases reported to the TOBY UK Cooling register approximately 50% of infants were reported to have clinical and/or EEG seizures within a few hours of birth and before cooling therapy was started. The occurrence of seizures before cooling did not exclude a potential benefit from cooling, but in the CoolCap trial, there was no evidence of benefit with cooling in the subgroup of infants with the combination of electrical seizures and severe EEG suppression before cooling [1]. It may be that this specific combination of severely suppressed cerebral electrocortical activity with seizures heralds the occurrence of secondary energy failure signifying that treatment is too late, but this needs to be confirmed. In experimental studies the occurrence of transient epileptic potentials in the phase before paroxysmal activity defined a distinct period when neuroprotective intervention was possible [13]; this also needs to be examined in clinical studies.

In summary, cerebral electrocortical activity monitoring is strongly qualified as a biomarker of hypoxic–ischaemic injury but at present there are insufficient data regarding its role as a biomarker of treatment effect. The use of cerebral electrocortical activity monitoring in therapeutic hypothermia is discussed more fully elsewhere (see Chapter 13).

# Neuroimaging as a biological marker and surrogate endpoint

Cranial ultrasound scans are routinely carried out as part of clinical care in infants with HIE. Major cerebral abnormalities or complications such as haemorrhage or infarction can be identified and cranial ultrasound may suggest an alternative diagnosis to HIE. When carried out by highly experienced examiners, cranial ultrasound correlates well with standard magnetic resonance imaging (MRI) in infants with moderate/severe encephalopathy but mild/moderate abnormalities on MRI may be missed on cranial ultrasound. Cranial ultrasound imaging is too imprecise for use as a marker of disease severity; its role for assessing response to neuroprotective treatments has not been evaluated so far.

Cerebral haemodynamics can be assessed by repeated cranial doppler ultrasonography. It may be possible to identify the different phases of the cerebral vascular response following asphyxia, especially the onset of hyperperfusion which may be a marker of secondary energy failure, but this has not been examined systematically. Repeated measurements of cerebral blood flow velocities may be helpful in assessing prognosis but a single measurement soon after birth is not very informative. Computed tomography scanning has been superseded by magnetic resonance imaging and has a very limited clinical or research role following HIE.

Magnetic resonance techniques can reliably and non-invasively assess anatomy and physiology in infants with HIE and are commonly used to direct clinical care. Magnetic resonance techniques may, therefore, have a role in early phase studies of candidate neuroprotective therapies. The most likely role(s) are as early stage surrogate endpoints, but potentially as biomarkers of underlying processes. However, candidate neuroprotective therapies must ultimately be shown to improve long-term neurological outcomes by adequately sized randomized trials.

# Magnetic resonance spectroscopy

Magnetic resonance spectroscopy (MRS) enables *in vivo* quantitative analysis of cerebral metabolites. For more than two decades, phosphorus-31 ($^{31}$P) and proton ($^{1}$H) MRS have been used to investigate cerebral metabolism following perinatal asphyxia. The initial pioneering studies using $^{31}$P MRS defined the biphasic pattern of impairment of cerebral energy metabolism in infants with HIE: impairment of cerebral metabolism occurred following a delay of several hours after resuscitation in moderately or severely encephalopathic infants [14,15]. A close relationship was observed between the severity of cerebral energy impairment assessed by MRS in the first 7 days after birth and brain growth and neurological outcomes in the following months (Figure 20.1) [15,16]. These studies were critically important because they showed that there was a window of opportunity lasting several hours to attempt neuroprotective intervention. Further clinical studies using $^{1}$H MRS helped characterize the cerebral biochemical changes that occur in infants with HIE, such as elevation of cerebral lactate and intracellular pH, and demonstrated that these abnormalities persist for a considerable period after birth [17,18].

These early clinical studies rapidly led to experimental studies using both $^{31}$P and $^{1}$H MRS that confirmed the clinical observations and explored potential therapies following asphyxia [19–21]. Experimental studies in neonatal animal models of asphyxia using repeated MRS measurements carried out over 72 hours showed that prolonged mild hypothermia prevented the characteristic secondary depletion in cerebral high-energy phosphates, reduced cerebral lactate levels and lessened cerebral injury, confirming that MRS is a bridging biomarker of disease for asphyxia in animal studies [22–24]. These results had a strong influence on clinical research and directly led to the randomized trials that have now confirmed therapeutic hypothermia as the first effective treatment in newborns with HIE.

Most MRS studies employ $^{1}$H MRS because the greater sensitivity of the $^{1}$H nucleus allows more accurate regional measurements. Within the $^{1}$H spectrum, using appropriate scanning parameters, peaks can be assigned to N-acetyl aspartate (NAA), choline containing compounds (Cho), creatine plus phosphocreatinine (Cr), lactate (Lac), myo-inositol (mI) and alanine, glutamine and glutamate (Glu). In agreement with the cerebral metabolic disturbance that occurs with asphyxia, characteristic changes in these spectral peaks may be observed in infants with HIE, especially elevation of lactate which indicates tissue ischaemia and hypoxia and a fall in NAA, which is present primarily in neurons and reflects neuronal injury [17,18,25,26].

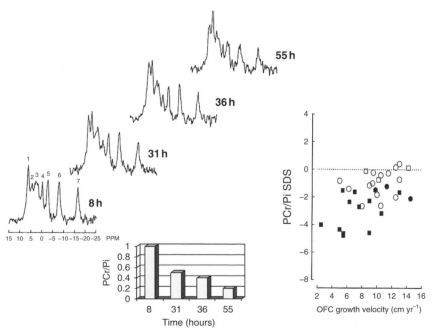

**Figure 20.1.** Changes in $^{31}$P magnetic resonance spectra following neonatal hypoxic ischaemic encephalopathy and relation to head growth. Adapted in part from reference [15].

**Table 20.2.** Accuracy of prediction of neurological outcome following hypoxic ischaemic encephalopathy by $^1$H magnetic resonance spectroscopy

| MRS measurement | Median cut off (range) | Sensitivity | Specificity |
| --- | --- | --- | --- |
| Lac/NAA | 0.29 (0.24–0.4) | 0.82 (0.74–0.89) | 0.95 (0.88–0.99) |
| Lac/Cr | 0.39 (0.32–0.95) | 0.77 (0.64–0.86) | 0.94 (0.85–0.98) |
| Lac/Cho | 0.25 (0.2–0.25) | 0.84 (0.71–0.93) | 0.81 (0.65–0.91) |
| NAA/Cho | 0.72 (0.6–1.0) | 0.59 (0.46–0.71) | 0.72 (0.50–0.83) |
| NAA/Cr | 1.2 (0.84–1.45) | 0.61 (0.51–0.70) | 0.71 (0.61–0.80) |

*Note:* Adapted from Thayyil [29].

A rise in myo-inositol, a marker for glia and glutamate, a major brain excitatory neurotransmitter, may also be observed with scanning parameters optimised to demonstrate these peaks [27,28]. Although absolute concentrations can be obtained most studies measure metabolite ratios from peak areas or peak heights.

Several studies have shown a significant relationship between several metabolite ratios and neurological outcome following asphyxia. The prognostic accuracy of MRS metabolite ratios has recently been assessed in a meta-analysis which found the Lac/NAA ratio to be most predictive, with a sensitivity of 0.82 (95% CI 0.74–0.89) and specificity 0.95 (0.88–0.99) (Table 20.2) [29]. The results were not influenced by the age at scanning during the first 30 days after birth. This indicates that the Lac/NAA ratio might be a suitable biomarker outcome in the neonatal period for use in early-phase neuroprotective studies in infants with HIE.

No clinical study so far has evaluated the effect of neuroprotective therapy on MRS metabolite concentrations in infants with HIE. Although MRS has not been formally qualified as a biomarker of treatment effect in human infants it is a qualified biomarker of disease with a strong physiological evidence base and it is rational to accept it as a bridging biomarker of treatment effect. However, further clinical studies which demonstrate this formally would be valuable.

Continuous variables such as metabolite ratios or concentrations are generally efficient outcome measures as a smaller study size is required to detect significant differences between treatment groups. However, sample size is dependent on the variance of the measurements. Clinical studies following asphyxia have studied small numbers of infants and the results show wide variance. Variance is reduced when data from several studies are combined, but it is still substantial and estimates of

sample size using these data indicate that a sample size greater than 100 infants is required to detect differences in metabolite ratios, including the Lac/NAA ratio, between experimental and control groups with standard levels of statistical significance (Figure 20.2). Improved scanning protocols with more precise sampling and analysis are required to reduce variance and improve the efficiency of MRS as a biological marker in neonatal neuroprotective studies.

# Magnetic resonance imaging

Magnetic resonance imaging (MRI) has become the preferred neuroimaging method following HIE because of its sensitivity for detection of hypoxic ischaemic injury. Following moderate/severe HIE abnormal signal intensity is most commonly detected in the basal ganglia and thalami, corticospinal tracts, the white matter and cortex [30,31]. These abnormalities correlate closely with pathology at autopsy and with the pattern of neurological abnormalities that develop in survivors and have high predictive values for detecting adverse outcomes [32–35]. Conventional T1 and T2 weighted MRI is, therefore, a valuable clinical assessment tool in infants with HIE.

Several studies have examined the prognostic accuracy of MRI following HIE. The timing of scanning is important since the characteristic abnormalities on conventional MRI occur progressively over several days and the severity of injury may be underestimated during the first few days after birth. Several methods of classifying the distribution and severity of lesions have been described, but the prognostic accuracy of visual MRI assessment may be less than with MRS and is dependent on the experience of the assessor since visual assessment is necessarily subjective. In a nested

223

sub-study comprising 131 infants from the TOBY randomised trial of cooling, expert visual assessment demonstrated a reduction in lesions in the basal ganglia and thalami, the posterior limb of the internal capsule and white matter but not the cortex following therapeutic hypothermia [11]. The presence of an abnormal signal in the posterior limb of the internal capsule, moderate or severe basal ganglia or thalami or severe white matter abnormalities was strongly predictive of subsequent serious neurological abnormalities, even in infants treated with cooling (Table 20.3).

**Table 20.3.** Accuracy of prediction of neurological outcome following hypoxic ischaemic injury by magnetic resonance imaging in infants treated with or without hypothermia

| Major MRI abnormalities | Cooled (95% confidence intervals) | Non-cooled (95% confidence intervals) |
| --- | --- | --- |
| Sensitivity | 0.88 (0.79–0.97) | 0.94 (0.88–1.0) |
| Specificity | 0.82 (0.72–0.92) | 0.68 (0.56–0.80) |
| Positive predictive value | 0.76 (0.65–0.87) | 0.74 (0.63–0.85) |
| Negative predictive value | 0.91 (0.83–0.99) | 0.92 (0.85–0.99) |

*Note:* Major MRI abnormalities were defined as the presence of moderate/severe abnormal signal intensity in basal ganglia or thalami, abnormal signal intensity in posterior limb of the internal capsule, or moderate/severe abnormal signal intensity in white matter. Adapted from Rutherford [11].

These data show that conventional MRI provides a qualified biomarker of disease and treatment effect for studies of neuroprotective therapies. The sample size required to show a treatment effect was considerably smaller than in pragmatic trials, but remains substantial.

Diffusion weighted imaging (DWI) refers to MRI that is made sensitive to water molecular diffusion. DWI can, therefore, provide information about tissue microstructure. DWI will typically show changes following ischaemia earlier than conventional MRI but may underestimate the extent of tissue injury during the first 24 hours [36–39]. Although DWI is complementary to conventional MRI, visual analysis of DWI does not seem to improve the prognostic accuracy of MRI in infants with HIE. However, quantitative analysis of DWI data is possible.

Quantitation of the "apparent diffusion coefficient" (ADC) is performed by voxelwise analysis of the information contained within DWI (mainly water diffusivity but also perfusion, motion and other factors). In infants with HIE, ADC values may be reduced in white matter and, less consistently, in basal ganglia and thalami, but they are influenced by the age at scanning: ADC values are typically reduced during the first week but then return to normal and rise further after approximately 2 weeks, so the postnatal age at scanning needs to be taken into account when assessing ADC values [38,40,41]. In a meta-analysis, the sensitivity and specificity for prediction of neurological outcome by measurement of ADC were 0.6 (0.55–0.9) and 0.66 (0.52–0.79), respectively, lower than that of MRS or visual analysis of MRI [29],

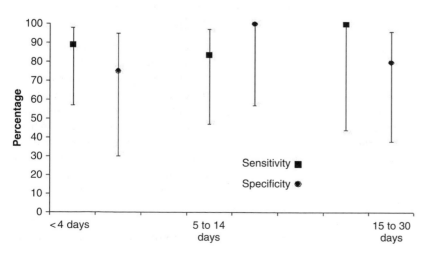

**Figure 20.2.** Postnatal age and sensitivity and specificity (95% CI) of Lac/NAA peak area ratios for predicting adverse outcome following perinatal asphyxia. Adapted from reference [29].

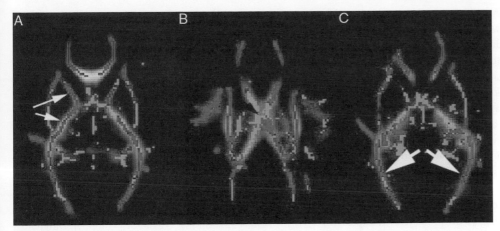

**Figure 20.3.** Axial images of mean FA of white matter tracts of infants with HIE. The group mean FA skeleton is shown in pink. Areas where the non-cooled group with HIE has a statistically lower FA than the cooled group are shown in blue: (a) internal capsules and external capsules (small white arrows), (b) body of the corpus callosum (black arrow), (c) optic radiations (large white arrows). Reproduced with permission from reference [49]. Please see plate section for colour version.

It is not known if ADC measurements are qualified to detect a treatment effect in human infants.

The directional diffusivity within a tissue is called anisotropy and can be measured by diffusion tensor imaging. Fractional anisotropy (FA) may be a more reproducible quantitative measure of tissue microstructure than the ADC but few studies have been carried out so far in infants [42–44]. Reduction of FA occurs in infants with HIE and correlates better than the ADC with visual analysis of MRI. Accuracy of FA for prediction of abnormality on visual analysis of MRI was best in the posterior limb of the internal capsule, but follow-up studies are needed to examine the relationship between FA and later neurological outcome.

Previous studies of changes in diffusivity using DWI or tensor imaging have all used an operator defined region of interest-based approach, which is time consuming and potentially introduces observer error. However, a newly described technique, Tract Based Spatial Statistics (TBSS), is an automated voxel and group-wise observer-independent whole-brain approach which aligns FA images from multiple subjects [45–47]. This allows statistically powerful comparisons of FA data without the need for subjectively defined regions or features of interest.

TBSS was used to examine differences in white matter FA between healthy infants and infants from one centre participating in the TOBY randomized trial of whole body cooling [48]. Despite a small sample size statistically significant differences in FA were detected in several white matter tracts, between the healthy and HIE infants even in regions with no visible abnormalities on MRI. FA was also

significantly reduced (indicating tissue microstructure injury) in the anterior and posterior limbs of the internal capsule, the optic radiations and the corpus callosum in the non-cooled compared with the cooled groups (Figure 20.3). Further studies to support these observations are needed but these data indicate that FA analysis by TBSS is a powerful tool for comparing tissue integrity between groups and is potentially an efficient biomarker in early stage investigation of neuroprotective therapies.

There is also some evidence that computational anatomical analysis might detect treatment effects. In a small study of infants entered into the National Institutes of Health Trial of Whole Body Hypothermia a difference in cerebral volume was found in cooled and non-cooled infants; however, this approach needs further study [49].

## Standardization of magnetic resonance studies

Moderate or severe HIE occurs relatively infrequently in centres with good obstetric care so multicentre studies are needed even for preliminary small sized studies of neuroprotective therapies. However, MRS and MRI data differ when acquired with different scanners, even when the same scanning protocol is used. This introduces inconsistencies, increases variance and hinders the use of magnetic resonance techniques as biomarkers. There is a need to develop methods of standardizing magnetic resonance data acquired with different scanners to facilitate multicentre studies.

In summary, cerebral MRS and MRI have an important role in the evaluation of candidate neuroprotective therapies. The Lac/NAA ratio and other cerebral metabolites measured by MRS and visual analysis of MRI during the first 30 days after birth accurately predict later neurological outcome and are valid biomarkers of pathology and physiology in neonatal HIE. Visual assessment of MRI is also a biomarker of the effect of neuroprotective therapy but current methods of MRS or MRI evaluation are relatively inefficient for use in early phase, first in human infant studies of novel neuroprotective therapies. However, if the initial results are confirmed, diffusion tensor imaging with TBSS analysis of FA promises to be a highly efficient biomarker and surrogate outcome for rapid preliminary evaluation of promising neuroprotective therapies for neonatal hypoxic ischaemic injury.

# References

1. Gluckman PD, Wyatt JS, Azzopardi D, et al. Selective head cooling with mild systemic hypothermia after neonatal encephalopathy: multicentre randomised trial. *Lancet* 2005;**365**:663–70.

2. Shankaran S, Laptook AR, Ehrenkranz RA, et al. Whole-body hypothermia for neonates with hypoxic-ischemic encephalopathy. *N Engl J Med* 2005;**353**:1574–84.

3. Azzopardi DV, Strohm B, Edwards AD, et al. Moderate hypothermia to treat perinatal asphyxial encephalopathy. *N Engl J Med* 2009;**361**:1349–58.

4. Baker M. In biomarkers we trust? *Nat Biotechnol* 2005;**23**:297–304.

5. Biomarkers Definitions Working Group. Biomarkeres and surrogate endpoints: preferred definitions and conceptual framework. *Clin Pharmacol Ther* 2001;**69**:89–95.

6. Casey BM, McIntire DD, Leveno KJ. The continuing value of the Apgar score for the assessment of newborn infants. *N Engl J Med* 2001;**344**:467–71.

7. Malin GL, Morris RK, Khan KS. Strength of association between umbilical cord pH and perinatal and long term outcomes: systematic review and meta-analysis. *BMJ* 2010;**340**:c1471.

8. Ramaswamy V, Horton J, Vandermeer B, et al. Systematic review of biomarkers of brain injury in term neonatal encephalopathy. *Pediatr Neurol* 2009;**40**:215–26.

9. Roka A, Kelen D, Halasz J, et al. Serum S100B and neuron-specific enolase levels in normothermic and hypothermic infants after perinatal asphyxia. *Acta Paediatr* 2012;**101**:319–23.

10. Massaro AN, Chang T, Kadom N, et al. Biomarkers of brain injury in neonatal encephalopathy treated with hypothermia. *J Pediatr* 2012;**116**:434–40.

11. Rutherford M, Ramenghi LA, Edwards AD, et al. Assessment of brain tissue injury after moderate hypothermia in neonates with hypoxic-ischaemic encephalopathy: a nested substudy of a randomised controlled trial. *Lancet Neurol* 2010;**9**:39–45.

12. Spitzmiller RE, Phillips T, Meinzen-Derr J, Hoath SB. Amplitude-integrated EEG is useful in predicting neurodevelopmental outcome in full-term infants with hypoxic-ischemic encephalopathy: a meta-analysis. *J Child Neurol* 2007;**22**:1069–78.

13. Bennet L, Dean JM, Wassink G, Gunn AJ. Differential effects of hypothermia on early and late epileptiform events after severe hypoxia in preterm fetal sheep. *J Neurophysiol* 2007;**97**:572–8.

14. Hope PL, Costello AM, Cady EB, et al. Cerebral energy metabolism studied with phosphorus NMR spectroscopy in normal and birth-asphyxiated infants. *Lancet* 1984;**2**:366–70.

15. Azzopardi D, Wyatt JS, Cady EB, et al. Prognosis of newborn infants with hypoxic-ischemic brain injury assessed by phosphorus magnetic resonance spectroscopy. *Pediatr Res* 1989;**25**:445–51.

16. Roth SC, Edwards AD, Cady EB, et al. Relation between cerebral oxidative metabolism following birth asphyxia and neurodevelopmental outcome and brain growth at one year. *Dev Med Child Neurol* 1992;**34**:285–95.

17. Robertson NJ, Cowan FM, Cox IJ, Edwards AD. Brain alkaline intracellular pH after neonatal encephalopathy. *Ann Neurol* 2002;**52**:732–42.

18. Robertson NJ, Cox IJ, Cowan FM, et al. Cerebral intracellular lactic alkalosis persisting months after neonatal encephalopathy measured by magnetic resonance spectroscopy. *Pediatr Res* 1999;**46**:287–96.

19. Penrice J, Amess PN, Punwani S, et al. Magnesium sulfate after transient hypoxia-ischemia fails to prevent delayed cerebral energy failure in the newborn piglet. *Pediatr Res* 1997;**41**:443–7.

20. Greenwood K, Cox P, Mehmet H, et al. Magnesium sulfate treatment after transient hypoxia-ischemia in the newborn piglet does not protect against cerebral damage. *Pediatr Res* 2000;**48**:346–50.

21. Penrice J, Lorek A, Cady EB, et al. Proton magnetic resonance spectroscopy of the brain during acute hypoxia-ischemia and delayed cerebral energy failure in the newborn piglet. *Pediatr Res* 1997;**41**:795–802.

22. Thoresen M, Penrice J, Lorek A, et al. Mild hypothermia after severe transient hypoxia-ischemia ameliorates delayed cerebral energy failure in the newborn piglet. *Pediatr Res* 1995;**37**:667–70.

23. Amess PN, Penrice J, Cady EB, et al. Mild hypothermia after severe transient hypoxia-ischemia reduces the delayed rise in cerebral lactate in the newborn piglet. *Pediatr Res* 1997;**41**:803–8.

24. Laptook AR, Corbett RJ, Sterett R, et al. Modest hypothermia provides partial neuroprotection when used for immediate resuscitation after brain ischemia. *Pediatr Res* 1997;**42**:17–23.

25. Barkovich AJ, Baranski K, Vigneron D, et al. Proton MR spectroscopy for the evaluation of brain injury in asphyxiated, term neonates. *AJNR Am J Neuroradiol* 1999;**20**:1399–405.

26. Cheong JL, Cady EB, Penrice J, et al. Proton MR spectroscopy in neonates with perinatal cerebral hypoxic-ischemic injury: metabolite peak-area ratios, relaxation times and absolute concentrations. *AJNR Am J Neuroradiol* 2006;**27**:1546–54.

27. Groenendaal F, Roelants-Van Rijn AM, van der GJ, Toet MC, de Vries LS. Glutamate in cerebral tissue of asphyxiated neonates during the first week of life demonstrated in vivo using proton magnetic resonance spectroscopy. *Biol Neonate* 2001;**79**:254–7.

28. Robertson NJ, Lewis RH, Cowan FM, et al. Early increases in brain myo-inositol measured by proton magnetic resonance spectroscopy in term infants with neonatal encephalopathy. *Pediatr Res* 2001;**50**:692–700.

29. Thayyil S, Chandrasekaran M, Taylor A, et al. Cerebral magnetic resonance biomarkers in neonatal encephalopathy: a meta-analysis. *Pediatrics* 2010;**125**:e382–95.

30. Rutherford M. The asphyxiated term infant. In: Rutherford M, editor. *MRI of the neonatal brain*. Philadelphia: WB Saunders; 2002. p. 99–123.

31. Rutherford M, Ramenghi LA, Edwards AD, et al. Assessment of brain tissue injury after moderate hypothermia in neonates with hypoxic-ischaemic encephalopathy: a nested substudy of a randomised controlled trial. *Lancet Neurol* 2010;**9**:39–45.

32. Cowan FM, de Vries LS. The internal capsule in neonatal imaging. *Semin Fetal Neonatal Med* 2005;**10**:461–74.

33. Rutherford M, Ward P, Allsop J, Malamatentiou C, Counsell S. Magnetic resonance imaging in neonatal encephalopathy. *Early Hum Dev* 2005;**81**:13–25.

34. Rutherford M, Srinivasan L, Dyet L, et al. Magnetic resonance imaging in perinatal brain injury: clinical presentation, lesions and outcome. *Pediatr Radiol* 2006;**36**:582–92.

35. Barkovich AJ. MR imaging of the neonatal brain. *Neuroimaging Clin N Am* 2006;**16**:117–ix.

36. Vermeulen RJ, van Schie PE, Hendrikx L, et al. Diffusion-weighted and conventional MR imaging in neonatal hypoxic ischemia: two-year follow-up study. *Radiology* 2008;**249**:631–9.

37. Bydder GM, Rutherford MA. Diffusion-weighted imaging of the brain in neonates and infants. *Magn Reson Imaging Clin N Am* 2001;**9**:83–98, viii.

38. Rutherford M, Counsell S, Allsop J, et al. Diffusion-weighted magnetic resonance imaging in term perinatal brain injury: a comparison with site of lesion and time from birth. *Pediatrics* 2004;**114**:1004–14.

39. Soul JS, Robertson RL, Tzika AA, du Plessis AJ, Volpe JJ. Time course of changes in diffusion-weighted magnetic resonance imaging in a case of neonatal encephalopathy with defined onset and duration of hypoxic-ischemic insult. *Pediatrics* 2001;**108**:1211–4.

40. Hunt RW, Neil JJ, Coleman LT, Kean MJ, Inder TE. Apparent diffusion coefficient in the posterior limb of the internal capsule predicts outcome after perinatal asphyxia. *Pediatrics* 2004;**114**:999–1003.

41. Boichot C, Walker PM, Durand C, et al. Term neonate prognoses after perinatal asphyxia: contributions of MR imaging, MR spectroscopy, relaxation times and apparent diffusion coefficients. *Radiology* 2006;**239**:839–48.

42. Barkovich AJ, Miller SP, Bartha A, et al. MR imaging, MR spectroscopy and diffusion tensor imaging of sequential studies in neonates with encephalopathy. *AJNR Am J Neuroradiol* 2006;**27**:533–47.

43. Ward P, Counsell S, Allsop J, et al. Reduced fractional anisotropy on diffusion tensor magnetic resonance imaging after hypoxic-ischemic encephalopathy. *Pediatrics* 2006;**117**:e619–30.

44. Malik GK, Trivedi R, Gupta RK, et al. Serial quantitative diffusion tensor MRI of the term neonates with hypoxic-ischemic encephalopathy (HIE). *Neuropediatrics* 2006;**37**:337–43.

45. Smith SM, Jenkinson M, Johansen-Berg H, et al. Tract-based spatial statistics: voxelwise analysis of multi-subject diffusion data. *Neuroimage* 2006;**31**:1487–505.

46. Smith SM, Johansen-Berg H, Jenkinson M, et al. Acquisition and voxelwise analysis of multi-subject diffusion data with tract-based spatial statistics. *Nat Protoc* 2007;**2**:499–503.

47. Anjari M, Srinivasan L, Allsop JM, et al. Diffusion tensor imaging with tract-based spatial statistics reveals local white matter abnormalities in preterm infants. *Neuroimage* 2007;**35**:1021–7.

48. Porter EJ, Counsell SJ, Edwards AD, Allsop J, Azzopardi D. Tract-based spatial statistics of magnetic resonance images to assess disease and treatment effects in perinatal asphyxial encephalopathy. *Pediatr Res* 2010;**68**:205–9.

49. Parikh NA, Lasky RE, Garza CN, et al. Volumetric and anatomical MRI for hypoxic-ischemic encephalopathy: relationship to hypothermia therapy and neurosensory impairments. *J Perinatol* 2009;**29**:143–9.

# Index

N-acetyl aspartate (NAA) 222–4
N-acetylcysteine (NAC) 212–13
acidosis 2–3, 87
adaptive behaviour assessment 177–8
ADC (apparent diffusion coefficient) 160–2, 224–5
adults, therapeutic hypothermia 166–7
adverse effects
  of AEDs 184, 209
  of anaesthetics 18, 202–3, 214
    mitigated by hypothermia 214
  of dexmedetomidine 213
  of EPO 197–8
  of hypothermia 41, 46–8, 120–1
    in low- and mid-income countries 128
AEDs see antiepileptic drugs
aEEG (amplitude-integrated EEG) see electroencephalography
aetiology of brain injury 16–24, 85
  see also risk factors for brain injury
Alberta Infant Motor Scale 176
alertness, at 7 days 173–4
allopurinol 22, 212–13
alpha-2 adrenoceptor agonists (dexmedetomidine) 18–19, 201, 202, 213
American Academy of Pediatrics/ ACOG consensus statement on diagnosis of perinatal asphyxia (1996) 131
American College of Obstetrics and Gynecology consensus statement on diagnosis of perinatal asphyxia (2003) 131
AMPA (α-amino-3-hydroxy-5-methyl-4-isoxazole-propionic acid) receptors 17–19
  ampakines 25
amplitude-integrated EEG (aEEG) see electroencephalography
anaesthetics
  as cause of neuroapoptosis 18, 202–3, 214

in combination with hypothermia 211–14
  neuroprotective effects 200–2
angiogenesis 196
angiography 155
animal models
  cooling of newborn miniature swine 107
  hypoxic–ischaemic injury in 7 day old rats 210
antiepileptic drugs (AEDs)
  adverse effects 184, 209
  in combination with hypothermia 24, 210–11, 215
  EEG and 147, 150
  for neonatal seizures 209
  prophylactic 186, 211
antioxidants 22, 196, 212–13
Apgar score 2–3, 88
apoptosis
  anaesthetics as cause 18, 202–3, 214
  anti-apoptotic effects
    EPO 195
    hypothermia 79, 214
    xenon 202
  discovery 34
  mechanisms 19–21, 75–6
apoptosis-inducing factor (AIF) 20
apparent diffusion coefficient (ADC) 160–2, 224–5
argon 202
Attention Deficit Hyperactivity Disorder (ADHD) 7
autistic spectrum disorder 7, 177
autophagy 21–2
axillary temperature, variability 101
Azzopardi, Denis 36

basal ganglia and thalamic (BGT) lesions, on MRI 159
  after hypothermia 160
  DTI 161
  DWI 159, 160–1
  mild, 156
  moderate, 157
  severe, 157–8

Bayley Scales of Infant and Toddler Development (Bayley III) 176–7
Bcl-2 protein family 21, 202
Behavioral Rating Inventory of Executive Function (BRIEF-II) 178–9
Behaviour Assessment System for Children (BASC-2) 178
behavioural problems 7
  assessment 177–9
BGT lesions see basal ganglia and thalamic lesions
bias in registry data 191
biomarkers 219
  biochemical markers 11, 220
  metabolites identified by MRS 222–3
  see also electroencephalography, magnetic resonance imaging
blood pressure (BP)
  effect of hypothermia 40–1, 184
  physiological response to hypoxia 85–6
brachial plexus injury 174
bradycardia, associated with dexmedetomidine 213
  hypothermia 40–1, 47, 120
brain injury
  risk factors 86–7, 129–31, 188
  traumatic
    adult 167
    paediatric 168
  see also pathogenesis of brain injury
brain-derived neurotrophic factor (BDNF) 25
brief rhythmic discharges (BRD) 148
N-tert-butyl-(2-sulphophenyl)-nitrone (S-PBN) 212

calcium, intracellular 19
calpains 21
carbonic acid 87
cardiac arrest, paediatric 168
cardio respiratory failure, neonatal 168–9

cardiopulmonary resuscitation
  hypothermia after 108–9, 168
  in low- and mid-income countries 134
  outcome 88
cardiovascular system
  cardiac arrest 168
  dexmedetomidine and 213
  hypothermia and 40–1, 47, 120
  junctional ectopic tachycardia 168
  response to fetal hypoxia 85–6
caspases 20, 79
causes of brain injury 16–24, 85
  see also risk factors for brain injury
cell-based therapy 26, 198–200
cerebral blood flow (CBF)
  in the latent phase of brain injury 78
  response to fetal hypoxia 85–6
  velocity measured by ultrasound 11, 221
cerebral function monitoring see electroencephalography
cerebral palsy (CP) 4
  BGT lesions on MRI 159
  diagnosis 176
  therapy 176–7
China, clinical trials 43–4, 139
chloral hydrate 153
chondroitinase 199
choreoretinitis 173
chorioamnionitis 131
clinical trials
  consent and communication with parents 65, 67–71
  economic evaluation as part of 53, 55
  meta-analysis 45–6
  pilot studies 35, 40–2, 135–9
  post hoc analysis 48–50
  randomized 35–6, 42–5, 139
  surrogate markers 215–16, 219–26
  see also Cool Cap trial, NICHD trial, TOBY trial
coagulopathy 41, 47, 49, 120–1
cognitive impairment
  anaesthetics as a cause 202–3
  assessment 178
  in HIE 5–7
  in mild/silent asphyxia 9
  white matter lesions 159–60
combination therapies, with hypothermia 185–6, 208–9, 215–16
  AEDs 24, 210–11, 215
  alpha-2-adrenoceptor agonists 213
  anaesthetics 213–14
    xenon 211–12
  antioxidants 212–13
  EPO 214
  magnesium sulphate 213

melatonin 213
  nutritional factors 214
  pharmacokinetics 215
communication with the parents 65–71
  about the possibility of disability 66–7, 175–6
  about the treatment 67
    research procedures 65, 67–71
  timing issues 66–9
communication skills in the affected child 7, 177, 178
complications see adverse effects
consent
  continuous 68, 70–1
  deferred/waived 71
  pre-randomized 71
  to hypothermia as an approved treatment 103
  to research procedures 65, 68–9, 71
Cool Cap system 96, 122
  FDA approval 36, 184
Cool Cap trial 35, 42–3, 50, 89, 121
  hyperthermia in controls 111
cost-benefit analysis (CBA) 55
cost-effectiveness acceptability curve (CEAC) 55
cost-effectiveness analysis (CEA) 54
cost-effectiveness (CE) plane 55
cost-minimization analysis (CMA) 54
cost-utility analysis (CUA) 54–5
CP see cerebral palsy
CritiCool system 96–7, 101–2
CSZ (Cincinnati Sub-Zero) Blanketrol II Hypo-Hyperthermia system 110, 112
cytochrome C 20
cytokines 23–4, 79, 220

decision analytic modelling 53–5
depth of hypothermia 77, 112, 122, 166
dermatological effects of hypothermia 47, 120–1
desflurane 202
developmental assessments 176–7
Developmental Coordination Disorder 178
dexmedetomidine 18–19, 201–2, 213
diagnosis
  cerebral palsy 176
  consensus statements 131
  HIE 3, 89, 103, 221
  perinatal asphyxia 2–3, 87–8, 129, 145–6
  seizures 145, 147–8, 209
diffusion tensor imaging (DTI) 155, 161, 225

diffusion weighted imaging (DWI) 155, 156, 160–1, 224–5
disability-free life year (DFLY) 59
Doppler ultrasound (cerebral) 11, 221
drug abuse, maternal 173
duration of hypothermia 75

EAAs see excitatory amino acids
ear protection, during MRI 154
early intervention programmes 176
ECMO (extracorporeal membrane oxygenation) 168–9
economic costs and benefits
  neonatal resuscitation 134
  perinatal asphyxia 1
  principles of economic evaluation 53–5
  therapeutic hypothermia 50, 55–61
educational performance 7–8, 178–9
Edwards, David 34
efficacy and effectiveness, registry data 182–3, 185, 190
electroclinical dissociation 147
electroencephalography (EEG) 142–51
  AEDs and 147, 150
  amplitude-integrated (aEEG), description 88–9, 144
  background activity 143–5
  conventional (cEEG) 142–3
  electrode positions 142, 145, 148
  electrode types 142–3
  monitoring during selective head cooling 121–2
  not needed by transport team 104
  in perinatal asphyxia 11, 46, 88–9, 145–7, 221
  predictive of outcome of hypothermia 89, 148–51, 221
  seizures 145, 147–50, 209
  sleep–wake cycles 143–6
eligibility criteria see selection criteria for treatment with hypothermia
embryonic stem (ES) cells 200
encephalopathy
  hepatic 167, 169
  neonatal
    definition 128, 188
    hypoxic see hypoxic-ischaemic encephalopathy
    VON registry 186–90
endocannabinoids 19
energy metabolism
  after hypoxia 16–17, 19, 222
  in normal labour 1, 86
  physiological response to hypothermia 109
  and therapeutic hypothermia 77–8, 120

epidemiology
  epilepsy 7
  neonatal encephalopathy 4, 128–33
  neonatal mortality worldwide 129, 131
  perinatal asphyxia 1
epigenetic mechanisms 26–7
epilepsy see seizures
erythropoietin (EPO) 26, 195–8
  in combination with hypothermia 214
  mimetic peptides 197
evidence-based medicine, therapeutic hypothermia as the standard of care 36, 134–5
excessive cooling 49–50, 96, 99, 104, 109
excitatory amino acids (EAAs) (excitotoxicity)
  anaesthetics and 201–2
  hypothermia and 78–9
  primary phase of brain injury 73, 78
  secondary phase of brain injury 17–19, 34
extracorporeal membrane oxygenation (ECMO) 168–9

facial tone 174
fat necrosis, subcutaneous 47, 121
fathers see parents
FDA (Food and Drug Administration) approvals 36, 184
feeding difficulties 174–5
Ferriero, Donna 35
fetal cell grafts 198
fetal heart rate monitoring 87
First Breath Study 134
follow-up after hypothermia 172–3
  at 7 days 173–5
  if 7 day assessment is abnormal 175–6
  at 6 months 176–7
  18 to 24 months 177
  at 4 to 5 years 177–8
  at school age 178–9
fractional anisotropy (FA) 161, 225
free radicals 22–3
  scavengers 22, 212–13
fructose-1,6-biphosphate 24
fullband EEG 143

gel packs used for cooling 96, 104
gender differences 215
Ginsberg, Myron 34
Gluckman, Peter 33–5
glucose, hyperglycaemia 120
glutamate see excitatory amino acids
glutamate receptors see NMDA receptors
glutathione 22

grasp reflex 175
growth factors 25, 199–200
  see also erythropoietin
Gunn, Alistair 34–5

Hammersmith Infant Neurological Examination 176
hats, use during whole body cooling 114
head circumference measurement 175
head injuries
  adult 167
  paediatric 168
hearing impairment 7, 174, 176
heart rate
  bradycardia
    dexmedetomidine and 213
    hypothermia, and 40–1, 47, 120
  junctional ectopic tachycardia 168
Helping Babies Breathe (HBB) programme 134
hepatic encephalopathy 167, 169
HIE see hypoxic-ischaemic encephalopathy
HIF-1α (hypoxia-inducible factor) 201
history of research into hypothermia 33–6
Horner's syndrome 174
human umbilical cord blood cells 198–9
hyperactivity 7
hyperammonaemia 169
hyperglycaemia 120
hyperthermia 48–9, 77
  avoidance of 91–2, 111
hypotension 40–1, 184
hypotonia, 7-day examination 174
hypoxanthine 22
hypoxia, physiological response 1, 85–6, 95
hypoxic-ischaemic encephalopathy (HIE)
  definitions 128, 172
  diagnosis/grading 3, 89, 103, 173, 221
  in low- and mid-income countries 128
  mechanisms causing brain injury 16–24
  outcome 4–8, 11, 133
  prediction of outcome 10–11, 87–90, 158–60, 223–4

ICE (Infant Cooling Evaluation) trial 43, 45
  outborn infants 97–8
incremental cost-effectiveness ratio (ICER) 54–5
incubators used for transport 100, 104
India 131, 137–8

infarctions, cerebral
  hypothermia (in adults) 166
  MRI (neonatal) 156, 160
infections
  chorioretinitis 173
  neonatal morbidity/mortality 131
  and risks of hypothermia 120, 135
inflammation in brain injury 23–5, 212
  effect of hypothermia 79–80
iNICQ programme (Improving Care for Neonatal Encephalopathy) 189
interleukins (IL) 23–4, 220
International Cerebral Palsy Task Force consensus statement on diagnosis of perinatal asphyxia (1999) 131
intracranial haemorrhage 47, 120–1
intracranial pressure 167
intrapartum care, importance of 134
intrapartum risk factors for brain injury 86–7, 129–31
IQ
  anaesthetics may affect 202, 203
  assessment 178
  in HIE 5
  in mild/silent asphyxia 9
  white matter lesions in cognitive impairment 159–60
isoflurane 202

JNK3 (C-Jun N-terminal kinase 3) 21
junctional ectopic tachycardia (JET) 168

Kathmandu study (NE outcome) 133

labour, problems during
  implications for parental communication 66
  importance of good obstetric care 134
  risk factors for brain injury 86–7, 129–31
lactate
  in the blood 2, 3, 87
  in the brain 155, 222–3
lactate dehydrogenase (LDH) 11
language difficulties 7, 177–8
legal liability, and communication with the parents 67
less developed countries see low- and mid-income countries
levetiracetam 210–11
limited channel EEG 144
liver, hepatic encephalopathy 167, 169
low- and mid-income countries
  clinical trials results 135–9

low- and mid-income countries (cont.)
difficulties in implementing
hypothermia 128, 135, 139
epidemiology of NE 128, 129–33
prevention of perinatal asphyxia
133–4, 139
Lucey, Jerry 35
lung disorders 47–8

macrophages see microglia
magnesium sulphate 34, 213
magnetic resonance imaging (MRI)
153, 225–6
injury patterns 155, 158–61, 223–5
delayed 162
following hypothermia 160, 225
normal neonates 154
practicalities 153–4, 225
sequences 154–5
timing 155–8
magnetic resonance spectroscopy
(MRS) 155, 161, 222–3
mechanism of action of hypothermia
77–80, 214–15
mechanisms of brain injury 16–24, 34,
85
apoptosis 19–21, 75–6
anaesthetic-induced 202
as a multiphase process 16, 73–4, 86
seizures 210
meconium-stained liquor 87
melatonin 25, 213
membrane depolarization during brain
injury 19
effect of hypothermia 77–8
memory deficits 7
mesenchymal stem cells (MSCs)
199–200
cord-blood derived 199
microcephaly 175
microglia
hypothermia 79–80
mechanisms of brain injury 18,
23–4
neuroprotective forms 24–5
mitochondria
hypothermia 78
hypoxia 19–21
Moro reflex 175
mortality rates
in clinical trials 46, 48
neonatal encephalopathy 4, 133
neonatal (worldwide) 129, 131
mothers see parents
motor development, assessment 174,
176–8
motor disorders see cerebral palsy
Movement Assessment Battery for
Children (M-ABC-2) 178
MRI see magnetic resonance imaging

MRS (magnetic resonance
spectroscopy) 155, 161,
222–3
multipotent progenitor cells 200
muscle tone, 7 day examination 174
myo-inositol 223

NAA (N-acetyl aspartate) 222–3
NAC (N-acetylcysteine) 212–13
National Institute for Health and
Clinical Excellence (NICE)
135
necroptosis 21, 79
necrotizing enterocolitis, neonatal 169
neonatal encephalopathy (NE)
definition 128, 188
in low- and mid-income countries
128
VON registry 186–90
see also hypoxic-ischaemic
encephalopathy
neo.nEURO (systemic hypothermia
after neonatal encephalopathy)
trial 43–5
Nepal (study on NE outcome) 133
NEPSY II (NEuroPSYchology) test
178
neural stem cells 198–9
neurological assessment
7 days 173–5
action to be taken if assessment is
abnormal 175–6
6 months 176–7
18 to 24 months 177
at 4 to 5 years 177–8
at school age 178–9
predicting outcome 10–11, 89–90
neuron specific enolase 220
neuronal injury see brain
injury
NICHD trial (National Institute for
Child Health and Human
Development) 35–6
cooling equipment 112
enrolment criteria 90
hyperthermia in controls 111
induction of hypothermia 112, 113
maintenance of hypothermia 114
results 42–3, 50, 90
rewarming protocol 115
NICQ programme (Neurointensive
Care Group) 189
NICQpedia 190
nitric oxide (NO) 23
effect of hypothermia 78–9
NMDA receptors (N-methyl-D-
aspartate)
anaesthetics acting on 200
antagonists 18, 201–2
in mechanisms of brain injury 17–19

nursing care required to maintain
hypothermia 96
nutrition 214

obstetric care, importance of 134
oligodendrocyte precursor cells (OPCs)
18
oligodendrocytes 195
Olympic Medical 35
optic nerve dysfunction 173
outborn infants
communication issues 68
cooling techniques/devices 95–7, 109
hypothermia in clinical practice
97–102, 109–11, 123
management protocols 91–2, 102–4,
111
need for early initiation of
hypothermia 86, 95
registry data 186
outcomes
7 day assessment 173–5
if 7 day assessment is abnormal
175–6
6 month assessment 176–7
18 to 24 month assessment 177
4 to 5 year assessment 177–8
school age assessment 178–9
of HIE 4–8, 11, 133
of mild/silent asphyxia 9–11
of neonatal seizures + hypoxia
209–10
prediction of 10–11
after hypothermia 89, 148–51, 221
by acid–base status 87–8
by EEG 11, 46, 88–9, 146–7, 221
by MRI/MRS 158–60, 223–4
by ultrasound 11, 221
problems with the literature 3–4,
10–13
overcooling 49–50, 96, 99, 104,
109
oxidative stress 22–3, 196, 212–13

p53, in apoptosis 21
parents
communication with 65–71
impact of diagnosis 175–6
maternal substance abuse 173
passive cooling 95–6, 98–101, 103–4
pathogenesis of brain injury 85
apoptosis 19–21, 75–6
anaesthetic-induced 202
effect of hypothermia on 77–80,
214–15
latent phase 74
as a multiphase process 16, 73–4, 86
primary phase 73–4, 77–8
secondary phase 16–24, 34, 74
seizures 210

perinatal asphyxia
  costs 1
  diagnosis 2–3, 87–8, 129, 145–6
  epidemiology 1, 128–33
  mechanisms of brain injury 16–24, 34, 85
  outcome
    of HIE 4–8, 11, 133
    of mild/silent disease 9–11
    problems with the literature 3–4, 11–13
  prevention in low- and mid-income countries 133–4, 139
  prognosis see prognosis
  terminology 1
periodic lateralized epileptiform discharges (PLED) 148
pharmacokinetics 215
pharmacotherapy 25–6
  anaesthetics 200–3, 211–14
  early failures 34
  EPO 26, 195–8
  see also antiepileptic drugs, combination therapies, with hypothermia
phase changing material mattresses 97, 137
phenobarbital 150, 186, 209–11
physiological response
  to hypothermia 109
  to hypoxia 1, 85–6, 95
platelets 49
posterior limb of the internal capsule (PLIC) 158
postnatal hypoxia 185
potassium channels 201
prediction of outcome see prognosis
premature infants 86, 169, 185
probabilistic tractography 161
prognosis 10–11
  enrolment criteria for clinical trials 41–2, 46, 219–20
  as predicted by acid–base status 87–8
  as predicted by EEG 11, 46, 88–9, 146–7, 221
    after hypothermia 89, 148–51, 221
  as predicted by MRI/MRS 158–60, 223–4
  as predicted by ultrasound 11, 221
psychiatric disorders 7, 10
pulmonary complications 47–8
pyrexia 48–9, 77
  avoidance of 91–2, 111

QT interval prolongation 120
quality adjusted life years (QALY) 55, 59
quality improvement, VON registry experience 189–90

rat model of hypoxic-ischaemic injury 210
reactive oxygen species (ROS) 22–3
rectal temperature
  monitoring 101, 103
  relationship to BP/heart rate 40–1
referring hospitals
  cooling techniques/devices 95–7, 109
  hypothermia in clinical practice 97–102, 109–11, 123
  management protocols 91–2, 102–4, 111
  need for early initiation of hypothermia 95
  registry data 186
registries 182
  assessment of efficacy/effectiveness 182–3, 185, 190
  improving treatment protocols 185–6
  improving/monitoring neonatal care 186, 189–90
  limitations 191
  monitoring adverse effects 183–5, 189, 190
  monitoring therapeutic drift 183, 188–9, 190
  TOBY 190–1
  VON NER 186–90, 191
respiratory failure, neonatal 168–9
resuscitation
  hypothermia after 108–9, 168
  in low- and mid-income countries 134
  outcome 88
retinal examination 173
retinopathy of prematurity (ROP) 197–8
rewarming 115, 123, 166
risk factors for brain injury 86–7, 130
  in low- and mid-income countries 129–31
  VON registry data 188
ROS (reactive oxygen species) 22–3
rtPA (recombinant tissue plasminogen activator) 166
Russia (as USSR) 33

S-PBN (N-tert-butyl-(2-sulphophenyl)-nitrone) 212
SAFEKIDS (Safety of Key Inhaled Anesthetics in Children) 203
safety
  of MRI 154
  of treatment see adverse effects
Sarnat grading of encephalopathy 3, 89–90, 173
scalp oedema 119–20
school performance 7–8, 178–9
sedation, for MRI 153

seizures
  diagnosis 145, 147–8, 209
  EEG patterns 145, 147–50, 209
  effects on the brain 209–10
  epidemiology 7
  hypothermia and 78, 149–50
    refractory status epilepticus 167–8
  treatment 186, 209
  VON registry data 188
selection criteria for treatment with hypothermia 85, 86–91, 103
  enrolment criteria used in clinical trials 41–2, 46, 90, 121
  sentinel biomarkers 219–20
selective head cooling 119–25
  adverse effects 119–20, 184
  clinical trials
    Chinese studies 43–4, 139
    Cool Cap 35, 42–3, 50, 89, 121
    pilot studies 40
  compared with whole body cooling 35, 45, 124
  and infant size/age 123–4
  initiation 122
  maintenance 122–3
  medical procedures and 123
  monitoring EEG 121–2
  preparation for the procedure 122
  rewarming 123
  temperature gradients 119, 124
servo-controlled cooling devices 96, 109, 116
set point temperature 77, 112, 122, 166
sevoflurane 202
sex hormones 215
sight, problems with 7, 173–4
  EPO and 197–8
skin, effects of hypothermia 47, 120–1
sleep wake cycles, EEG patterns 143–6
social functioning
  assessment 177
  in HIE 8
  in mild/silent asphyxia 9
South Africa 138–9
speech difficulties 7, 177–8
spinal cord injury, adult 167
STAIR group 40
status epilepticus 147–8
  refractory
    adult 167
    paediatric 168
stem cell therapy 26, 198–200
Strengths and Difficulties Questionnaire (SDQ) 179
stroke
  in adults, hypothermia 166
  perinatal, MRI scans 156, 160

substance abuse, maternal 173
sucking and swallowing reflexes 174–5
superoxide radical (O2.-) 22
swallowing reflex 174–5

TBSS (tract based spatial statistics) 161, 225
Tecotherm Total Body Cooling System 96, 110
temperature
    control of hypothermia 114, 122–3
    gradients
        during selective head cooling 119, 124
        during whole body cooling 107–8, 124
        physiological 119, 124
    monitoring 101, 103
    target 77, 112, 122, 166
terminology 1, 128
thalamic lesions see basal ganglia and thalamic (BGT) lesions
therapeutic drift 183, 188–9, 190
therapeutic window 50, 75–6, 86, 91, 112
    extension of 24, 208
    implications for parental communication 66–9
    registry data 185
    speeding up decision-making 91
Thoresen, Marianne 34
thrombocytopenia 49
thrombolysis 166
timing of interventions 50, 75–7, 86, 112
    extension of the therapeutic window 24, 208
    implications for parental communication 66–9
    registry data 185
    speeding up decision-making 91
tissue plasminogen activator 166
TOBY register 190–1
    guidelines for cooling during retrieval of outborn infants 100, 110

TOBY trial (Total Body Hypothermia for Neonatal Encephalopathy) 36, 43–4
    cooling equipment 112
    economic evaluation based on 58–60
    enrolment criteria 90
    hyperthermia in controls 111
    induction of hypothermia 112–13
    maintenance of hypothermia 114
    MRI scans 160
    outborn infants 97
    results 43, 44, 89, 90
    rewarming protocol 115
TOBY-QUAL study (TQ) 66–9
topiramate 24, 210, 211, 215
'tracé alternant' EEG pattern 143
'tracé discontinu' EEG pattern 143
tract-based spatial statistics (TBSS) 161, 225
transport of infants
    cooling techniques/devices 95–7, 109
    hypothermia in clinical practice 97–102, 109–11, 123
    management protocols 104, 111
    need for hypothermia during 95
    registry data 186
traumatic brain injury
    adult 167
    paediatric 168
traumatic spinal cord injury, adult 167
tumour necrosis factor-α (TNFα) 79

Uganda (Mulago Hospital, Kampala) 131, 135–7
ultrasound (cerebral) 11, 221
umbilical cord blood cells 198, 199
Union of Soviet Socialist Republics (USSR) 33
urea cycle disorders 169

venography 155
ventilation artefacts on EEG 146
Vermont Oxford Network Neonatal Encephalopathy Registry (VON NER) 186–91
    compared with the TOBY register 190

VHE Study (Views of Hypothermia and ECMO) 65–9
visual impairment 7, 173–4
    EPO and 197–8

water bottles used for cooling 97, 136
Wechsler Individual Achievement Test (WIAT-II) 178
Wechsler Preschool and Primary Scale of Intelligence (WPPSI-III) 178
Weiler, Ted 35
white matter lesions 156, 159–60
    after hypothermia 160
    delayed appearance 162
    on DTI 161, 225
    on DWI 159, 160
    protective effect of EPO 195
whole body cooling
    adverse effects 41, 46–8, 120–1
    care of the head during 114–15
    clinical trials
        in low- and mid-income countries 135–9
        pilot studies 40–2
        see also NICHD trial, TOBY trial
    compared with selective head cooling 35, 45, 124
    initiation 112–14
    maintenance 114–15
    outside specialized centres see outborn infants
    overcooling 49–50, 96, 99, 104, 109
    rewarming 115
    techniques/devices used 96–7, 109, 112, 136, 137
        not FDA-approved 184
    temperature gradients 107–8, 124
    troubleshooting 115
Wyatt, John 34, 35

xenon 201–2
    in combination with hypothermia 211–12

Zhou trial (selective head cooling) 43, 44, 139